Managing Pain in Children and Young People

Managing Pain in Children and Young People

A Clinical Guide

Third Edition

Edited by

Alison Twycross
*Honorary Associate Professor, School of Nursing and Midwifery,
University of Birmingham, UK; Editor-in-Chief, Evidence
Based Nursing*

Jennifer Stinson
*Department of Anesthesia and Pain Medicine and Child Health Evaluative Sciences,
Research Institute, The Hospital for Sick Children; and Lawrence S. Bloomberg Faculty of Nursing,
University of Toronto, Toronto, Ontario, Canada*

William T. Zempsky
*Professor of Pediatrics, University of Connecticut School of Medicine and Head of the Division of
Pain and Palliative Medicine at Connecticut Children's Medical Center, Storrs, Connecticut, USA*

and

Abbie Jordan
*Reader in the Department of Psychology and member of the Centre for Pain
Research at the University of Bath, Bath, UK*

WILEY Blackwell

This edition first published 2024
© 2024 John Wiley & Sons Ltd

Edition History
Blackwell Publishing Ltd. (1e, 2009); John Wiley & Sons, Ltd. (2e, 2014)

The right of Alison Twycross, Jennifer Stinson, William T. Zempsky, and Abbie Jordan to be identified as the authors of the editorial material in this work has been asserted in accordance with law.

Registered Offices
John Wiley & Sons, Inc., 111 River Street, Hoboken, NJ 07030, USA
John Wiley & Sons Ltd, The Atrium, Southern Gate, Chichester, West Sussex, PO19 8SQ, UK

For details of our global editorial offices, customer services, and more information about Wiley products visit us at www.wiley.com.

Wiley also publishes its books in a variety of electronic formats and by print-on-demand. Some content that appears in standard print versions of this book may not be available in other formats.

Limit of Liability/Disclaimer of Warranty
The contents of this work are intended to further general scientific research, understanding, and discussion only and are not intended and should not be relied upon as recommending or promoting scientific method, diagnosis, or treatment by physicians for any particular patient. In view of ongoing research, equipment modifications, changes in governmental regulations, and the constant flow of information relating to the use of medicines, equipment, and devices, the reader is urged to review and evaluate the information provided in the package insert or instructions for each medicine, equipment, or device for, among other things, any changes in the instructions or indication of usage and for added warnings and precautions. While the publisher and authors have used their best efforts in preparing this work, they make no representations or warranties with respect to the accuracy or completeness of the contents of this work and specifically disclaim all warranties, including without limitation any implied warranties of merchantability or fitness for a particular purpose. No warranty may be created or extended by sales representatives, written sales materials or promotional statements for this work. This work is sold with the understanding that the publisher is not engaged in rendering professional services. The advice and strategies contained herein may not be suitable for your situation. You should consult with a specialist where appropriate. The fact that an organization, website, or product is referred to in this work as a citation and/or potential source of further information does not mean that the publisher and authors endorse the information or services the organization, website, or product may provide or recommendations it may make. Further, readers should be aware that websites listed in this work may have changed or disappeared between when this work was written and when it is read. Neither the publisher nor authors shall be liable for any loss of profit or any other commercial damages, including but not limited to special, incidental, consequential, or other damages.

Library of Congress Cataloging-in-Publication Data
Names: Twycross, Alison, editor. | Stinson, Jennifer, 1963– editor. |
    Zempsky, William T., editor. | Jordan, Abbie, editor.
Title: Managing pain in children and young people : a clinical guide /
    edited by Alison Twycross, Jennifer Stinson, William
    Zempsky, Abbie Jordan.
Other titles: Managing pain in children.
Description: Third edition. | Hoboken, NJ : Wiley-Blackwell, 2024. |
    Preceded by: Care planning in children : a clinical guide for nurses and
    healthcare professionals / edited by Alison Twycross, Stephanie Dowden,
    and Jennifer Stinson. 2nd edition. 2014. | Includes bibliographical
    references and index.
Identifiers: LCCN 2023040793 (print) | LCCN 2023040794 (ebook) | ISBN
    9781119645320 (paperback) | ISBN 9781119645689 (adobe pdf) | ISBN
    9781119645672 (epub)
Subjects: MESH: Pain Management | Child | Adolescent
Classification: LCC RJ365 (print) | LCC RJ365 (ebook) | NLM WL 704.6 |
    DDC 616/.0472083–dc23/eng/20231031
LC record available at https://lccn.loc.gov/2023040793
LC ebook record available at https://lccn.loc.gov/2023040794

Cover Design: Wiley
Cover Image: © ljubaphoto/Getty Images; Paul Burns/Getty Images; Caia Image/Getty Images

Set in 11.5/13.5pt STIXTwoText by Straive, Pondicherry, India

Printed and bound by CPI Group (UK) Ltd, Croydon, CR0 4YY

C9781119645320_260324

For Isabella, Joseph, Dexter, Io, Tallulah, Winston, Isodora, Zinnia and Elodie
For my daughters Hayley and Sara and my grandson Lowen
For Ava, Ophelia and Evangeline
For my OG pain colleagues Neil Schechter, Nancy Bright and Barbara Rzepski

Contents

Poh Heng Chong and Hwee Hsiang Liow

16 Knowledge Implementation and Dissemination: Effectively Moving Forward 291

Bonnie Stevens, Amelia Swift, and Denise Harrison

Contributors

Julia Ambler
Umduduzi – Hospice Care for Children, and
Department of Paediatrics, Nelson Mandela
Medical School, University of KwaZulu-Natal,
Durban, South Africa

Britney Benoit
Rankin School of Nursing, St Francis Xavier
University, Antigonish, Nova Scotia, Canada

Krista Baerg
Associate Professor General Pediatrics,
University of Saskatchewan, Saskatoon,
Saskatchewan, Canada

Kathryn A. Birnie
Assistant Professor, Departments of
Anesthesiology, Perioperative and Pain
Medicine and Community Health Sciences,
University of Calgary; Associate Scientific
Director, Solutions for Kids in Pain (SKIP);
and Psychologist, Alberta Children's Hospital,
Calgary, Alberta, Canada

Line Caes
Division of Psychology, Faculty of Natural
Sciences, University of Stirling, Stirling, UK

Marsha Campbell-Yeo
School of Nursing and Departments of
Pediatrics, Psychology and Neuroscience,
Dalhousie University, and IWK Health,
Halifax, Nova Scotia, Canada

Christine T. Chambers
Professor, Departments of Psychology and
Neuroscience and Pediatrics, Dalhousie
University, and Scientific Director,
Solutions for Kids in Pain (SKIP), Halifax,
Nova Scotia, Canada

Karen Chiu
Physiotherapist, Chronic Pain Program and
Department of Rheumatology, The Hospital for
Sick Children, Toronto, Ontario, Canada

Poh Heng Chong
Medical Director, HCA Hospice Ltd,
Singapore

Jacqui Clinch
Department of Paediatric Rheumatology,
Bristol Royal Children's Hospital and Bath
Centre for Pain Services, UK

Kaytlin Constantin
Department of Psychology, University of
Guelph, Guelph, Ontario, Canada

Stephanie Dowden
NursePrac Australia, Fremantle, Western
Australia, Australia

Julia Downing
Chief Executive, International Children's
Palliative Care Network (ICPCN), Bristol,
UK; and Honorary Professor in
Palliative Care, Makerere University,
Kampala, Uganda

Mats Eriksson
Örebro University, School of Health Sciences,
Örebro, Sweden

Paula Forgeron
School of Nursing, Faculty of Health Sciences,
University of Ottawa and Children's Hospital
of Eastern Ontario, Ottawa; and Research
Institute and Department of Anesthesia,
Dalhousie University, Halifax,
Nova Scotia, Canada

Liesbet Goubert
Faculty of Psychology and Educational Sciences, Department of Experimental-Clinical and Health Psychology, Ghent University, Ghent, Belgium

Denise Harrison
Professor, Department of Nursing, School of Health Sciences, Faculty of Medicine, Dentistry and Health Services, University of Melbourne, and Honorary Fellow, Murdoch Children's Research Institute and Royal Children's Hospital, Melbourne, Victoria, Australia; and Adjunct Professor, School of Nursing, Faculty of Health Sciences, University of Ottawa, Ontario, Canada

Jennifer Hunt
Independent Palliative Care Consultant, Harare, Zimbabwe

Lindsay Jibb
Child Health Evaluative Sciences, Research Institute, The Hospital for Sick Children, and Lawrence S. Bloomberg Faculty of Nursing, University of Toronto, Toronto, Ontario, Canada

Deepa Kattail
Department of Anesthesiology, McMaster University, Hamilton, Ontario, Canada

Sara Klein
Physiotherapist, Chronic Pain Program, Hospital for Sick Children, Toronto, Ontario, Canada

Charlie H.T. Kwok
Hotchkiss Brain Institute, University of Calgary, Calgary, Alberta, Canada

Christina Liossi
School of Psychology, University of Southampton, Southampton, and Pain Control Service, Great Ormond Street Hospital NHS Foundation Trust, London, UK

Hwee Hsiang Liow
Child Life Therapist, Children's Cancer Foundation, Singapore

Nicole E. MacKenzie
Department of Psychology and Neuroscience, Dalhousie University, Halifax, Nova Scotia, Canada

C. Meghan McMurtry
Department of Psychology, University of Guelph, Guelph; Pediatric Chronic Pain Program, McMaster Children's Hospital, Hamilton; and Children's Health Research Institute, Department of Paediatrics, Schulich School of Medicine and Dentistry, Western University, London, Ontario, Canada

Giulia Mesaroli
Physiotherapist, The Hospital for Sick Children, Toronto and PhD student in Clinical Epidemiology, The University of Toronto

Sueann Penrose
Children's Pain Management Service, Royal Children's Hospital, Melbourne, Victoria, Australia

Brittany N. Rosenbloom
Child Health Evaluative Sciences, The Hospital for Sick Children, Toronto, Ontario, Canada

Cate Sinclair
Vital Connections Allied Health, Albert Park, Victoria, Australia

Bonnie Stevens
Professor Emeritus, Lawrence S. Bloomberg Faculty of Nursing, University of Toronto, and Senior Scientist Emeritus, The Hospital for Sick Children, Toronto, Ontario, Canada

Jennifer Stinson
Department of Anesthesia and Pain Medicine and Child Health Evaluative Sciences, Research Institute, The Hospital for Sick Children, and Lawrence S. Bloomberg Faculty of Nursing, University of Toronto, Toronto, Ontario, Canada

Janice E. Sumpton
Pharmacist Emeritus, London, Ontario, Canada

Naiyi Sun
Department of Anesthesia and Pain Medicine, The Hospital for Sick Children, University of Toronto, Toronto, Ontario, Canada

Amelia Swift
Reader in Health Professional Education, School of Nursing and Midwifery, College of Medical and Dental Sciences, University of Birmingham, Edgbaston, Birmingham, UK

Anna Taddio
Leslie Dan Faculty of Pharmacy, University of Toronto, Toronto, Ontario, Canada

Tuan Trang
Hotchkiss Brain Institute, University of Calgary, Calgary, Alberta, Canada

Perri R. Tutelman
Division of Psychosocial Oncology, Department of Oncology, Cancer Care Alberta and University of Calgary Calgary, Alberta, Canada

Alison Twycross
Honorary Associate Professor, School of Nursing and Midwifery, University of Birmingham, UK; Editor-in-Chief, *Evidence-Based Nursing*

Foreword

I have had the extreme pleasure of working with hospitalised children and young people for over three decades. In my early years as a paediatric nurse at the bedside, I was struck by the pain that children and young people endured as part of their diagnosis and treatment and how helpless healthcare professionals and family members felt in trying to comfort them. We did not know the impact of pain on these children and young people, but we did have an intuitive sense that it was harmful both physically and emotionally and needed to be prevented, reduced or eliminated.

I was fortunate to be part of a growing body of research focused on generating pain assessment measures and prevention and evaluating treatment strategies that were pharmacological, behavioural, physical and environmental. Yet there were still broad gaps remaining on how to prevent and treat pain in children and young people. In addressing these gaps, we needed a diverse set of skills from basic and clinical sciences and pain-relieving strategies that integrated children, young people and families, healthcare professionals and organisational needs within the context of inter-professional pain care. The voice of individuals with lived pain experiences was also needed, as was the exploration of the underlying mechanisms of pain and its treatment.

In addition, the dawning comprehension that even though we were generating evidence on effective pain prevention and treatment strategies, we did not always effectively disseminate or implement this new knowledge into practice. This lack of understanding of implementation and dissemination as critical components of implementation science is perhaps our greatest challenge and the one that needs the most attention moving forward.

This book serves to present and synthesise new knowledge, re-igniting our commitment to solving the puzzle of pain in children and young people and to explore why treating and preventing pain matters. We will see what we have learned about the anatomy and physiology of pain and how this has influenced the clinical pain practices of assessment and treatment. There is a renewed focus on prevention, but where this is not possible, on the most up-to-date strategies on relieving acute nociceptive pain, procedural pain, neuropathic and visceral pain, chronic musculoskeletal pain, headaches and both acute and chronic postsurgical pain. As well, there is attention to special populations including neonates, children receiving palliative care, and children in low- and middle-income countries. Finally, the challenges of implementation and dissemination of new knowledge are addressed in summarising the effective ways of moving forward.

We have an abundance of evidence that underlies effective prevention and treatment of pain in children and young people. However, the failure to effectively implement and disseminate this evidence results in the continued pain and suffering of children. We need to consider not only the effectiveness of the pain-relieving intervention but the effectiveness of the implementation strategies across multiple populations and contexts. The new knowledge presented in this book will increase our awareness and knowledge of both pain prevention and treatment but also of how to best implement pain practice change that will improve child health outcomes.

Bonnie Stevens, RN, PhD

Acknowledgements

This edition has taken much longer to write than planned, at least in part due to an ongoing global pandemic. There are several people without whom this book would not have been completed:

- The authors, for delivering chapters despite the immense pressure the last few years has brought, and particularly those who stepped up at the last minute.
- Abbie Jordan and William (Bill) Zempsky, for agreeing to join the editorial team due to other members stepping down.

- My wonderful editorial assistant, Toni McIntosh.
- MSc Health Psychology students Amy Parkinson, Holly Waring and Jenny Corser, all of whom supported development of some of the chapters.

Long Covid means I have had to take early retirement and so this will be the last edition of the book I am involved with. Given this, I would also like to thank Jennifer Stinson for being such a great writing partner over the years.

Alison Twycross

1 Introduction

Alison Twycross

Honorary Associate Professor, School of Nursing and Midwifery, University of Birmingham, UK; Editor-in-Chief, Evidence-Based Nursing

Welcome to the third edition of *Managing Pain in Children and Young People: A Clinical Guide*. In this edition we have done things a little differently. Our aim remains to pull together current evidence for managing pain in children and young people (CYP) in an easily accessible format. However, we wanted the book to be seen as relevant to students and to members of interdisciplinary teams involved in managing children's pain around the globe. To reflect this broader focus, the editorial line-up now includes a medic (physician), a psychologist and two nurses. We have also extended the range of contributors, again drawing on international expertise across the multidisciplinary team. A new chapter has been added to ensure the book is applicable to those working in low- to middle-income countries (Chapter 15).

The first few chapters set the scene for effective multimodal pain management by focusing on the following:

- Why managing pain in children and young people is important.
- The anatomy and physiology of pain.
- Pain as a biopsychosocial phenomenon.
- Pharmacology of analgesic drugs.
- Pain assessment.

Given the new International Classification of Diseases (ICD)-11 definition of chronic pain, we have decided to include three shorter chapters in this edition rather than one longer one. These chapters focus on the prevention and treatment of chronic postsurgical pain, musculoskeletal pain, and headaches.

Other chapters pull together the current evidence for the prevention and treatment of nociceptive pain, neuropathic and visceral pain, procedural pain, neonatal pain, and paediatric palliative care.

Despite the extensive research that has been carried out over the past 25 years, CYP still do not receive evidence-based pain care. To address this issue, the final chapter covers how to effectively move forward with knowledge dissemination and implementation.

Multimodal Pain Management

Pain is a biopsychosocial phenomenon (see Chapter 4) and often has a spiritual element (Friedrichsdorf and Goubert 2020). Given this, the prevention and treatment of pain requires a multimodal approach (Figure 1.1). To make

Managing Pain in Children and Young People: A Clinical Guide, Third Edition. Edited by Alison Twycross, Jennifer Stinson, William T. Zempsky, and Abbie Jordan.
© 2024 John Wiley & Sons Ltd. Published 2024 by John Wiley & Sons Ltd.

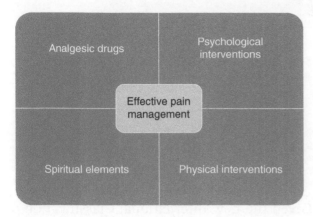

Figure 1.1 Components of effective multimodal pain management.

this explicit, one of the changes we have made to this edition is to integrate the evidence for physical and psychological pain-relieving interventions into the chapters focusing on the prevention and treatment of pain. A brief description of physical and psychological pain-relieving interventions is provided in Tables 1.1 and 1.2. Physical and psychological strategies used with neonates are outlined in Chapter 13.

World Health Organization Pain Ladder

An integral part of multimodal pain management is the use of analgesic drugs to prevent and treat pain. The World Health Organization (WHO) (2020) has devised a two-step pain ladder to help guide decision-making in this context (Figure 1.2). The 2020 WHO ladder takes into account the fact that codeine is no longer recommended for use in CYP (Box 1.1).

Table 1.1 Physical pain-relieving interventions.

Active physical interventions	
Activity pacing and energy conservation	▪ Pacing involves reaching a balanced pattern of varied activity that is achievable on good and bad days without causing 'crashes' or increases in symptoms ▪ The Royal College of Occupational Therapy provides useful advice about how to pace: https://www.rcot.co.uk/conserving-energy ▪ Energy conservation is identified as a strategy for chronic pain management in the Canadian Pediatric Pain Management Standards (HSO 2023)
Physiotherapy and daily exercise	▪ Identified as a key strategy for chronic pain management by the Scottish Government (2018) and in the Canadian Pediatric Pain Management Standards (HSO 2023) ▪ Seen as a key component of managing chronic pain in CYP (Caes et al. 2018; Harrison et al. 2019) ▪ Involves individualised exercise programmes aimed at increasing muscle strength and flexibility ▪ Likely to be more effective when combined with psychological therapies, e.g. cognitive behavioural therapy, and goal setting (Caes et al. 2018)
Relaxation	▪ Identified as a strategy for acute and chronic pain management in the Canadian Pediatric Pain Management Standards (HSO 2023) ▪ The Scottish Government (2018) suggests relaxation is a low-risk intervention that should be considered in the management of chronic pain in CYP
Yoga	▪ Some evidence to support its use in chronic pain management (Harrison et al. 2019)

Table 1.1 (Continued)

Passive physical interventions	
Acupuncture	▦ Identified as a strategy for acute pain management in the Canadian Pediatric Pain Management Standards (HSO 2023) ▦ The Scottish Government (2018) recommends the use of acupuncture for CYP with back pain or headache
Ice and heat	▦ Thermal applications identified as a strategy for chronic pain management in the Canadian Pediatric Pain Management Standards (HSO 2023)
Massage	▦ Identified as a strategy for chronic pain management in the Canadian Pediatric Pain Management Standards (HSO 2023)
Transcutaneous electrical nerve stimulation (TENS)	▦ Identified as a strategy for acute pain management in the Canadian Pediatric Pain Management Standards (HSO 2023) ▦ The Scottish Government (2018) suggests that TENS is a low-risk intervention that should be considered in the management of chronic pain in CYP
Sensory and brain-based strategies	
Graded motor imagery and mirror therapy	▦ The process of thinking and moving without actually moving ▦ Has been shown to be particularly effective when moving the injured body part is too painful (Ramsey et al. 2017)
Tactile stimulation or desensitisation	▦ Desensitisation techniques help to restore normal sensitivity and include varied exercises to increase tolerance to the feel of different tactile and thermal sensations on the affected body part (Ayling Campos et al. 2011) ▦ The start of desensitisation can be difficult, as CYP experience increased discomfort during the application of sensory techniques (Ayling Campos et al. 2011) ▦ No evidence to support its use in practice

Table 1.2 Psychological pain-relieving strategies.

Strategy	Description
Acceptance and commitment therapy (ACT)	▦ A type of psychotherapy that promotes acceptance to deal with negative thoughts, feelings, symptoms or circumstances ▦ ACT also encourages increased commitment to healthy constructive activities that uphold CYP's values or goals ▦ More information is available at Glashofer (2022)
Biofeedback	The Institute for Chronic Pain (2017) describes biofeedback as: ▦ Enabling individuals to learn how to change physiological activity for the purposes of improving health and performance ▦ Using precise instruments to measure physiological activity, e.g. brainwaves, heart function, breathing, muscle activity and skin temperature ▦ Using this feedback to support the desired physiological changes ▦ Over time, these changes endure without continued use of an instrument (Schwartz and Andrasik 2016) ▦ More information about biofeedback can be found in this video: `https://www.facebook.com/watch/?v=638866001271911&extid=NS-UNK-UNK-UNK-IOS_GK0T-GK1C&ref=sharing`

(Continued)

Table 1.2 (Continued)

Strategy	Description
Cognitive behavioural therapy (CBT)	◼ MIND (2022) describes CBT as a type of talking therapy that teaches coping skills for dealing with different problems (pain, mood, etc.) ◼ CBT is not a single type of treatment; rather it is a class of multi-component therapies based in the cognitive behavioural theoretical model (Palsson and Ballou 2020) ◼ CBT focuses on how your thoughts, beliefs and attitudes affect your feelings and actions ◼ Can be delivered face to face or online (Fisher et al. 2019) ◼ More information about CBT can be seen in this video: `https://www.youtube.com/watch?v=9c_Bv_FBE-c`
Distraction	◼ Great Ormond Street Hospital (2020) define distraction as: An approach that helps a child or young person cope with an invasive procedure or if they are facing a difficult experience in the hospital. It can also be helpful if a child is in pain or discomfort. ◼ More information is available on their website: `https://www.gosh.nhs.uk/conditions-and-treatments/procedures-and-treatments/distraction/` ◼ Nowadays digital distraction is often used, e.g. virtual reality or video games (Gates et al. 2020)
Exposure-based therapies	◼ A type of CBT ◼ Based on the concept that avoidance behaviours can exacerbate symptoms ◼ Through exposure CYP are encouraged to face sensations and situations that cause them pain or make them fearful, therefore alleviating their distress (Person and Keefer 2021)
Hypnotherapy	◼ Relies on a special mental state (hypnosis) induced with the help of verbal guidance from the therapist to facilitate receptivity to therapeutic suggestions ◼ While the patient is in a receptive state, the therapist uses *deepening techniques* and then delivers post-hypnotic suggestions that help facilitate changes in emotions, thoughts and physical symptoms (Palsson and Ballou 2020)
Mindfulness	◼ Involves focusing on bringing attention to the present moment (Harrison et al. 2019)
Psychotherapy (counselling)	Psychotherapy can help someone in pain to: ◼ Express their feelings and process them in a safe and supportive relationship ◼ Gain deeper insight into the issues they face ◼ Talk about things in a confidential environment that they might not feel able to discuss with anyone else ◼ Find better ways to cope with feelings and fears ◼ Change the way they think and behave to improve their mental and emotional well-being ◼ Improve relationships in their life, including with themselves ◼ Make sense of any clinical diagnoses they have been given by understanding what has happened to them ◼ Heal from trauma ◼ For more information, see `https://www.psychotherapy.org.uk/seeking-therapy/what-is-psychotherapy/`

Sleep hygiene strategies	◼ Many young people with chronic pain report disturbed sleep (Badawy et al. 2019)
	◼ Sleep hygiene is an important component of managing chronic pain
	◼ More information can be found on the following two websites:
	    ◼ `https://www.gosh.nhs.uk/conditions-and-treatments/procedures-and-treatments/sleep-hygiene-children/`
	    ◼ `https://www.sleepfoundation.org/sleep-hygiene`

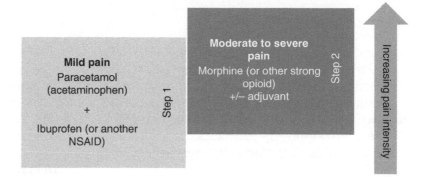

Figure 1.2 WHO (2020) two-step pain ladder.

Physical Pain-relieving Interventions

Physical pain-relieving interventions are an integral part of managing CYP pain (Figure 1.1) and particularly useful when managing chronic pain. They are defined as:

Interventions intended to help the body function physically (Health Standards Organization [HSO] 2023, p. XVI).

However, there is very little evidence of their effectiveness (Caes et al. 2018; Birnie et al. 2020). Despite this, WHO (2020) recommends the use of physical therapies either alone or in combination with other treatments for CYP with chronic pain. The commonly used physical interventions used in CYP are outlined in Table 1.1.

Psychological Pain-relieving Interventions

Psychological pain-relieving interventions are an important part of preventing and treating pain (Figure 1.1) and have been described as:

Interventions to harness the connection between mind and body by addressing thoughts (cognition), emotions and behaviours/actions to help the child and their family directly or indirectly influence the experience of pain (HSO 2023, p. XVI).

While these techniques are widely used in practice, the results of several systematic reviews all conclude that there is minimal and low-quality evidence to support their use (Birnie et al. 2018; Caes et al. 2018; Fisher et al. 2018, 2019). Evidence suggests that these interventions can be delivered online or face-to-face (Fisher 2019; WHO 2020). Some of the psychological strategies used with CYP are defined in Table 1.2.

References

Ayling Campos, A., Amaria, K., Campbell, F. and McGrath, P.A. (2011) Clinical impact and evidence base for physiotherapy in treating childhood chronic pain. *Physiotherapy Canada* 63(1), 21–33.

Badawy, S.M., Law, E.F. and Palermo, T.M. (2019) The interrelationship between sleep and chronic pain in adolescents. *Current Opinion in Physiology* 11, 25–28.

Birnie, K.A., Noel, M., Chambers, C.T., Uman, L.S. and Parker, J.A. (2018) Psychological interventions for needle-related procedural pain and distress in children and adolescents. *Cochrane Database of Systematic Reviews* (10), CD005179.

Birnie, K.A., Ouellette, C., Do Amaral, T. and Stinson, J.N. (2020) Mapping the evidence and gaps of interventions for pediatric chronic pain to inform policy, research, and practice: a systematic review and quality assessment of systematic reviews. *Canadian Journal of Pain* 4(1), 129–148.

Caes, L., Fisher, E., Clinch, J. and Eccleston, C. (2018) Current evidence-based interdisciplinary treatment options for pediatric musculoskeletal pain. *Current Treatment Options in Rheumatology* 4(3), 223–234.

Fisher, E., Law, E., Dudeney, J., Palermo, T.M., Stewart, G. and Eccleston, C. (2018) Psychological therapies for the management of chronic and recurrent pain in children and adolescents. *Cochrane Database of Systematic Reviews* (9), CD003968.

Fisher, E., Law, E., Dudeney, J., Eccleston, C. and Palermo, T.M. (2019) Psychological therapies (remotely delivered) for the management .of chronic and recurrent pain in children and adolescents. *Cochrane Database of Systematic Reviews* (4), CD011118.

Friedrichsdorf, S.J. and Goubert, L. (2020) Pediatric pain treatment and prevention for hospitalized children. *Pain Reports* 5(1), e804.

Gates, M., Hartling, L., Shulhan-Kilroy, J. et al. (2020) Digital technology distraction for acute pain in children: a meta-analysis. *Pediatrics* 145(2), e20191139.

Glashofer, D.R. (2022) What is acceptance and commitment therapy (ACT)? Available at https://www.verywellmind.com/acceptance-commitment-therapy-gad-1393175 (accessed 15 December 2022).

Great Ormond Street Hospital (2020) Distraction. Available at https://www.gosh.nhs.uk/conditions-and-treatments/procedures-and-treatments/distraction/ (accessed 16 May 2023).

Harrison, L.E., Pate, J.W., Richardson, P.A., Ickmans, K., Wicksell, R.K. and Simons, L.E. (2019) Best-evidence for the rehabilitation of chronic pain. Part 1: pediatric pain. *Journal of Clinical Medicine* 8(9), 1267.

Health Standards Organization (HSO) (2023) *Pediatric Pain Management*. HSO, Ottawa, Canada. Available at https://store.health-standards.org/products/pediatric-pain-management-can-hso-13200-2023-e (accessed 26 May 2023).

Institute for Chronic Pain (2017) Biofeedback. Available at https://www.institute-forchronicpain.org/treating-common-pain/what-is-pain-management/biofeedback#:~:text=Biofeedback%20is%20a%20treatment%20used%20for%20a%20variety,computer%20screen%20or%20other%20monitor%20in%20real%20time (accessed 15 December 2022).

Kelly, L.E., Reider, M., van den Anker, J., et al. (2012) More codeine fatalities after tonsillectomy in North American children. *Pediatrics* 129(5), e1343–e1347.

Medicines and Healthcare products Regulatory Agency (MHRA) (2013). Codeine: restricted use as analgesic in children and adolescents after European safety review. Available at https://www.gov.uk/drug-safety-update/codeine-restricted-use-as-analgesic-in-children-and-adolescents-after-european-safety-review (accessed 31 May 2023).

MIND (2022) Cognitive behavioural therapy (CBT). Available at https://www.mind.org.uk/information-support/drugs-and-treatments/talking-therapy-and-counselling/cognitive-behavioural-therapy-cbt/ (accessed 15 December 2022).

Palsson, O.S. and Ballou, S. (2020) Hypnosis and cognitive behavioral therapies for the management of gastrointestinal disorders. *Current Gastroenterology Reports* 22(7), 31.

Person, H. and Keefer, L. (2019) Brain–gut therapies for pediatric functional gastrointestinal disorders and inflammatory bowel disease. *Current Gastroenterology Reports* 21(4), 12.

Ramsey, L.H., Karlson, C.W. and Collier, A.B. (2017) Mirror therapy for phantom limb pain in a 7-year-old male with osteosarcoma. *Journal of Pain and Symptom Management* 53(6), e5–e7.

Schwartz, M.S. and Andrasik, F. (2016) *Biofeedback: A Practitioner's Guide*, 4th edn. Guildford Press, New York.

Scottish Government (2018) *Management of Chronic Pain in Children and Young People. A National Clinical Guideline.* Scottish Government, Edinburgh. Available at https://www.gov.scot/publications/management-chronic-pain-children-young-people/ (accessed 16 May 2023).

World Health Organization (WHO) (2020) *Guidelines for the Management of Chronic Pain in Children*, pp. 1–11. WHO, Geneva. Available at https://apps.who.int/iris/bitstream/handle/10665/337999/9789240017870-eng.pdf (accessed 16 May 2023).

2 Why Treating and Preventing Pain Matters

Nicole E. MacKenzie, Perri R. Tutelman, Christine T. Chambers, and Kathryn A. Birnie

Pain is a universal experience for children and young people (CYP). Undermanaged and preventable pain can have significant short- and long-term consequences for CYP and their families. This chapter provides an introduction to pain in CYP, including an overview of the definition, types and prevalence of pain experienced by children from infancy to adolescence. Factors that make pain in CYP unique, such as developmental changes and family involvement, are reviewed. The history of CYP pain and its development as a discipline is discussed. An overview of the biological, psychological and social sequelae of undermanaged acute and chronic pain in CYP is provided. Finally, the ethical imperative of managing pain in CYP is discussed.

What is Pain?

From everyday aches to medical procedures, illnesses and injuries, pain is a sensation experienced by all CYP from a young age. Despite the ubiquitous experience of pain, its subjective and individualised nature makes it difficult to define. The most widely accepted definition of pain is that of the International Association for the Study of Pain (IASP). Initially adopted in 1979, the definition was revised for the first time in 2020 to align with research and theoretical advancements in the field. According to the IASP, pain is broadly defined as (Raja et al. 2020):

> *An unpleasant sensory and emotional experience associated with, or resembling that associated with, actual or potential tissue damage.*

By definition, pain is more than a bodily sensation; it is a multidimensional *experience* that is inextricably linked to one's psychological and social functioning and context (see Chapter 4 for further information on the biopsychosocial model of pain). The IASP definition is accompanied by six supplemental notes that highlight key features of pain (Box 2.1), several of which have direct implications for the understanding of pain in CYP; e.g., pain as a concept learned throughout one's life experiences, and the importance of behavioural pain assessment for young children or others who cannot communicate verbally (Craig and MacKenzie 2021). This definition must therefore be actively integrated into the pain care and management of CYP (Jordan et al. 2021).

Managing Pain in Children and Young People: A Clinical Guide, Third Edition. Edited by Alison Twycross, Jennifer Stinson, William T. Zempsky, and Abbie Jordan.

BOX 2.1   ACCOMPANYING NOTES FOR THE REVISED IASP DEFINITION OF PAIN

- Pain is always a personal experience that is influenced to varying degrees by biological, psychological and social factors.
- Pain and nociception are different phenomena. Pain cannot be inferred solely from activity in sensory neurons.
- Through their life experiences, individuals learn the concept of pain.
- A person's report of an experience as pain should be respected.
- Although pain generally serves an adaptive role, it may have adverse effects on function and social and psychological well-being.
- Verbal description is only one of several behaviours to express pain; inability to communicate does not negate the possibility that a human or a non-human animal experiences pain.

Taken from Raja et al. (2020).

Table 2.1 Common types, and examples of, nociceptive pain.

Procedural pain (see Chapter 12)	Pain due to vaccination, venepuncture or lumbar puncture
Postoperative pain (see Chapter 7)	Pain after surgery
Pain due to injuries	Pain from a playground or sports-related injury
Visceral pain (see Chapter 8)	Appendicitis
Acute exacerbations of chronic conditions (see Chapters 8–11)	Sickle cell vaso-occlusive crises, juvenile idiopathic arthritis flares

Sources: Eccleston et al. (2021); Stevens and Zempsky (2021).

Nociceptive Pain

At its most fundamental level, pain serves a critical evolutionary purpose. Pain is a sensation associated with the body's protection system; it is a warning sign of bodily threat and serves as an alert to take action to avoid harm. Nociceptive (acute) pain refers to the often sudden, time-limited pain experienced in response to noxious stimuli that motivates behaviours to avoid tissue injury (Kent et al. 2017). CYP experience various types of nociceptive pain; some of the most common are described in Table 2.1.

The prevention and treatment of nociceptive pain is described in more detail in Chapter 7. When nociceptive pain persists for an extended period of time (i.e. beyond three months; Treede et al. 2015), it no longer serves a protective role, at which time it is considered chronic.

Chronic Pain

With the 2019 release of the 11th revision of the International Classification of Diseases (ICD-11), chronic pain was systematically defined and classified for the first time. According to the ICD-11, chronic pain is pain that persists or recurs for longer than three months (Treede et al. 2015). The cut-off of three months or longer was selected by the ICD-11 taskforce to allow for a clear and measurable definition and to align with temporal cut-offs of other chronic conditions (Finnerup et al. 2018).

Much like nociceptive pain, there are various types of chronic pain that are grouped based on aetiology and pathophysiology. In the ICD-11, chronic pain disorders are classified into two overarching categories with several subcategories (Table 2.2).

However, several chronic pain conditions in CYP have established diagnostic criteria that deviate from the ICD-11 definition of chronic pain. For instance, according to the Rome IV criteria

Table 2.2 Classification of chronic pain disorders.

Category	Definition	Main subcategories
Chronic primary pain	Chronic pain in one or more locations associated with significant emotional distress and/or functional impairment that is not accounted for by another chronic pain condition. Importantly, chronic primary pain conditions are considered health conditions in and of themselves	1. Chronic widespread pain (e.g. fibromyalgia) 2. Complex regional pain syndrome 3. Chronic primary headache or orofacial pain (e.g. chronic migraine) 4. Chronic primary visceral pain (e.g. irritable bowel syndrome) 5. Chronic primary musculoskeletal pain (e.g. chronic primary low back pain)
Chronic secondary pain	Chronic pain linked to other diseases as the underlying cause	1. Chronic cancer-related pain (e.g. pain during or after cancer due to the disease or its treatments) 2. Chronic postsurgical (e.g. after thoracotomy) or post-traumatic (e.g. after burn injury) pain 3. Chronic neuropathic pain (e.g. pain due to diabetic neuropathy) 4. Chronic secondary headache or orofacial pain (e.g. chronic headache due to seizures) 5. Chronic secondary visceral pain (e.g. pain due to inflammatory bowel disease) 6. Chronic secondary musculoskeletal pain (e.g. pain due to joint inflammation from juvenile idiopathic arthritis)

Sources: Nicholas et al. (2019); Treede et al. (2019).

for CYP functional abdominal pain disorders, symptoms are only required to be present for a duration of two months or longer for diagnosis (Hyams et al. 2016). A degree of flexibility and prudent clinical judgement is therefore necessary in clinical practice when it comes to the diagnosis and treatment of CYP with chronic pain (see Chapters 9–11).

What is Unique about Pain in Children and Young People?

CYP have unique biological, psychological and social factors that influence their experience of pain. For instance, there are clear anatomical and physiological differences between CYP and adults that are relevant to how pain is managed pharmacologically in CYP (see Chapter 5).

However, there are numerous other considerations that make pain a distinct experience for CYP. These are outlined in Table 2.3.

The Historical Context of Children and Young People's Pain

Today, CYP's pain management is considered a fundamental human right (Brennan et al. 2019). However, it was not always this way. As recently as 35 years ago, it was widely believed that children, particularly infants, were not neurologically mature enough to feel pain (Unruh and McGrath 2013). This thinking was questioned in the early 1980s when Anand and colleagues began a series of clinical trials comparing the outcomes of premature infants who received standard surgical

Table 2.3 Factors that make pain a distinct experience for children and young people.

The concept of pain develops throughout childhood

- CYP's understanding of pain develops as they mature cognitively and as their experience with pain (e.g. vaccinations, injuries, illnesses) grows in terms of contextual experiences (Jaaniste et al. 2016)
- CYP's cognitive and social development may influence how pain is remembered later in life (Noel et al. 2015)
- The ongoing development of CYP's understanding of pain highlights the importance of taking a developmental approach to pain assessment and treatment across childhood

The challenge of self-report

- Self-report is considered optimal for pain assessment given the subjective nature of pain (see Chapter 6)
- The ability for a CYP to reliably self-report on their pain begins at age three years in a limited capacity. More advanced skills (e.g. ability to provide visual analogue and numerical ratings) emerges around age six or seven years in typically developing children (Birnie et al. 2019a)

The role of parents

- Parental behaviours that attend to the pain (e.g. reassurance, empathy, protectiveness) contribute to worsened pain (Neville et al. 2020)
- Behaviours that direct attention away from pain (e.g. distraction, coping strategies) are associated with the ability to regulate distress related to pain (Russell and Park 2018)
- Degree of family cohesion, distress and social environment may also impact CYP's perceptions of pain and subsequent responses (Meints and Edwards 2018)

The lifelong impact of pain in childhood

- CYP are uniquely at risk for long-term effects of pain given the early stage of the developing somatosensory and central nervous systems (Walker 2019)
- Nociceptive pain in early life has documented effects on sensory thresholds, pain sensitisation and neurodevelopment observed into adulthood (Vinall et al. 2014; Walker et al. 2019)
- Upwards of 19% of CYP with chronic pain continue to report chronic pain in adulthood (Larsson et al. 2018), which can influence mental health and vocational prospects later in life (Groenewald et al. 2019; Murray et al. 2020)

pain care (i.e. no pain management) with premature infants who received anaesthesia. These trials found that infants did, in fact experience pain and infants who did not receive anesthesia experienced poorer outcomes than those who did (e.g. Anand et al. 1987; Anand & Hickey 1992).

Meaningful change in CYP's surgical pain practices were achieved only after a mother, Jill Lawson, brought lived experience of this research into the public eye (Rovner 1986). In 1985, Jill's prematurely born son, Jeffrey Lawson, underwent major surgery at Children's National Hospital (Washington, DC) soon after birth, and in line with standard care at the time received no anaesthesia. Jill spoke out about Jeffrey's experience, and her advocacy efforts, coupled with Dr Anand's landmark research, drew public

attention to the issue of pain management in children and catalysed the development of the field of paediatric pain management.

In 1987, the American Academy of Pediatrics and American Society of Anesthesiologists released a joint statement recognising infants' sense of pain and proclaiming that it was no longer ethical to perform surgery on preterm babies without anaesthesia (American Academy of Pediatrics 1987; American Society of Anesthesiologists 1987). The history of CYP pain provides important context to the advancement of the discipline, which required a combination of both science and parental advocacy (McGrath 2011). As was true with Jill Lawson's early efforts, public awareness and changes to policy remain necessary to continue to move the field forward.

The Current Context of Children and Young People's Pain

While progress has been made in paediatric pain management, CYP continue to experience pain in a variety of circumstances. In 2021, the Lancet Child and Adolescent Health Commission released a report on the state of pain in childhood, identifying that the global recognition, assessment and treatment of children's pain lag behind the wealth of available research evidence on effective pain management practices in adults (Eccleston et al. 2021). The Commission proposed four transformative goals that researchers, clinicians, policy-makers and funders must collaboratively address to move the field of CYP's pain management forward in partnership with CYP and their families (Box 2.2).

The Commission also highlighted the importance of understanding what is most important to patients, both in clinical assessment and in research priorities. In a recent Priority Setting Partnership, young people with chronic pain, family members and health professionals identified patient-oriented research priorities, which included topics such as the relative efficacy of physical, psychological and pharmacological treatments, chronic pain care delivery, access and coordination, academic and vocational support, and clinician training (Birnie et al. 2019a). However, a review of the published literature on paediatric chronic pain found that most of these patient-oriented priorities had little to no available evidence, suggesting a gap between what has been researched and what is important to patients (Birnie et al. 2020).

There is a critical need for new research to inform best practice in dissemination and implementation of pain management (Chambers 2018), and creative approaches to knowledge mobilisation that address the needs of patients, health professionals, policy-makers and other groups. Examples of such initiatives include the Solutions for Kids in Pain (SKIP) network (kidsinpain.ca), whose mission is to improve CYP's pain management through coordination and collaboration (SKIP 2021). The importance of knowledge translation in pain has been recognised by IASP, naming 2022 the Global Year for Translating Pain Knowledge to Practice, providing researchers and clinicians with resources to support knowledge translation of pain research (https://www.iasp-pain.org/advocacy/global-year/translating-pain-knowledge-to-practice/). See also Chapter 16 for more information about knowledge implementation and dissemination.

BOX 2.2   TRANSFORMATIVE GOALS TO MOVE CYP PAIN MANAGEMENT FORWARD

To make CYP's pain:

1. *matter* (e.g. to clinicians, policy-makers, healthcare executives)
2. *understood* (e.g. further knowledge generation of the biopsychosocial aspects of pain in childhood is needed)
3. *visible* (e.g. implementation of regular, validated pain assessment practices for all children)
4. *better* (e.g. more research on pharmacological, psychological and personalised treatment approaches).

Source: Lancet Commission (Eccleston et al. 2021).

Children and Young People Continue to Experience Undermanaged and Preventable Nociceptive Pain

Nociceptive pain (acute) remains one of the most common causes of CYP pain and is a ubiquitous experience regardless of whether CYP are healthy or ill. Everyday pains, procedural pain and postoperative pain are common types of nociceptive pain CYP experience and are highly problematic (Tomblin Murphy et al. 2016; Noel et al. 2018; see Table 2.4). The various types of nociceptive pain are discussed in detail in Chapter 7. Despite the prevalence of nociceptive pain, pain management strategies continue to be underused in both hospital and primary care settings (Taddio et al. 2009; Birnie et al. 2014; Friedrichsdorf et al. 2015). This is coupled with evidence that CYP's reports of pain are not consistently acted upon (Bui and Lima 2021). Consistent efforts must be made to ensure CYP's nociceptive pain is properly managed.

Table 2.4 Common types of nociceptive pain.

Everyday pains
- 81% of CYP experience minor bumps, bruises or scrapes while engaging in play (Noel et al. 2018)

Procedural pain
- Needle pain is the most common type of nociceptive pain experienced in CYP (Postier et al. 2018)
- Over 75% of hospitalised children will experience painful procedures during their stay in hospital, with an average of 6.3 painful procedures administered daily (Stevens et al. 2014; Friedrichsdorf et al. 2015)
- CYP with a chronic illness (e.g. juvenile idiopathic arthritis, cancer, other conditions with visceral or exacerbations of pain) experience additional procedural pain due to needle procedures associated with treatment (Guzman et al. 2014; Tutelman et al. 2018)

Postoperative pain
- Chronic pain develops in 20% of children who undergo surgery (Rabbitts et al. 2017)
- The effects of postsurgical pain differ on the basis of the child's age as well as the pain management modality used (i.e. opioids or another analgesic (Ferland et al. 2018)

Children and Young People Continue to Experience Undermanaged Chronic Pain

With increased recognition of chronic pain in CYP, greater understanding has developed in terms of the impacts and factors that influence its development. Prevalence of chronic pain in children ranges from 4 to 88% (King et al. 2011; Liao et al. 2022); common types include *chronic secondary* and *acute to chronic* pain. Chronic secondary pain is problematic in CYP with chronic illnesses, as pain may be a symptom of the illness and also be associated with treatment (e.g. juvenile idiopathic arthritis is associated with significant secondary musculoskeletal pain).

The progression from nociceptive to chronic pain is an area of developing interest, given the importance of preventing chronic pain. Early research has shown that 20% of patients report significant pain three months after their surgery (i.e. meeting the temporal criteria for a diagnosis of chronic pain), while 50% report disability related to their pain (Rabbitts et al. 2017; Horn-Hofmann et al. 2018). The various types of chronic pain are discussed in detail in Chapters 9–11.

Despite its prevalence, chronic pain remains widely undermanaged in children (Palermo et al. 2019). This is associated with:

- lack of access to care (Palermo et al. 2019)
- presence of negative psychosocial factors (e.g. trauma; Meints and Edwards 2018)
- limited practitioner knowledge (Shipton et al. 2018), as well as resources and evidence available on chronic pain management in paediatrics (Birnie et al. 2019b, 2020).

It is imperative to address these barriers and shortcomings to ensure that the negative consequences of undermanaged chronic pain do not negatively impact CYP's development.

Consequences of Undermanaged Pain in Children and Young People

Suboptimal management of CYP's pain has detrimental consequences of a psychosocial and physiological nature. The experience of pain and its impacts on CYP in the short term ultimately lays the groundwork for their health and well-being for the rest of their lives.

Consequences of Undermanaged Nociceptive Pain in Childhood

Nociceptive pain has the capacity to have negative consequences in the short and long term, as outlined in Table 2.5.

Consequences of Undermanaged Chronic Pain in Childhood

In the context of chronic pain, where an individual experiences pain over a prolonged time, CYP are at risk for numerous short-term (e.g. increased sensitisation) and long-term (e.g. functional impairments) consequences. Table 2.6 provides some examples of the negative consequences of undermanaged chronic pain in CYP.

Ethical Imperative of Managing Pain in Children

Children have a right to pain management, as stated in the United Nations Declaration on the Rights of the Child (United Nations 1989):

Children should in all circumstances be among the first to receive protection

Table 2.5 Negative consequences of undermanaged nociceptive pain.

Physiological changes	▪ Elevated stress hormones and biomarkers (Eriksson and Campbell-Yeo 2019) ▪ Abnormalities in brain structure and development (Duerden et al. 2018) ▪ Lower pain thresholds in later childhood and adulthood (Walker et al. 2018; Eriksson and Campbell-Yeo 2019)
Psychological and social impacts	▪ Poor sleep quality (Evans et al. 2017) ▪ Low mood and self-esteem (Grasaas et al. 2020) ▪ Development of needle fears (McMurtry et al. 2015)
Prolonged hospitalisation and healing after a painful major procedure	▪ Increased duration of hospitalisation (Coffelt et al. 2013) ▪ Elevated hospital readmission rate (Coffelt et al. 2013) ▪ Prolonged and more painful healing period (Rabbitts et al. 2015)
Experience of future medical procedures	▪ Negative expectations and experiences of future procedural pain (Noel et al. 2017) ▪ Weakened effect of analgesia for future painful procedures and prolonged stress responses to pain (Weisman et al. 1998; McPherson et al. 2020) ▪ Greater reports of pain during future medical procedures (Noel et al. 2017)
Avoidance of healthcare	▪ Fear of pain accounts for 8% of self-reported vaccine refusal in children (Taddio et al. 2012) ▪ Avoidance of vaccinations later in life is associated with fear of needles developed in childhood (Zimlich 2018) ▪ 25% of adults who feared needle pain in childhood remain fearful in adulthood (Taddio et al. 2012)

Table 2.6 Negative consequences of undermanaged chronic pain.

Changes in brain structure	■ Disrupted neural connectivity (Walker 2019) ■ Increased stress and nociceptive brain activity (Jones et al. 2017) ■ Alterations in somatosensory functioning (Kersch et al. 2020)
Functional and psychosocial impairments	■ Impaired cognitive functioning (Valeri et al. 2015) ■ Impaired sleep quality (Murphy et al. 2020) ■ Reduced school attendance and self-efficacy in school (Logan et al. 2017) ■ Reduced physical activity (Rabbitts et al. 2016)
Increased healthcare utilisation	■ Increased healthcare utilisation (Tian et al. 2018) ■ Higher medical costs associated with care (Tian et al. 2018) ■ Increased economic burden (Health Canada 2021)
Worsened mental health and familial outcomes	■ Elevated risk of lifetime anxiety and depressive disorders (Vinall et al. 2016) ■ Worsened mental health persists from childhood into adulthood (Noel et al. 2016) ■ Chronic pain may negatively influence family functioning and well-being (Leeman et al. 2016)
Presence of chronic pain throughout the lifespan	■ Persistence of chronic pain from childhood into adulthood in upwards of 20–30% of children (Larsson et al. 2018)

and relief, and should be protected from all forms of neglect, cruelty and exploitation.

Despite the imperative to implement this, children's pain remains undertreated and they continue to experience moderate to severe pain (Birnie et al. 2014; Friedrichsdorf et al. 2015). When children's pain is left unmanaged, this infringes on their rights and is not considered to meet adequate standards of care (Friedrichsdorf and Goubert 2019). This is particularly problematic when the physiological, psychological and social consequences of undermanaged pain are considered.

Since the UN declaration, the Declaration of Montreal (IASP 2010) furthered the discussion of these rights and outlined the importance of these rights by highlighting the ethical imperative of managing pain. It specifies that pain management is a right of all humans, specifically stating that individuals:

■ should have access to pain management without discrimination
■ have the right to have one's pain acknowledged and receive information about pain and pain management
■ have the right to access pain assessment and treatment, delivered by appropriately trained health professionals.

These rights call on health professionals, policy makers and institutions to consider how pain management is prioritised and delivered, particularly for their youngest patients. Incorporating these standards is an essential step towards improving health and developmental outcomes for CYP who experience pain.

Summary

- Pain is a common experience in childhood and can be nociceptive (acute) or chronic in nature.
- Pain in childhood is unique given the developmental influences of this time of life impacting conceptualisation, assessment and treatment of pain.
- Despite growing research into paediatric pain, it continues to be undertreated in both nociceptive and chronic contexts.
- When CYP's pain is undermanaged, the biopsychosocial consequences are both immediate and long-lasting throughout the lifespan.
- The assessment and treatment of pain must be considered in the unique context of each individual CYP, including their developmental stage and psychosocial context.
- Pain management is a right of all humans, including CYP, to ensure they receive adequate care and their development is supported.

Multiple Choice Questions

1. Which of the following is *not* a reason that accounts for the undermanagement of children and young people's chronic pain?
   a. Limited practitioner knowledge of pain management
   b. Inadequate resources to implement pain management evidence
   c. Lack of family desire to engage in the child's care
   d. Lack of access to care for pain management

2. What is the most common type of pain experienced by children and young people?
   a. Visceral pain
   b. Needle pain
   c. Chronic pain
   d. Pain from chronic illness

3. On average, how many children and young people will go on to develop chronic pain following major surgery?
   a. 20%
   b. 45%
   c. 60%
   d. 80%

4. What is a common consequence of mismanaged pain in infancy?
   a. Changes in family functioning
   b. Significant alterations in physical activity
   c. Alterations in somatosensory development
   d. Development of a sleep disorder

5. Which of the following is *not* a factor that makes pain a distinct experience for children and young people as compared with adults?
   a. The ongoing development of the concept of pain
   b. The challenge of reliance on self-report
   c. The role of parents in children and young people's pain management
   d. The risk of developing chronic pain because of illness and/or surgical intervention

References

American Academy of Pediatrics Comittee on Fetus and Newborn (1987) Neonatal anesthesia. *Pediatrics* 80(3), 446.

American Society of Anesthesiologists (1987) Neonatal anesthesia. *ASA Newsletter* 15(2).

Anand, K., Sippell, W. and Aynsley-Green, A. (1987) Randomised trial of fentanyl anaesthesia in preterm babies undergoing surgery: effects on the stress response. *Lancet* 329, 62–66.

Anand, K. J. S., & Hickey, P. R. (1992). Halothane-Morphine Compared with High-Dose Sufentanil for Anesthesia and Postoperative Analgesia in Neonatal Cardiac Surgery. New England Journal of Medicine, 326(1), 1–9. https://doi.org/10.1056/NEJM199201023260101

Birnie, K.A., Chambers, C.T., Fernandez, C.V., et al. (2014) Hospitalized children continue to report undertreated and preventable pain. *Pain Research and Management* 19, 614784.

Birnie, K.A., Dib, K., Ouellette, C., et al. (2019a) Partnering for pain: a priority setting partnership to identify patient-oriented research priorities for pediatric chronic pain in Canada. *CMAJ Open* 7(4), E654–E664.

Birnie, K.A., Hundert, A.S., Lalloo, C., Nguyen, C. and Stinson, J.N. (2019b) Recommendations for selection of self-report pain intensity measures in children and adolescents: a systematic review and quality assessment of measurement properties. *Pain* 160(1), 5–18.

Birnie, K.A., Ouellette, C., Do Amaral, T. and Stinson, J.N. (2020) Mapping the evidence and gaps of interventions for pediatric chronic pain to inform policy, research, and practice: a systematic review and quality assessment of systematic reviews. *Canadian Journal of Pain* 4(1), 129–148.

Brennan, F., Lohman, D. and Gwyther, L. (2019) Access to pain management as a human right. *American Journal of Public Health* 109(1), 61–65.

Bui, M.V. and Lima, S. (2021) Parental preference for treatment location and inclusion in decision making in painful pediatric procedures: towards an evidence-based clinical guideline. *Journal of Pediatric Nursing* 59, 70–74.

Chambers, C.T. (2018) From evidence to influence: dissemination and implementation of scientific knowledge for improved pain research and management. *Pain* 159(Suppl.), S56–S64.

Coffelt, T.A., Bauer, B.D. and Carroll, A.E. (2013) Inpatient characteristics of the child admitted with chronic pain. *Pediatrics* 132(2), e422–e429.

Craig, K.D. and MacKenzie, N.E. (2021) What is pain: are cognitive and social features core components? *Paediatric and Neonatal Pain* 3(3), 106–118.

Duerden, E.G., Grunau, R.E., Guo, T., et al. (2018) Early procedural pain is associated with regionally-specific alterations in thalamic development in preterm neonates. *Journal of Neuroscience* 38(4), 878–886.

Eccleston, C., Fisher, E., Howard, R.F., et al. (2021) Delivering transformative action in paediatric pain: a *Lancet Child and Adolescent Health* Commission. *Lancet Child and Adolescent Health* 5(1), 47–87.

Eriksson, M. and Campbell-Yeo, M. (2019) Assessment of pain in newborn infants. *Seminars in Fetal and Neonatal Medicine* 24(4), 101003.

Evans, S., Djilas, V., Seidman, L.C., Zeltzer, L.K. and Tsao, J.C.I. (2017) Sleep quality, affect, pain, and disability in children with chronic pain: is affect a mediator or moderator? *Journal of Pain* 18(9), 1087–1095.

Ferland, C.E., Vega, E. and Ingelmo, P.M. (2018) Acute pain management in children: challenges and recent improvements. *Current Opinion in Anesthesiology* 31(3), 327–332.

Finnerup, N.B., Scholz, J., First, M.B., et al. (2018) Chronic pain as a symptom or a disease. *Pain* 160(1), 19–27.

Friedrichsdorf, S.J. and Goubert, L. (2019) Pediatric pain treatment and prevention for hospitalized children. *Pain Reports* 5(1), e804.

Friedrichsdorf, S.J., Postier, A., Eull, D., et al. (2015) Pain outcomes in a US children's hospital: a prospective cross-sectional survey. *Hospital Pediatrics* 5(1), 18–26.

Grasaas, E., Helseth, S., Fegran, L., Stinson, J., Småstuen, M. and Haraldstad, K. (2020) Health-related quality of life in adolescents with persistent pain and the mediating role of self-efficacy: a cross-sectional study. *Health and Quality of Life Outcomes* 18(1), 19.

Groenewald, C.B., Law, E.F., Fisher, E., Beals-Erickson, S.E. and Palermo, T.M. (2019) Associations between adolescent chronic pain and prescription opioid misuse in adulthood. *Journal of Pain* 20(1), 28–37.

Guzman, J., Oen, K., Huber, A.M., et al. (2014) The risk and nature of flares in juvenile idiopathic arthritis: results from the reACCh-Out cohort. *Pediatric Rheumatology* 12(Suppl. 1), O9.

Health Canada (2021) *An Action Plan for Pain in Canda*. Health Canada, Ottawa. Available at https://www.canada.ca/content/dam/hc-sc/documents/corporate/about-health-canada/public-engagement/external-advisory-bodies/canadian-pain-task-force/report-2021-rapport/report-rapport-2021-eng.pdf

Horn-Hofmann, C., Scheel, J., Dimova, V., et al. (2018) Prediction of persistent post-operative pain: pain-specific psychological variables compared with acute post-operative pain and general psychological variables. *European Journal of Pain* 22(1), 191–202.

Hyams, J.S., Di Lorenzo, C., Saps, M., Shulman, R.J., Staiano, A. and Van Tilburg, M. (2016) Childhood functional gastrointestinal disorders: child/adolescent. *Gastroenterology* 150(6), 1456–1468.e2.

International Association for the Study of Pain (2010) Access to pain management: Declaration of Montreal. https://www.iasp-pain.org/advocacy/iasp-statements/access-to-pain-management-declaration-of-montreal/

Jaaniste, T., Noel, M. and von Baeyer, C.L. (2016) Young children's ability to report on past, future, and hypothetical pain states: a cognitive-developmental perspective. *Pain* 157(11), 2399–2409.

Jones, E., Lattof, S.R. and Coast, E. (2017) Interventions to provide culturally-appropriate maternity care services: factors affecting implementation. *BMC Pregnancy and Childbirth* 17(1), 1–10.

Jordan, I., Martens, R. and Birnie, K.A. (2021) Don't tell me, show me: reactions from those with lived experience to the 2020 revised IASP definition of pain. *Paediatric and Neonatal Pain* 3(3), 119–122.

Kent, M.L., Tighe, P.J., Belfer, I., et al. (2017) The ACTTION-APS-AAPM Pain Taxonomy (AAAPT) multidimensional approach to classifying acute pain conditions. *Pain Medicine* 18(5), 947–958.

Kersch, A., Perera, P., Mercado, M., et al. (2020) Somatosensory testing in pediatric patients with chronic pain: an exploration of clinical utility. *Children* 7(12), 275.

King, S., Chambers, C.T., Huguet, A., et al. (2011) The epidemiology of chronic pain in children and adolescents revisited: a systematic review. *Pain* 152(12), 2729–2738.

Larsson, B., Sigurdson, J.F. and Sund, A.M. (2018) Long-term follow-up of a community sample of adolescents with frequent headaches. *Journal of Headache and Pain* 19, 79.

Leeman, J., Crandell, J.L., Lee, A., Bai, J., Sandelowski, M. and Knafl, K. (2016) Family functioning and the well-being of children with chronic conditions: a meta-analysis. *Research in Nursing and Health* 39(4), 229–243.

Liao, Z.W., Le, C., Kynes, J.M., et al. (2022) Paediatric chronic pain prevalence in low- and middle-income countries: a systematic review and meta-analysis. *EClinicalMedicine* 45, 101296.

Logan, D.E., Gray, L.S., Iversen, C.N. and Kim, S. (2017) School self-concept in adolescents with chronic pain. *Journal of Pediatric Psychology* 42(8), 892–901.

McGrath, P.J. (2011) Science is not enough: the modern history of pediatric pain. *Pain* 152(11), 2457–2459.

McMurtry, C.M., Riddell, R.P., Taddio, A., et al. (2015) Far from 'just a poke': common painful needle procedures and the development of needle fear. *Clinical Journal of Pain* 31(10 Suppl.), S3–S11.

McPherson, C., Miller, S.P., El-Dib, M., Massaro, A.N. and Inder, T.E. (2020) The influence of pain, agitation, and their management on the immature brain. *Pediatric Research* 88(2), 168–175.

Meints, S.M. and Edwards, R.R. (2018) Evaluating psychosocial contributions to chronic pain outcomes. *Progress in Neuropsychopharmacology and Biological Psychiatry* 87, 168–182.

Murphy, L.K., Palermo, T.M., Tham, S.W., et al. (2020) Comorbid sleep disturbance in adolescents with functional abdominal pain. *Behavioral Sleep Medicine* 19(4), 471–480.

Murray, C.B., Groenewald, C.B., de la Vega, R. and Palermo, T.M. (2020) Long-term impact of adolescent chronic pain on young adult educational, vocational, and social outcomes. *Pain* 161(2), 439–445.

Neville, A., Griep, Y., Palermo, T.M., et al. (2020) A 'dyadic dance': pain catastrophizing moderates the daily relationships between parent mood and protective responses and child chronic pain. *Pain* 161(5), 1072–1082.

Nicholas, M., Vlaeyen, J.W.S., Rief, W., et al. (2019) The IASP classification of chronic pain for ICD-11: chronic primary pain. *Pain* 160(1), 28–37.

Noel, M., Palermo, T.M., Chambers, C.T., Taddio, A. and Hermann, C. (2015) Remembering the pain of childhood: applying a developmental perspective to the study of pain memories. *Pain* 156(1), 31–34.

Noel, M., Groenewald, C.B., Beals-Erickson, S.E., Gebert, J.T. and Palermo, T.M. (2016) Chronic pain in adolescence and internalizing mental health disorders: a nationally representative study. *Pain* 157(6), 1333–1338.

Noel, M., Rabbitts, J.A., Fales, J., Chorney, J. and Palermo, T.M. (2017) The influence of pain memories on children's and adolescents' post-surgical pain experience: a longitudinal dyadic analysis. *Health Psychology* 36(10), 987–995.

Noel, M., Chambers, C.T., Parker, J.A., et al. (2018) Boo-boos as the building blocks of pain expression: an observational examination of parental responses to everyday pain in toddlers. *Canadian Journal of Pain* 2(1), 74–86.

Palermo, T.M., Slack, M., Zhou, C., Aaron, R., Fisher, E. and Rodriguez, S. (2019) Waiting for a pediatric chronic pain clinic evaluation: a prospective study characterizing waiting times and symptom trajectories. *Journal of Pain* 20(3), 339–347.

Postier, A.C., Eull, D., Schulz, C., et al. (2018) Pain experience in a US children's hospital: a point prevalence survey undertaken after the implementation of a system-wide protocol to eliminate or decrease pain caused by needles. *Hospital Pediatrics* 8(9), 515–523.

Rabbitts, J.A., Zhou, C., Groenewald, C.B., Durkin, L. and Palermo, T.M. (2015) Trajectories of postsurgical pain in children: risk factors and impact of late pain recovery on long-term health outcomes after major surgery. *Pain* 156(11), 2383–2389.

Rabbitts, J.A., Holley, A.L., Groenewald, C.B. and Palermo, T.M. (2016) Association between widespread pain scores and functional impairment and health-related quality of life in clinical samples of children. *Journal of Pain* 17(6), 678–684.

Rabbitts, J.A., Fisher, E., Rosenbloom, B.N. and Palermo, T.M. (2017) Prevalence and predictors of chronic postsurgical pain in children: a systematic review and meta-analysis. *Journal of Pain* 18(6), 605–614.

Raja, S.N., Carr, D.B., Cohen, M., et al. (2020) The revised International Association for the Study of Pain definition of pain: concepts, challenges, and compromises. *Pain* 161(9), 1976–1982.

Rovner, S. (1986) Surgery without anesthesia: can preemies feel pain? *Washington Post*, 13 August 1986. https://www.washingtonpost.com/archive/lifestyle/wellness/1986/08/13/surgery-without-anesthesia-can-preemies-feel-pain/54d32183-8eed-49a8-9066-9dc7cf0afa82/

Russell, B.S. and Park, C.L. (2018) The role of emotion regulation in chronic pain self-management. *Topics in Pain Management* 33(6), 1–10.

Shipton, E.E., Bate, F., Garrick, R., Steketee, C., Shipton, E.A. and Visser, E.J. (2018) Systematic review of pain medicine content, teaching, and assessment in medical school curricula internationally. *Pain and Therapy* 7(2), 139–161.

Solutions for Kids in Pain (2021) *Solutions for Kids in Pain.* https://kidsinpain.ca/#

Stevens, B.J. and Zempsky, W.T. (2021) Prevalence and distribution of pain in children. In *Oxford Textbook of Paediatric Pain*, 2nd edn (eds B.J. Stevens, G. Hathway and W.T. Zempsky), pp. 11–20. Oxford University Press, Oxford.

Stevens, B.J., Yamada, J., Promislow, S., Stinson, J., Harrison, D. and Victor, J.C. (2014) Implementation of multidimensional knowledge translation strategies to improve procedural pain in hospitalized children. *Implementation Science* 9(1), 120.

Taddio, A., Ilersich, A.L., Ipp, M., Kikuta, A. and Shah, V. (2009) Physical interventions and injection techniques for reducing injection pain during routine childhood immunizations: systematic review of randomized controlled trials and quasi-randomized controlled trials. *Clinical Therapeutics* 31(Suppl. B), S48–S76.

Taddio, A., Ipp, M., Thivakaran, S., et al. (2012) Survey of the prevalence of immunization non-compliance due to needle fears in children and adults. *Vaccine* 30(32), 4807–4812.

Tian, F., Guittar, P., Moore-Clingenpeel, M., et al. (2018) Healthcare use patterns and economic burden of chronic musculoskeletal pain in children before diagnosis. *Journal of Pediatrics* 197, 172–176.

Tomblin Murphy, G., Birch, S., MacKenzie, A., Bradish, S. and Elliott Rose, A. (2016) A synthesis of recent analyses of human resources for health requirements and labour market dynamics in high-income OECD countries. *Human Resources for Health* 14(1), 1–16.

Treede, R.D., Rief, W., Barke, A., et al. (2015) A classification of chronic pain for ICD-11. *Pain* 156(6), 1003–1007.

Treede, R.D., Rief, W., Barke, A., et al. (2019) Chronic pain as a symptom or a disease: the IASP classification of chronic pain for the International Classification of Diseases (ICD-11). *Pain* 160(1), 19–27.

Tutelman, P.R., Chambers, C.T., Stinson, J.N., et al. (2018) Pain in children with cancer: prevalence, characteristics, and parent management. *Clinical Journal of Pain* 34(3), 198–206.

United Nations (1989) *Convention on the Rights of the Child.* https://www.unicef.org.uk/what-we-do/un-convention-child-rights/

Unruh, A.M. and McGrath, P.J. (2013) History of pain in children. In *Oxford Textbook of Paediatric Pain* (eds P.J. McGrath, B.J. Stevens, S.M. Walker and W.T. Zempsky), pp. 3–11. Oxford University Press, Oxford.

Valeri, B.O., Holsti, L. and Linhares, M.B.M. (2015) Neonatal pain and developmental outcomes in children born preterm: a systematic review. *Clinical Journal of Pain* 31(4), 355–362.

Vinall, J., Miller, S.P., Bjornson, B.H., et al. (2014) Invasive procedures in preterm children: brain and cognitive development at school age. *Pediatrics* 133(3), 412–421.

Vinall, J., Pavlova, M., Asmundson, G.J.G., Rasic, N. and Noel, M. (2016) Mental health comorbidities in pediatric chronic pain: a narrative review of epidemiology, models, neurobiological mechanisms and treatment. *Children* 3(4), 40.

Walker, S.B., Rossi, D.M. and Sander, T.M. (2019) Women's successful transition to motherhood during the early postnatal period: a qualitative systematic review of postnatal and midwifery home care literature. *Midwifery* 79, 102552.

Walker, S.M. (2019) Long-term effects of neonatal pain. *Seminars in Fetal and Neonatal Medicine* 24(4), 101005.

Walker, S.M., Melbourne, A., O'Reilly, H., et al. (2018) Somatosensory function and pain in extremely preterm young adults from the UK EPICure cohort: sex-dependent differences and impact of neonatal surgery. *British Journal of Anaesthesia* 121(3), 623–635.

Weisman, S.J., Bernstein, B. and Schechter, N.L. (1998) Consequences of inadequate analgesia during painful procedures in children. *Archives of Pediatrics and Adolescent Medicine* 152(2), 147–149.

Zimlich, R.B. (2018) New study urges clinicians to consider needle fears. *Contemporary Pediatrics.* https://www.contemporarypediatrics.com/view/new-study-urges-clinicians-consider-needle-fears

3 Anatomy and Physiology of Pain

Charlie H.T. Kwok and Tuan Trang

Nociceptive (acute) pain serves as a warning system and protects from harm, whereas chronic pain is a debilitating condition in which pain signalling and processing may have gone awry. Knowledge of the anatomy and physiology of pain is crucial to understanding its presentation and management. This chapter describes the neural circuits and cellular mechanisms involved in pain perception, with relevance to the management of pain in children and young people.

What is Pain?

The International Association for the Study of Pain (IASP) defines pain as 'an unpleasant sensory and emotional experience associated with, or resembling that associated with, actual or potential tissue damage'. Some key pain terminologies are summarised in Table 3.1.

The Nervous System

The nervous system is subdivided into the central nervous system (CNS) and peripheral nervous system (PNS), comprising neurons and glia that form the neural circuitry for communicating and relaying information from the brain, spinal cord and peripheral organs. Important nervous system structures and terms are presented in Table 3.2.

- The PNS includes all nervous tissues (nerves, ganglia, enteric plexuses and sensory receptors) outside the CNS. It transmits information to the CNS (via sensory or afferent neurons) and from the CNS (via motor or efferent neurons).
- The CNS consists of the brain and spinal cord, and is responsible for interpreting sensory information and determining a response.
- The dorsal horn of the spinal cord acts as a sensory relay between the brain and site of injury.

Pain Mechanisms

Nociception is a complex biological phenomenon that can be broadly classified into four key processes: transduction, transmission, perception and modulation.

Managing Pain in Children and Young People: A Clinical Guide, Third Edition. Edited by Alison Twycross, Jennifer Stinson, William T. Zempsky, and Abbie Jordan.
© 2024 John Wiley & Sons Ltd. Published 2024 by John Wiley & Sons Ltd.

Table 3.1 Key pain terminology.

	Term	Definition
Type of pain	Acute pain	Pain of short duration attributed to injury or disease, generally considered to be protective as it triggers behaviours that remove us from harm and promote recovery. Pain arising from activation of nociceptors is known as *nociceptive pain* (the term used in this book)
	Chronic pain	Pain that persists beyond the expected time of healing and may occur in the absence of tissue damage. As a result, it serves no protective function and may become a health problem in itself
	Neuropathic pain	Pain caused by a lesion or disease of the nervous system
	Postsurgical chronic pain	Pain which arises after surgical procedure(s), lasting for three months or longer, with no other causes or underlying pathology associated with such pain
	Visceral pain	Pain that results from the activation of nociceptors of the thoracic, pelvic or abdominal viscera (organs). Pain perceived at a site other than the damaged viscera is known as referred pain, e.g. pain felt in the back when the pancreas is damaged
	Nociplastic pain	Chronic and widespread pain, e.g. fibromyalgia
	Total pain	Suffering that encompasses all of an individual's physical, psychological, social, spiritual and practical struggles
Pain symptom	Hypoalgesia	Diminished pain in response to a normally painful stimulus
	Sensitisation	Increased responsiveness of nociceptive neurons to their normal or subthreshold afferent input
	Wind-up	An increase in the excitability of spinal cord neurons provoked by repetitive stimulation of C fibres
	Allodynia	Pain due to a stimulus that does not generally provoke pain
	Hyperalgesia	Increased pain from a stimulus that generally provokes pain. Can be further described as *primary hyperalgesia* (enhanced responses at the site of injury) and *secondary hyperalgesia* (enhanced responses in areas adjacent to original injury)

Sources: Melzack and Wall (1983); IASP (2011).

Transduction

Transduction is the conversion of noxious (pain-inducing) stimulation to nerve impulses. In the presence of an injury, an inflammatory response is triggered when the damaged cells release chemicals (e.g. potassium, hydrogen ions, leukotrienes and prostaglandins) that activate nociceptors. Nociceptors are specialised sensory nerve endings, and encode information relating to the intensity, duration and location of noxious stimulations. They are found in somatic tissues (i.e. skin, cornea, mucous membranes, bones, joints and blood vessels) and visceral tissues (i.e. gastrointestinal tract and organs). Their concentration is highest in areas most prone to

Table 3.2 Key nervous system terminology.

	Term	Definition
Cellular organisation	Glia	Non-neuronal cells including astrocytes, microglia, ependymal cells, oligodendrocytes and Schwann cells
	Neuron	Excitable nerve cell (capable of transmitting an impulse and processing information) made up of cell body, dendrites and an axon
	Nociceptor	A sensory nerve ending capable of responding to noxious (painful) stimulation
	Synapse	The junction between two or more neurons
	Nerve	Bundle of axons in the PNS
	Ganglion	Cluster of neuronal cell bodies in the PNS
	Grey matter	Comprises neuronal cell bodies, dendrites, unmyelinated axons, axon terminals and neuroglia
	White matter	Comprises myelinated axons
	Tract	Bundle of axons in the CNS
Anatomy of a neuron	Axon	Single long process of a neuron that conducts nerve impulses towards another neuron
	Dendrite	Receiving, input portion of neuron
	Myelin sheath	Lipid and protein covering that insulates the axon, enabling faster electrical transmission
Anatomy of sensory pathways	Afferent (*sensory*) neurons	Neurons that carry sensory information *to* the CNS
	Efferent (*motor*) neurons	Neurons that carry motor information *from* the CNS
	Interneurons	Form connections between sensory and motor neurons in the CNS
	Substantia gelatinosa	Superficial area of the spinal dorsal horn where primary afferents of the spinothalamic tract synapse
	Enteric plexuses	Networks of neurons in organs and gastrointestinal tract
	Cranial nerves	Twelve pairs of nerves emerging from the brain
	Dorsal horn	Found in all spinal cord levels and comprising sensory nuclei that receive and process somatic information
Pain signalling processes	Action potential (nerve impulse)	Electrical signal created by changes in electrochemical energy across the membrane of the neuron
	Descending modulation	Mechanisms that modulate nociception (may be facilitatory or inhibitory) via nerve impulses transmitted from the brain to the spinal cord
	Myelination	Process of forming the myelin sheath, performed by oligodendrocytes in the CNS and Schwann cells in the PNS
	Neurotransmitters	Chemicals that influence the transmission of the impulse across the synapse by inhibition or excitation

Sources: Melzack and Wall (1965); Almeida et al. (2004); Clancy and McVicar (2009); Macintyre et al. (2010); Tortora and Derrickson (2018).

injuries (i.e. hands and feet) or in regions of the body needing additional protection (i.e. corneal, dental and some visceral tissues) (Charlton 2005). Importantly, the inflammatory response can be further enhanced by the release of mediators from inflammatory cells (e.g. histamine, serotonin and bradykinin) and nerve terminals (e.g. substance P) within the site of injury. Nociceptors have specific receptor sites to many of these substances and upon sufficient receptor binding, the nerve terminal becomes depolarised and firing of action potential(s) is triggered.

Under normal physiological conditions, inflammation increases local blood flow to produce local redness and warmth. In acute pain episodes this promotes healing by prompting us to protect the affected area. In contrast, persistent inflammation sensitises nociceptors by allowing the transmission of nerve impulses at lower thresholds (see definition in Table 3.1), a phenomenon known as *peripheral sensitisation*. Under these conditions, non-noxious touch or movement could be interpreted as painful. Sensitisation at the injury site is referred to as *primary hyperalgesia*. The sensitive area that extends beyond the area of tissue damage (i.e. secondary hyperalgesia) is the result of changes in pain processing within the CNS (Wall et al. 1999).

Transmission

Transmission involves conveying noxious impulses to the CNS. Somatosensory information encoded by nociceptors is passed on to the CNS via primary afferent fibres (PAFs). These fibres innervate the body and originate from cell bodies in the trigeminal (facial regions) and dorsal root ganglia. PAFs are classified into three main subtypes: $A\alpha/\beta$, $A\delta$ and C, based on degree of myelination, axon diameter and action potential conduction velocity (Table 3.3).

Myelination and Transmission Speed

Myelin allows impulses to be transmitted more quickly, but transmission occurs even when there is no myelin. There are two sensations of pain: fast, sharp pain (via myelinated $A\delta$ fibres), which is followed by slower, dull pain (via unmyelinated C fibres). In the spinal dorsal horn, small-diameter nociceptive fibres (C and $A\delta$) terminate in the superficial lamina known as the substantia gelatinosa, whereas large-diameter $A\beta$ fibres terminate in the deeper lamina.

PRACTICE POINT

The human body is divided into zones known as dermatomes. A dermatome represents the area of the body served by a particular spinal nerve. Knowledge of dermatomes assists in the management of spinal and epidural analgesia. This type of analgesia works by blocking transmission along a specific spinal nerve or group of nerves. Additional information about dermatomes and spinal/epidural analgesia can be found in Chapter 7.

Table 3.3 Conduction speed of nerve fibres.

Type of nerve fibre	Axon diameter (μm)	Myelinated	Conduction speed (m/s)
$A\alpha/\beta$	5–14	Yes	80–120
$A\delta$	2–5	Yes	5–40
C	0.4–1.2	No	0.5–2

Source: Adapted from *The Brain from Top to Bottom* (www.thebrain.mcgill.ca)

For action potentials to continue once they reach the spinal cord, they must be transmitted across the synapses between the PAFs and the second-order neurons that ascend the spinal cord. Several neurotransmitter systems are involved in the synaptic transmission of pain, some examples of which are summarised in Table 3.4.

Neurotransmitters are chemicals released in response to a nerve impulse reaching the presynaptic neuron (Figure 3.1). The neurotransmitters diffuse across the synaptic cleft and bind to receptor sites in postsynaptic neurons, leading to depolarisation of the neuronal membrane. When the threshold is reached, an action potential is generated that converts the chemical signal back to an electrical signal (Tortora and Derrickson 2018). Neurotransmitters interact with different receptors, which can result in either excitatory or inhibitory effects on nerve transmission.

PRACTICE POINT

Analgesics are designed to target neurotransmitter systems involved in pain processes. See Chapter 5 for more information about how analgesic medications work.

Table 3.4 Neurotransmitters important in pain pathways.

Function	Signalling molecule	Description
Excitatory	Glutamate	The principal excitatory neurotransmitter, acts via ionotropic (AMPA, NMDA, kainate) or metabotropic receptors (group I mGluR1 and mGluR5)
	Substance P	A pro-nociceptive neuropeptide found mostly in the spinal cord, but also in brain regions with direct projections to the spinal cord. Acts via the receptor neurokinin 1 (NK1)
Inhbitory	Gamma-aminobutyric acid (GABA)	The principal inhibitory neurotransmitter, acts via ionotropic $GABA_A$ or metabotropic $GABA_B$ receptors (of note, gabapentin does not act on GABA receptors)
	Opioids	Neuropeptides concentrated in the brainstem, act via mu, delta, kappa or nociceptin-like receptors
	Endocannabinoids	Lipid mediators ubiquitously expressed in many CNS regions, act mostly via CB1 and CB2 receptors
Modulator	Noradrenaline	Important for arousal and concentrated in the brainstem. It causes either inhibition or excitation of neurons depending on receptor subtype
	Serotonin	Concentrated in the brainstem and involved in the regulation of temperature, sensory perception, sleep and mood, and depending on the receptor subtype it interacts with, can have inhibitory or facilitatory effects
	Dopamine	Concentrated in the midbrain and involved in the regulation of emotional responses and subconscious movements of the skeletal muscles, also causes inhibition of neuronal receptors in dendrites

AMPA, α-amino-3-hydroxy-5-methyl-4-isoxazolepropionic acid; GABA, gamma-aminobutyric acid; NMDA, N-methyl-D-aspartate.
Source: Adapted from Smith (2009).

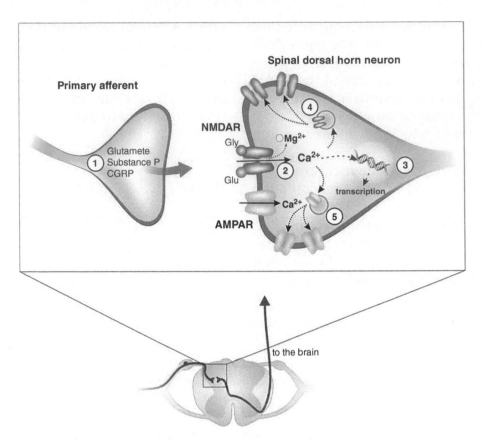

Figure 3.1 Synaptic events required for pain signalling in the spinal dorsal horn. (1) Incoming pain signals arriving at the primary afferent terminals lead to the release of neurotransmitters, including glutamate, substance P and calcitonin gene-related peptide (CGRP). (2) Upon receptor binding, the postsynaptic dorsal horn neuron becomes depolarised and allows the influx of calcium ions. (3) Secondary messenger signalling system of the receptor facilitates gene transcription and (4) protein trafficking for (5) insertion of additional receptors to the cell surface.

Once pain impulses succeed in overriding inhibitory mechanisms, they are transmitted across the spinal cord via projection neurons. Projection neurons carry sensory information to the brain via several ascending tracts, including the spinothalamic, spinoparabrachial, spinoreticular and spinomesencephalic tracts (Almeida et al. 2004). The efferent destinations of these tracts include cortical (e.g. prefrontal cortex, anterior cingulate cortex) and subcortical (e.g. thalamic nuclei, parabrachial nucleus and the red nucleus) structures of the brain. Activity in these brain regions underlies the sensory, emotional and cognitive experience of pain.

Perception

Perception occurs when the individual becomes consciously aware of pain: its intensity, nature and location. Conscious awareness of any sensation is generally considered to involve the cortex. Studies using advanced imaging techniques, e.g. magnetic resonance imaging (MRI) and positron emission tomography (PET), have revealed that perception of pain in the brain probably involves several areas of the cerebral cortex (prefrontal cortex, primary and secondary somatosensory cortices, anterior cingulate cortex and insular cortex), but also subcortical regions including the thalamus, basal ganglia and cerebellum (Schweinhardt and Bushnell 2010; Goksan et al. 2015; Duff et al. 2020).

Modulation

Modulation describes the neural processes that either inhibit or amplify pain. The periaqueductal grey (PAG), an area located in the midbrain, integrates descending sensory inputs from the cortex, thalamus and other regions involved in the perception of pain signals (Fields 2004). Herein, neurons in the PAG control nociceptive transmission via a spinobulbar loop by descending into the spinal dorsal horn via another midbrain nucleus, the rostroventral medial medulla (RVM). Under normal conditions, activation of the PAG–RVM–spinal dorsal horn pathway leads to anti-nociception (inhibition of pain). However, under pathological persistent pain, aberrant signalling can excite the spinal pain circuit, leading to an amplification of pain. A summary of ascending and descending pain modulatory pathways is shown in Figure 3.2.

Gate Control Theory of Pain

The gate control theory (Melzack and Wall 1965) posits that there is a *gating mechanism* in the spinal dorsal horn. When the gate is closed, impulses from nociceptors cannot travel up the spinal cord, and therefore painful inputs cannot be transmitted or perceived. Melzack and Wall also hypothesised that impulses descending from the brain could operate the pain gate. Diffuse noxious inhibitory control (DNIC) or conditioned pain modulation (CPM) represents this theory, whereby activity of nociceptive neurons innervating one location of the body may be inhibited by sensory (painful or innocuous) stimulation applied to another location. Examples of DNIC or CPM would be the perception that rubbing a bruise or pressure to skin areas adjacent to a wound alleviates pain.

ADDITIONAL INFORMATION

Illustrations that aid understanding of the gate control theory can be found at http://science.howstuffworks.com/environmental/life/human-biology/pain4.htm

Neuromatrix Theory of Pain

Melzack (1999) noted that the gate control theory could not explain the existence of phenomena such as phantom limb pain. The neuromatrix theory suggests that the mechanisms for interpreting and responding to pain are best viewed as a network of areas of the brain interacting with each other and with the gating mechanism in the spinal cord (Melzack 1999). Together these areas influence how we feel about a pain experience and how we interpret it, as well as determining our response. Collectively, the areas that contribute to the pain neuromatrix also ensure that information received from nociceptors is combined with other sensory information, memory, emotions and arousal states, a notion consistent with viewing pain as a biopsychosocial process (see Chapter 4). The neuromatrix theory adds to the gate control theory, emphasising that pain mechanisms are dynamic and capable of change.

The pain neuromatrix has since been used to explain a wide range of phenomena that influence pain experience, including placebo analgesics and the expectation/anticipation of pain (Ossipov et al. 2010; Eccleston et al. 2012). The potential influence of suggestion or expectation on pain experience is demonstrated by the following. In a study that monitored descending inhibition, one group of subjects were told that submerging their arm in cold water would reduce the intensity of a painful

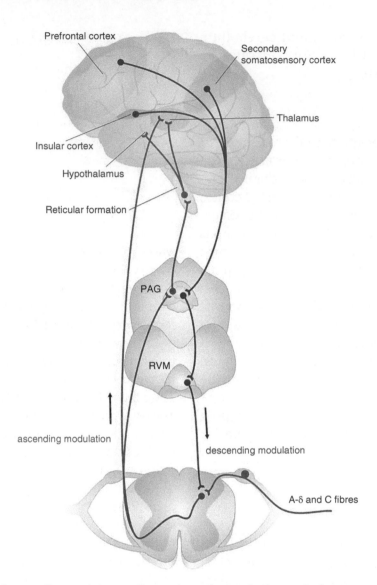

Figure 3.2 Schematic of ascending and descending pain pathways in the central nervous system. Noxious inputs into the CNS are generally encoded by Aδ and C fibres. They enter the spinal dorsal horn via the dorsal root ganglion and travel to the brain through ascending tracts. Once the signals reach the brain, a network of neurons involved in modulating pain signals descend back to the spinal dorsal horn. Key sites of pain modulation include the periaqueductal grey (PAG) and rostroventral medial medulla (RVM).

stimulus, and the second group were told that it would enhance it (Goffaux et al. 2007). Individuals expecting an analgesic effect experienced less pain and reduced spinal reflex activity in response to the painful stimulus. This reduction was not seen in those who were told to expect an increase in pain.

Biopsychosical Theory of Pain

The multitude of modulatory factors ultimately led to the creation of the biopsychosocial models of pain (*bio*, biological; *psych*, psychological; *social*, societal). This model highlights the mind–body relationship of pain transmission, wherein dynamic interactions between biological, psychological and social factors govern the overall pain experience. Of note, individual variability in pain experiences can be due to the differential influences of these factors. Examples of the biological, psychological and social factors that lead to either inhibition or amplification of pain are summarised in Table 3.5.

PRACTICE POINT

Expectations based on previous experiences and the confidence that CYP have in pain-reducing strategies enhance anti-nociceptive stimuli (i.e. modify descending inhibition).

Central Sensitisation in Chronic Pain

As the term suggests, the mechanisms for central sensitisation have been attributed to processes that occur within the CNS and are distinct from peripheral sensitisation or primary hyperalgesia, which originates within the region of tissue injury. Central sensitisation involves both a reduction in pain threshold and an amplification of the pain that is transmitted, which are critical for both the development and maintenance of chronic pain. Specifically, there are multiple mechanisms that contribute to nociceptive hyperexcitability within the CNS, including the following.

■ Recruitment of Aβ fibres, such that non-noxious stimuli are 'transferred' to the ascending spinothalamic tract and interpreted as pain.

Table 3.5 Factors influencing the experience of pain.

	Biological	Psychological	Societal
Inhibits pain	■ Analgesic drugs ■ Adjuvant analgesics ■ Counter-stimulation (e.g. massage, TENS, heat, acupuncture, acupressure) ■ Exercise ■ Endogenous analgesics	■ Hypnosis/imagery ■ Meditation ■ Cognitive behavioural therapy (CBT) ■ Suggestion of analgesic effect (placebo analgesics) ■ Positive thoughts ■ Relaxation ■ Biofeedback ■ Controlled breathing techniques ■ Distraction	■ Social support
Amplifies pain	■ Severity of illness or injury ■ Excessive activity ■ Re-injury ■ Sleep disturbance	■ Anxiety, fear or worry ■ Tension or stress ■ Depression ■ Focusing on pain ■ Catastrophising ■ Anticipation of severe pain	■ Stress in the home/school environment ■ Bereavement ■ Adverse childhood event

Source: Adapted from Smith (2009).

- An increase in the excitability of postsynaptic neurons in the spinal cord (meaning less stimulation is required to open the gate).
- Greater excitation at synapses between neurons carrying pain impulses (therefore more impulses pass through to be experienced as pain).
- Reduced inhibition in the spinal cord (meaning mechanisms that close the gate are not as effective).

Structural changes within the CNS may also occur that most likely result in chronic intractable pain (Kuner 2010). These changes include:

- a loss of grey matter resulting from the release of glutamate (Harris 2011)
- an increase in the number of connections that develop between synapses in pain pathways that are used repeatedly.

Recently, apart from neuronal targets, glia including microglia (resident immune cells of the CNS) and astrocytes (supporting cells, important for maintaining the integrity of the blood–brain barrier) have been shown to play a role in pain transmission. In particular, cytokines and chemokines – signalling molecules for communication between neuron and glia – are critically involved in the development and maintenance of chronic pain.

PRACTICE POINT

Central sensitisation is of interest to clinicians because:

- it helps illustrate the capacity of the nervous system to adapt to experience
- it is used to provide potential insight into chronic pain states (Woolf 2011)
- sensitisation may account for the increased risk of chronic pain in children and adults who experience abdominal pain early in their lives (Walker et al. 2010).

ADDITIONAL INFORMATION

- More information about central sensitisation can be found at http://junior-prof.wordpress.com/2008/07/07/what-is-central-sensitization/.
- A review of the role of glia cells in pain can be found at https://www.nature.com/articles/nrn2533.

Nociceptive Pain

Nociceptive pain is a response to tissue damage, which generally resolves as the injury heals. This type of pain is common in both children and adults; examples include bruises, sprains, burns or a reaction to an irritant such as a bee sting. The pain is typically well localised, may be constant, and often has an aching or throbbing quality. The severity of the pain can change with movement, position and the mechanical weight borne on the injured site. Throughout this book the term *nociceptive pain* is used.

Visceral Pain

Visceral pain is the pain of organs in the thoracic or abdominal cavities. This type of pain can evolve over time and is poorly localised and diffuse. Visceral pain is generally perceived in the midline of the body, at the lower sternum or upper abdomen, and is known as *referred pain*. The viscera are sensitive to distension (stretch), inflammation and ischaemia, but are less sensitive to cutting or heat. Visceral organs do not possess Aδ fibres but the C fibres carrying the pain information converge on the same area of spinal cord (substantia gelatinosa) where the Aδ fibres converge, so the brain localises the pain as if it were originating from the peripheral area instead of the visceral organ. Referred pain also occurs in areas supplied by cranial nerves.

Visceral pain can be accompanied by autonomic disturbances, such as pallor, sweating and nausea (Sikandar and Dickenson 2012). Persistent stimulation of visceral nociceptors can produce hyperalgesia, leading to central sensitisation and chronic pain states (Sikandar and Dickenson 2012).

Neuropathic Pain

Neuropathic pain is the consequence of injury or disease to the nervous system (Treede et al. 2015). This type of pain is generally chronic, as nerves do not heal well (Woolf and Mannion 1999). Neuropathic pain has a wide range of aetiologies and is common in hospitalised CYP. Trauma, spinal cord injury and chemotherapy-induced neuropathies are the more common entitities, but phantom limb pain, autoimmune and degenerative neuropathies, as well as neurodegenerative disorders, can also lead to neuropathic pain. This type of pain may overlap with nociceptive pain after surgery or injury (Macintyre et al. 2010). Central sensitisation is a key component of neuropathic pain, as aberrant signalling within the pain pathways can render nociceptive neurons hyperresponsive. Non-neuronal cell types, including astrocytes and microglia, also play a role by increasing the responsiveness of nociceptive neurons in the spinal cord (Scholz and Woolf 2007).

ADDITIONAL INFORMATION

Further information about the mechanisms and clinical management of neuropathic pain can be found at https://www.nature.com/articles/ncpneuro0113.

Chronic Postsurgical Pain

Chronic postsurgical pain (CPSP) is pain that lasts for more than two months after surgery (Macrae 2008). Surgery, by nature, involves the cutting of tissues and nerves, which induces an inflammatory response. The persistence of the inflammatory response can alter the activity of peripheral and central pain systems, which ultimately leads to chronic pain. Although all types of surgery can lead to postsurgical pain, some surgeries are at higher risk of causing nerve damage and these can transform into chronic neuropathic pain (e.g. thoracic surgery and coronary artery bypass surgery). Research has also suggested that a patient's emotional state can influence their susceptibility to CPSP (Page et al. 2013; Schug and Bruce 2017; Fischer et al. 2019). It has been recognised that perioperative pain management can reduce the risk of the development of CPSP. Current data indicate that around 20% of children develop CPSP after surgery (Rabbitts et al. 2017). It remains undertreated and individual variabilities represent a significant challenge in its management.

ADDITIONAL INFORMATION

Further information about the risk factors for and prevention of postsurgical pain can be found at https://www.science-direct.com/science/article/pii/S014067360668700X.

Physiology of Pain in Children and Young People

While the neural pathways responsible for pain processing are already present in premature infants, descending inhibition only develops in older children beyond infancy. The nervous system continues to develop from birth and, in parallel, pain processing undergoes significant postnatal maturation. The behavioural observations of immature nocifensive (reaction to painful stimulation) responses, such as an exaggerated withdrawal reflex and lower pain thresholds (Andrews and Fitzgerald 1999), highlight that pain is processed differently during early life. The literature relating to pain mechanisms in adults is arguably more comprehensive, due to the outdated misconception that an immature nervous system is less able to perceive pain. Children's vulnerability is also exemplified by the lack of effective verbal abilities in communicating their pain. Recent advances in developmental neurobiology have allowed us to better understand *how* pain is signalled in the immature nervous system, and *what* clinicians can do to better treat pain in infants and children. Some of the key differences identified by clinical and experimental animal studies in pain processing between adults and infants and children are presented in Table 3.6.

Postnatal Development of Pain Processing

The nervous system of infants and children is highly plastic, and the wiring of functional neuronal networks is shaped by activity. There is

Table 3.6 Key differences in the physiology of pain in infants and children.

Mechanistic difference	Functional outcome
Myelination is not complete at birth	Myelination progresses rapidly in the first few months of life (Benes et al. 1994). Pain is transmitted via both myelinated and unmyelinated nerve fibres. Impulse transmission can occur along Aδ fibres before they are fully myelinated but does so more slowly (Loizzo et al. 2009). Myelination is not necessary for conduction along C fibres
Postnatal refinement in termination of primary afferent fibres, large-diameter A fibres retract into deeper lamina of the spinal cord	Anatomical studies using experimental rodents discovered that large-diameter A fibres in the mature nervous system terminate in the deeper lamina of the spinal dorsal horn. During early life, A fibres also terminate in the superficial dorsal horn, which is critical for pain signalling. As a result, information transmitted via A fibres can also be interpreted as painful in the immature nervous system
Descending modulation of pain continues to develop until late adolescence	The ascending and descending pathways are present from birth. However, functional modulation requires an extended period of postnatal maturation, and descending inputs into the spinal dorsal horn are predominantly facilitatory during early life. As a result, inhibitory drive is weaker in young people compared to adults
Maturation of cortical representation of pain occurs postnatally	Cortical presentation is important in the perception of pain and influences the subsequent pain modulatory mechanisms. Non-invasive electroencephalogram (EEG) recording has revealed that neuronal encoding begins to discriminate between tactile and noxious stimulation at 35–37 weeks of gestation in humans (Fabrizi et al. 2011). A later study has also shown that noxious encoding in the cortex increases in clarity and response amplitude during early infancy (Verriotis et al. 2015)
Development of neurotransmitter signalling systems	Pharmacological studies in immature rodents have identified that inhibitory neurotransmitter signalling systems including GABA and glycine are functionally excitatory within the spinal pain circuit during early life (Koch et al. 2008). Also, descending modulation utilising opioid signalling is also facilitatory; the functional switch to inhibition occurs around pre-adolescence (Hathway et al. 2012; Kwok et al. 2014)

now ample evidence that early pain experiences can produce significant and persistent changes in the developing sensory nervous system, and these alter pain experiences later in life.

Infancy is a period of rapid nervous system development and is therefore a time when the nervous system is highly influenced by experiences such as pain (Grunau et al. 1994). Elegant studies suggest that the evolution from acute pain to persistent chronic pain in infants transpires through neuroplastic adaptation in the peripheral and central nervous systems, to the extent that they are more sensitive to pain (Beggs and Fitzgerald 2007; Bouza 2009; Loizzo et al. 2009).

The most striking example on how early life pain can prime future pain responses is shown in studies comparing development between premature and mature infants. Premature infants in the neonatal intensive care unit often experience multiple painful procedures daily during routine monitoring, as well as any surgical interventions necessary for their survival (Low and Schweinhardt 2012). Follow-up studies of premature children provide compelling evidence for the long-term effects of early pain experiences.

- The EPICure cohort, which followed extremely preterm infants born at less than 26 weeks of gestation up to the age of 20 years, found that children who were born preterm had significantly decreased sensitivity to thermal stimuli compared with age- and sex-matched term children at age 11 (Walker et al. 2009).
- At ages 18–20 years old, individuals born extremely prematurely had more episodes of moderate to severe recurring pain. In particular, females showed increased sensitivity to noxious cold, which correlated with smaller amygdala volume (Walker et al. 2018).
- A similar result was seen in a different cohort of premature children at age 9–12 years old who had neonatal cardiac surgery; subjects were significantly less sensitive than the control group to non-noxious mechanical and thermal stimuli at both the previously operated site and non-injured areas (Schmelzle-Lubiecki et al. 2007).

Also, experiencing pain is one factor associated with reduced growth of infants born before 32 weeks of gestation (Vinall et al. 2012). Slower postnatal growth is one of the predictors of adverse neurodevelopmental outcomes in infants born preterm. A later study revealed that impaired weight, length and head growth were associated with delayed microstructural development of the cortical grey matter, but not white matter (Vinall et al. 2013). Using experimental rodent models, it has also been reported that early life skin-breaking procedures (repetitive needle pricks) lead to persistent hyperexcitability of spinal dorsal horn neurons (van den Hoogen et al. 2018). This study showed that animals subjected to early life pain had a baseline increase in noxious processing, and enhanced responses to touch and noxious stimulations, after small incisional surgeries in adulthood.

Given the paramount consequences of early life pain on future pain sensitivity, neonatal pain treatment and prevention must incorporate strategies that mitigate the 'priming effects' of early pain to nociceptive circuits.

The cellular and molecular architecture for acute pain processing is present from birth and is highly plastic throughout postnatal development. It is well established that the experience of pain during infancy may produce structural and functional reorganisation of developing nociceptive pathways, which in turn may cause long-lasting alterations in pain processing that extend well into childhood and adulthood (Fitzgerald and Walker 2006). This mechanistic understanding underscores the importance of effective pain management in children and the consequences later in life.

Summary

- Structures involved in pain perception include peripheral and central nervous system components that perceive a sensation and generate feelings about the experience, as well as modulating incoming and outgoing impulses.
- The gate control theory remains useful in conceptualising nociceptive pain, but the neuromatrix theory and the biopsychosocial model provide a better framework for explaining the subjectivity of pain experiences and the development of chronic pain syndromes.
- Understanding the physiology of pain enables health professionals to appreciate the physical and psychological effects of pain, and to gain insight into how pain management strategies work.
- Recent advances in the science of pain have established that neonates, even those born prematurely, have the capacity to feel pain.
- Pain modulation undergoes significant postnatal maturation, and early life exposure to pain has a lifelong impact on sensory processing.
- More mechanistic understanding of immature pain processing will facilitate age-appropriate pain-relieving strategies.

Multiple Choice Questions

1. What is the definition of allodynia?
   a. Reduced pain sensation as a result of diseases
   b. Pain due to a stimulus that does not normally provoke pain
   c. Heightened response to a normally painful stimulus
   d. Pain sensed at a site distal to the injured area

2. What is the dorsal horn?
   a. Networks of neurons in the gastrointestinal tract
   b. A ventricle in the brain
   c. Sensory portion in the spinal cord that receives and processes somatic information
   d. Cell body of nerves entering the central nervous system

3. Which one of the following is a practical application of the gate control theory?
   a. Cognitive behavioural therapy
   b. Relaxation
   c. Mindfulness
   d. Conditioned pain modulation

4. What is the difference in pain experience between children and adults?
   a. Children cannot feel pain due to an immature nervous system
   b. Children are much more resilient compared to adults
   c. Adults have higher sensory thresholds and more coordinated responses to injuries
   d. Children are less affected by pain as they are more forgetful

5. What do children between the ages of 9 and 12 exhibit, after neonatal cardiac surgery?
   a. Changes in physical activity
   b. Reduced response to painful sensory stimulation
   c. Heightened response to painful sensory stimulation
   d. Changes in feeding behaviours

Acknowledgements

We would like to acknowledge Dr Churmy Fan for figures and Dr Nynke van den Hoogen for helpful discussions.

References

Almeida, T.F., Roizenblatt, S. and Tufik, S. (2004) Afferent pain pathways: a neuroanatomical review. *Brain Research* 1000, 40–56.

Andrews, K. and Fitzgerald, M. (1999) Cutaneous flexion reflex in human neonates: a quantitative study of threshold and stimulus–response characteristics after single and repeated stimuli. *Developmental Medicine and Child Neurology* 41, 696–703.

Beggs, S. and Fitzgerald, M. (2007) Development of peripheral and spinal nociceptive systems. In *Pain in Neonates and Infants*, 3rd edn (eds K.J.S. Anand, B.J. Stevens and P.J. McGrath), pp. 11–24. Elsevier, New York.

Benes, F.M., Turtle, M., Khan, Y. and Farol, P. (1994) Myelination of a key relay zone in the hippocampal formation occurs in the human brain during childhood, adolescence, and adulthood. *Archives of General Psychiatry* 51, 477–484.

Bouza, H. (2009) The impact of pain in the immature brain. *Journal of Maternal-Fetal and Neonatal Medicine* 22, 722–732.

Charlton, J.E. (ed.) (2005) *Core Curriculum for Professional Education in Pain*, 3rd edn. IASP Press, Seattle, WA.

Clancy, J. and McVicar, A. (2009) *Physiology and Anatomy for Nurses and Healthcare Practitioners: A Homeostatic Approach*, 3rd edn. Routledge, London.

Duff, E.P., Moultrie, F., van der Vaart, M., et al. (2020) Inferring pain experience in infants using quantitative whole-brain functional MRI signatures: a cross-sectional, observational study. *Lancet Digital Health* 2(9), e458–e467.

Eccleston, C., Fisher, E.A., Vervoort, T. and Crombez, G. (2012) Worry and catastrophizing about pain in youth: a reappraisal. *Pain* 153, 1560–1562.

Fabrizi, L., Slater, R., Worley, A., et al. (2011) A shift in sensory processing that enables the developing human brain to discriminate touch from pain. *Current Biology* 21, 1552–1558.

Fields, H. (2004) State-dependent opioid control of pain. *Nature Reviews Neuroscience* 5, 565–575.

Fischer, S., Vinall, J., Pavlova, M., et al. (2019) Role of anxiety in young children's pain memory development after surgery. *Pain* 160, 965–972.

Fitzgerald, M. and Walker, S. (2006) Infant pain traces. *Pain* 125, 204–205.

Goffaux, P., Redmond, W.J., Rainville, P. and Marchand, S. (2007) Descending analgesia: when the spine echoes what the brain expects. *Pain* 130, 137–143.

Goksan, S., Hartley, C., Emery, F., et al. (2015) fMRI reveals neural activity overlap between adult and infant pain. *Elife* 4, e06356.

Grunau, R.V., Whitfield, M.F. and Petrie, J.H. (1994) Pain sensitivity and temperament in extremely low-birth-weight premature toddlers and preterm and full-term controls. *Pain* 58, 341–346.

Harris, R.E. (2011) Central pain states: a shift in thinking about chronic pain. *Journal of Family Practice* 60(9 Suppl.), S37–S42.

Hathway, G.J., Vega-Avelaira, D. and Fitzgerald, M. (2012) A critical period in the supraspinal control of pain: opioid-dependent changes in brainstem rostroventral medulla function in preadolescence. *Pain* 153, 775–783.

International Association for the Study of Pain (2011) Pain terminology. https://www.iasp-pain.org/resources/terminology/

Koch, S.C., Fitzgerald, M. and Hathway, G.J. (2008) Midazolam potentiates nociceptive behavior, sensitizes cutaneous reflexes, and is devoid of sedative action in neonatal rats. *Anesthesiology* 108, 122–129.

Kuner, R. (2010) Central mechanisms of pathological pain. *Nature Medicine* 16, 1258.

Kwok, C.H., Devonshire, I.M., Bennett, A.J. and Hathway, G.J. (2014) Postnatal maturation of endogenous opioid systems within the periaqueductal grey and spinal dorsal horn of the rat. *Pain* 155, 168–178.

Loizzo, A., Loizzo, S. and Capasso, A. (2009) Neurobiology of pain in children: an overview. *The Open Biochemistry Journal* 3, 18–25.

Low, L.A. and Schweinhardt, P. (2012) Early life adversity as a risk factor for fibromyalgia in later life. *Pain Research and Treatment* 2012, 140832.

Macintyre, P.E., Scott, D.A., Schug, S.A., Visser, E.J. and Walker, S.M. (2010) *Acute Pain Management: Scientific Evidence*, 3rd edn. Australian and New Zealand College of Anaesthetists, Melbourne.

Macrae, W.A. (2008) Chronic post-surgical pain: 10 years on. *British Journal of Anaesthesia* 101, 77–86.

Melzack, R. (1999) From the gate to the neuromatrix. *Pain* 82(Suppl. 1), S121–S126.

Melzack, R. and Wall, P.D. (1965) Pain mechanisms: a new theory. *Science* 150, 971–979.

Melzack, R. and Wall, P.D. (1983) *The Challenge of Pain*. Basic Books, New York.

Ossipov, M.H., Dussor, G.O. and Porreca, F. (2010) Central modulation of pain. *Journal of Clinical Investigation* 120, 3779–3787.

Page, M.G., Stinson, J., Campbell, F., Isaac, L. and Katz, J. (2013) Identification of pain-related psychological risk factors for the development and maintenance of pediatric chronic postsurgical pain. *Journal of Pain Research* 6, 167–180.

Rabbitts, J.A., Fisher, E., Rosenbloom, B.N. and Palermo, T.M. (2017) Prevalence and predictors of chronic postsurgical pain in children: a systematic review and meta-analysis. *Journal of Pain* 18, 605–614.

Schmelzle-Lubiecki, B., Campbell, K.A., Howard, R., Franck, L. and Fitzgerald, M. (2007) Long-term consequences of early infant injury and trauma upon somatosensory processing. *European Journal of Pain* 11, 799–809.

Scholz, J. and Woolf, C.J. (2007) The neuropathic pain triad: neurons, immune cells and glia. *Nature Neuroscience* 10, 1361–1368.

Schug, S.A. and Bruce, J. (2017) Risk stratification for the development of chronic postsurgical pain. *Pain Reports* 2, e627.

Schweinhardt, P. and Bushnell, M.C. (2010) Pain imaging in health and disease: how far have we come? *Journal of Clinical Investigation* 120, 3788–3797.

Sikandar, S. and Dickenson, A.H. (2012) Visceral pain: the ins and outs, the ups and downs. *Current Opinion in Supportive and Palliative Care* 6, 17–26.

Smith, J. (2009) Anatomy and physiology of pain. In *Managing Pain in Children: A Clinical Guide* (eds A. Twycross, S.J. Dowden and E. Bruce), pp. 17–28. Wiley Blackwell, Chichester.

Tortora, G.J. and Derrickson, B.H. (2018) *Principles of Anatomy and Physiology*, 15th edn. John Wiley & Sons, Hoboken, NJ.

Treede, R.-D., Rief, W., Barke, A., et al. (2015) A classification of chronic pain for ICD-11. *Pain* 156, 1003–1007.

van den Hoogen, N.J., Patijn, J., Tibboel, D., Joosten, B.A., Fitzgerald, M. and Kwok, C.H.T. (2018) Repeated touch and needle-prick stimulation in the neonatal period increases the baseline mechanical sensitivity and postinjury hypersensitivity of adult spinal sensory neurons. *Pain* 159, 1166–1175.

Verriotis, M., Fabrizi, L., Lee, A., Ledwidge, S., Meek, J. and Fitzgerald, M. (2015) Cortical activity evoked by inoculation needle prick in infants up to one-year old. *Pain* 156, 222–230.

Vinall, J., Miller, S.P., Chau, V., Brummelte, S., Synnes, A.R. and Grunau, R.E. (2012) Neonatal pain in relation to postnatal growth in infants born very preterm. *Pain* 153, 1374–1381.

Vinall, J., Grunau, R.E., Brant, R., et al. (2013) Slower postnatal growth is associated with delayed cerebral cortical maturation in preterm newborns. *Science Translational Medicine* 5(168), 168ra8.

Walker, S.L., Dengler-Crish, C.M., Rippel, S. and Bruehl, S. (2010) Functional abdominal pain in childhood and adolescence increases risk for chronic pain in adulthood. *Pain* 150(3), 568–572.

Walker, S.M., Franck, L.S., Fitzgerald, M., Myles, J., Stocks, J. and Marlow, N. (2009) Long-term impact of neonatal intensive care and surgery on somatosensory perception in children born extremely preterm. *Pain* 141, 79–87.

Walker, S.M, Melbourne, A., O'Reilly, H., et al. (2018) Somatosensory function and pain in extremely preterm young adults from the UK EPICure cohort: sex-dependent differences and impact of neonatal surgery. *British Journal of Anaesthesia* 121, 623–635.

Wall, P.D., Melzack, R. and Bonica, J.J. (1999) *Textbook of Pain*. Churchill Livingstone, Edinburgh.

Woolf, C.J. (2011) Central sensitization: implications for the diagnosis and treatment of pan. *Pain* 152(3 Suppl), S2–S15.

Woolf, C.J. and Mannion, R.J. (1999) Neuropathic pain: aetiology, symptoms, mechanisms, and management. *Lancet* 353, 1959–1964.

4 Pain: A Biopsychosocial Phenomenon

Line Caes, Paula Forgeron, and Liesbet Goubert

Introduction

Pain is a complex phenomenon comprising biological, psychological and social factors. These factors influence and interact to shape the pain experience of children and young people (CYP) (Figure 4.1). For example, previous pain experiences contribute to pain memory and together with cognitive development influence future pain experience and expression. Pain expression is also influenced by how previous pain expression was received by caregivers (social environment). Physiological processing of pain can be altered by repeated painful stimulation as well as previous pain experiences. Notably, some factors that influence pain experience do not fit within one of these three broad factors. For instance, cognitive development and temperament have a biological basis but are influenced by psychological and social factors. We discuss these factors in this chapter.

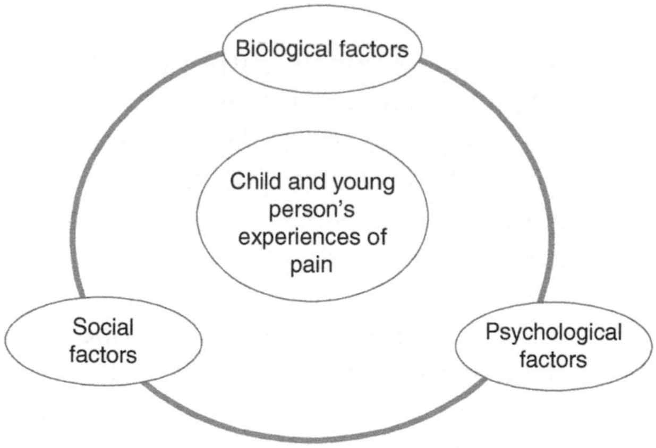

Figure 4.1 Pain as a biopsychosocial phenomenon.

Nociception

Nociception is the sensory nervous system's response to harmful (or potentially harmful) stimuli and has a protective function by motivating an individual to remove themselves from harm. The nociceptive system comprises multiple sites (e.g. nociceptors, spinal cord, brainstem and the brain), resulting in various patterns of activity that contribute to individual pain experiences. Over time, and in certain situations (e.g. exposure to repeated painful stimuli), pain processing can be altered. This can result in allodynia and hyperalgesia due to neuroplasticity, leading to a disruption of normal pain processing in CYP and adults (Woolf and Salter 2000; Fitzgerald 2009). See Table 4.1 for definitions of terms.

Managing Pain in Children and Young People: A Clinical Guide, Third Edition. Edited by Alison Twycross, Jennifer Stinson, William T. Zempsky, and Abbie Jordan.
© 2024 John Wiley & Sons Ltd. Published 2024 by John Wiley & Sons Ltd.

Table 4.1 Definitions of main terms used throughout the chapter.

Allodynia	Pain due to a stimulus that is not typically painful
Hyperalgesia	Increased pain due to a stimulus that typically provokes pain
Sex	A biological binary construct referring to 'the biological and physiological characteristics that define men and women' (World Health Organization (WHO) 2022)
Gender	A social construct referring to 'the roles, behaviours, activities, and attributes that any society considers appropriate for girls and boys, and women and men' (WHO, 2022)
Catastrophic thinking about pain	An exaggerated negative orientation towards actual or anticipated pain experiences (Sullivan et al. 1995)

Biological Factors

Age

At birth even very preterm infants process painful stimuli, as illustrated by cortical responses to heel lance (Slater et al. 2006). Variations in noxious stimuli responses throughout childhood are influenced by age, illness/stress and previous pain experience. Management of pain may also be impacted by age; neonates, seven days and younger, have been shown to require significantly less morphine than older neonates postoperatively (Bouwmeester et al. 2003). Age-related and genotype differences can also impact the metabolism of certain analgesics such as codeine (Williams et al. 2002).

Age has also been found to affect pain perception. At an early age, CYP recognise that pain is unpleasant. Perceptions and descriptions of pain in CYP are influenced by age, cognitive developmental stage and previous painful experiences (McGrath and Hillier 2003). Several studies have examined CYP's experiences of procedural pain, with McCarthy et al. (2010) for example demonstrating:

- age-related differences in reported pain intensity, with older CYP reporting less pain intensity
- differing levels of behavioural distress during procedures, with older CYP displaying less distress.

Decreases in pain perception with increase in age may be related to older CYP having:

- greater understanding of what is happening and subsequent reductions in anxiety
- developed coping strategies and methods to self-distract from procedural pain.

However, in relation to the effect of age on the experience of postoperative pain, research evidence is inconclusive.

- Age did not consistently predict pain-related outcomes among CYP aged 8–21 years on postoperative day three following spinal fusion (Kotzer 2000).
- No difference was found among young people aged 13–20 years undergoing oral surgery (Gidron et al. 1995).
- Older CYP reported more postoperative pain intensity when swallowing after tonsillectomy than children aged 7–13 years (Crandall et al. 2009).

Regarding chronic pain, prevalence rates increase with age; older children experience more headaches, musculoskeletal, back and non-specific or general pain, but less abdominal pain than younger children (King et al. 2011).

Sex and Gender

Despite clear definitions provided by the WHO (2022) (Table 4.1), confusion exists regarding the terminology of sex and gender in the context of CYP's pain experiences. Research evidence concerning the role of sex differences in explaining pain perceptions and behaviour is contradictory and inconclusive.

- Some studies have identified no sex difference in pain intensity during medical procedures (Bournaki 1997) or postoperatively (Crandall et al. 2009).
- Sex differences were found in the prevalence and response to chronic pain as well as the use of coping strategies. Girls use more social support-seeking behaviours while boys use more behavioural distraction techniques (Lynch et al. 2007; Martin et al. 2007).
- A systematic review on sex differences in experimentally induced pain responses found no sex difference unless age was taken into account. Female participants 12 years and older reported more pain intensity than males 12 years and older (Boerner et al. 2014).
- For chronic pain, prevalence rates for most types of pain are higher in girls than in boys after the onset of puberty (King et al. 2011), but mediating factors for the relationship between sex and pain are unclear.

Few studies have directed attention to *gender* differences in pain behaviours (Boerner et al. 2014, 2018).

- Gender differences have been attributed to social factors, such as parents responding differently due to societal factors (e.g. boys don't cry), suggesting it is more socially acceptable for girls to express pain than boys (Finley et al. 2009).

- Social factors could interact with biological differences between boys and girls, as there is evidence that females may be more susceptible to pain than males because of hormonal or neurobiological factors (Kuba and Quinones-Jenab 2005).
- Biological and psychosocial factors, and their interaction, are important in understanding sex and gender differences in pain perception (Boerner et al. 2018).

ADDITIONAL INFORMATION

For an overview of the effects of sex and gender, see Boerner, K.E., Schinkel, M. and Chambers, C.T. (2015) It is not as simple as boys versus girls: the role of sex differences in pain across the lifespan. *Pain Management* 5(1), 1–4.

Cognitive Development

Cognitive development results from a complex interaction of biological, psychological and social factors. Research has shown how CYP's level of cognitive development may influence their pain experiences by shaping their understanding of pain, the coping strategies they use and how they communicate about pain (McGrath and McAlpine 1993). Research has revealed how CYP's level of cognitive development impacts:

- their perception of pain (Hurley and Whelan 1988; Gaffney 1993)
- their ability to reliably report their pain (Chan and von Baeyer 2016)
- our communication with CYP in pain (Table 4.2 provides information on how to adapt communication about pain in accordance with cognitive development).

Table 4.2 How to adapt communication about pain in accordance with cognitive development.

Age	Developmental consideration	Useful communication techniques
0–12 months	▪ Stranger anxiety (6–12 months) ▪ Pre-verbal communication ▪ Beginning verbalisation	▪ Rapport through touch, feeding and simple communication ▪ Primary information exchange is with parents
13–35 months	▪ Increase in vocabulary and sentence complexity ▪ Separation anxiety ▪ Increasing ability to follow commands	▪ Rapport through play (physical and imaginary) ▪ Use simple commands in familiar terms ▪ Encourage family presence
3–6 years	▪ Ability to articulate experiences (e.g. pain) and emotions ▪ Awareness of body and body parts as well as sense of self	▪ Use play, books and stories to convey information ▪ Be honest ▪ Use familiar concepts for emotional expressions
7–12 years	▪ Increasing language and concept comprehension ▪ Knowledge of body parts and function	▪ Writing, drawing, storytelling and multimedia to convey information
13–18 years	▪ Increasing independence ▪ Broad range of emotional maturity	▪ Include in decision-making ▪ Respect need for privacy and confidentiality

Source: Adapted from Sheldon and Foust (2014).

Illustrating the complexity, while CYP with a cognitive impairment may function at a typically younger developmental stage compared with their chronological age, they can develop an understanding of some medical concepts typically only understood at a more advanced developmental stage. Nonetheless, it is important to note that such repeated exposure to painful medical procedures (e.g. bone marrow aspirations, lumbar punctures in the context of cancer treatment) can still provoke fear in the absence of adequate pain management (McMurtry et al. 2015).

Further, adolescence can be a particularly challenging time as this developmental stage represents a sensitive period for the development of higher-order cognitive skills such as executive functioning. Executive functions enable goal-directed thoughts and actions, including skills such as cognitive flexibility, planning, working memory and inhibition. Executive functioning improves from childhood into adulthood, with some aspects (e.g. working memory) showing a dip in performance during early adolescence due to rapid changes in brain structure and functioning (Blakemore and Choudhury 2006). The implications of developing executive functioning skills on CYP's abilities to perceive and manage pain remain unknown.

Genetics

Although genetic determinants of pain responses have been identified, Mogil et al. (2000) argue it is unlikely that a simple genetic basis explains variation in pain sensitivity and responses. Genes may affect how people respond to different types of pain relief.

- A single gene (catechol-*O*-methyltransferase, *COMT*) was found to affect how people tolerate pain. This gene produces an enzyme that regulates endorphin production in the body (Zubieta et al. 2003).
- Kleiber et al. (2007) found that a genotype predicted how effective topical anaesthetic was in CYP undergoing intravenous catheter insertion. Specifically, CYP who reported higher pain were more likely to have the endothelin receptor type A (EDNRA) TT genotype, suggesting that variation in genes involved in peripheral nociception may mediate responses to topical anaesthetic.
- No single nucleotide polymorphisms (out of three genes including *COMT*) were associated with pain tolerance (Patanwala et al. 2019).

Psychological Factors

Numerous psychological factors have been found to influence CYP's pain experiences. These include negative influences (e.g. fear, catastrophic thinking, negative memories about previous pain experiences), positive influences (e.g. optimism) and mixed influences (e.g. temperament).

Temperament

Temperament refers to the general nature, behavioural style or characteristic mood of an individual (Chess and Thomas 1986). Temperament is considered to have a strong heritable component, be present from infancy, and influenced by social and psychological factors.

Several studies have demonstrated that a CYP's temperament affects how that individual behaves when in pain. However, the relationship between temperament and various aspects of the pain experience is complex and multidimensional.

- Temperament has been shown to influence how CYP behave when they are in pain (e.g. cry and complain versus withdraw and feign sleep), and coping strategies used (Conte et al. 2003).
- Rocha et al. (2003) found that CYP low in the temperament dimension of adjustment or adaptability showed higher pain reactivity (as assessed by facial responses) during immunisations.
- A systematic review of CYP identified activity and mood as the most consistent temperamental factors influencing CYP's pain experiences (Ranger and Campbell-Yeo 2008).
- Prospective examinations identified a fearful temperament as a predictor of somatic complaints one year (Wolff et al. 2010) and seven years later than baseline assessment (Rocha and Prkachin 2007).

Temperament not only has the potential to influence the pain perception and experiences of CYP, but can moderate the impact of pain-relieving interventions.

- Chen et al. (2000) demonstrated that CYP's pain sensitivity influences the impact of a cognitive-behavioural intervention to reduce distress during lumbar puncture.
- Temperament can influence CYP's ability to pay attention to a stimulus; this could negatively impact their ability to engage with distractors to reduce nociceptive pain experiences (McCarthy and Kleiber 2006).

In summary, it is important that health professionals have a good understanding of the CYP's temperament to inform individualised treatment. Parents are most familiar with their CYP's temperament and critical to facilitating effective pain relief in CYP (Ranger and Campbell-Yeo 2008).

ADDITIONAL INFORMATION

For an overview of temperament and pain response, see Ranger, M. and Campbell-Yeo, M. (2008) Temperament and pain response: a review of the literature. *Pain Management Nursing* 9(1), 2–9.

Fear

Fear is commonly experienced by CYP in pain, impacting their perception of pain and predicting their responses to acute and chronic pain experiences (Huguet et al. 2011). Fear has been found to be strongly associated with avoiding activities assumed to further increase or induce pain, thereby contributing to muscle deconditioning and pain persistence (Wilson et al. 2011). Evidence also suggests that pain-related fear strongly influences pain-associated functional disability (Martin et al. 2007; Simons et al. 2011). Interestingly, Simons and colleagues found that a decline in pain-related fear over a month was associated with improved functioning and resumption of daily activities. Several tools have been developed to assess fear (Table 4.3).

Catastrophic Thinking

Catastrophic thinking about pain is characterised by three components: magnifying the pain experience, feeling helpless in dealing with the pain and ruminating about the pain experience (Sullivan et al. 1995). Numerous studies have shown how catastrophising about pain is related to negative pain outcomes in CYP, including:

- heightened experience of pain (Vervoort et al. 2006)
- academic, recreational, physical and psychosocial disability (Vervoort et al. 2006)
- transition from adult acute to chronic pain (Simons et al. 2015).

Although evidence supports the detrimental impact of catastrophic thinking on pain-related functioning, how to define and operationalise the concept in childhood is contested. Specifically, it is unclear to what extent catastrophic thinking should be considered as an independent construct or as an extreme version of worrying. It has been suggested that the standard measure for catastrophic thinking (the Pain Catastrophizing Scale for Children) reflects a measure of CYP's worry instead of assessing their catastrophic beliefs (Eccleston et al. 2012). Consequently, caution is advised in adopting and interpreting assessments of catastrophic thoughts or worries in CYP.

Table 4.3 Questionnaires assessing pain-related fears.

Measure	Context
Fear-Avoidance Beliefs Questionnaire (Wilson et al. 2011)	Chronic pain
Fear of Pain Questionnaire (FOPQ-C) (Simons et al. 2011)	Chronic pain
Children's Fear Scale (CFS) (McMurtry et al. 2011)	Acute pain situations (https://www.uoguelph.ca/pphc/childrens-fear-scale)

Optimism

While research investigating psychological factors influencing CYP's pain has typically focused on factors increasing pain experiences, recent studies have explored which factors boost CYP's resilience to pain (e.g. optimism). Of these few optimism-based studies, evidence suggests that higher levels of optimism are related to shorter pain duration, lower pain-related disability and better quality of life amongst CYP with chronic pain (Cousins et al. 2015). Expanding our understanding of the role of optimism will inform how pain management interventions can be enhanced with strategies to stimulate positive emotions, such as positive future thinking techniques (Cousins et al. 2016).

Pain Memories

CYP's previous experiences of pain influence how they react to subsequent painful events. Evidence shows how current pain experiences are modified by previous exposure to painful situations, and how assessment and management evaluations rely heavily on CYP's memory (Noel et al. 2012). Research found that CYP's negative pain memories were as important as their actual pain experiences in terms of increasing their risk for greater pain and distress at future painful procedures. Negative memories and pain experiences were also linked to reduced engagement with healthcare (Noel et al. 2012). Consequently, CYP's pain should be managed effectively from their first healthcare encounter.

ADDITIONAL INFORMATION

For an overview of pain memories, see Noel, M., Palermo, T.M., Chambers, C.T., et al. (2015) Remembering the pain of childhood: applying a developmental perspective to the study of pain memories. *Pain* 156(1), 31–34.

Social Factors

Culture

Culture is a widely used yet debated term, defined as a 'multidimensional phenomenon that encompasses processes, products, and results of human activity, material and spiritual, transmitted from generation to generation in a non-biological way' (Mironenko and Sorokin 2018, p. 338). Culture has also been described as a framework for learning behaviour and communication, which might shape a CYP's perspective on health and illness (Craig 1986), including pain.

Consequently, CYP's culture is likely to influence how they perceive, express and react to pain, as well as how they are assessed and treated for pain. The effect of culture on CYP's perception of, and responses to, pain is likely to be, at least in part, attributable to *social learning*. Social learning occurs when an individual learns something by observing another person doing it; essentially, learning by modelling (Bandura 1977). There is little evidence for cultural differences in nociception (sensation), or the perception of pain itself. Instead, studies suggest the following:

- CYP's *expressions* of pain may be influenced by their cultural background (Finley et al. 2009).
- Cultural factors influence non-verbal pain behaviours and coping strategies of CYP during painful procedures (Kristjansdottir et al. 2012).
- Country of residence (Canada, Iceland, Thailand) alone does not explain the effects of culture and was not associated with predictors (vertical individualism, horizontal individualism, collectivism), mediators (parenting style) or outcomes (parental use of solicitousness or discouraging behaviours) when predicting

parental responses to their CYP's pain (Kristjansdottir et al. 2018).

- Thai CYP defined pain as dispiriting, as *torture* and as *suffering*, and their expression of pain was influenced by cultural values of patience and endurance ('ot ton' in Thai). CYP may refrain from overt expressions of pain, believing parents and family members will look after them and value endurance in the face of pain (Jongudomkarn et al. 2006).

Parental, Family and Other Social Agents

Pain is experienced in a social context. The behaviour of others (e.g. parents, family members, peers and teachers) can affect a CYP's pain. Evidence reveals the following (see Brown et al. 2018 for an overview):

- Parental responses can teach CYP how to behave in a manner acceptable to their family (which is influenced by their culture as well as the society in which they live).
- Protective responses (reassuring, soothing, asking about the pain and providing physical comfort) are associated with increased CYP's pain, distress and functional disability.
- Coping/promoting responses (distraction, encouraging deep breathing or using humour) are related to positive CYP's outcomes.

ADDITIONAL INFORMATION

For an overview, see Brown, E.A., De Young, A., Kimble, R., et al. (2018) Review of a parent's influence on pediatric procedural distress and recovery. *Clinical Child and Family Psychology Review* 21(2), 224–245.

Acknowledging the important role that parental cognitive, emotional and behavioural responses play in understanding CYP's pain experiences, Goubert and Simons (2013) developed the Interpersonal Fear Avoidance Model (IFAM). The IFAM underscores the bidirectional influence between parental and CYP's fear, catastrophic thinking and protective, avoidant behaviours in the context of pain. Preparing parents appropriately for nociceptive painful medical procedures and including them in chronic pain management programmes is important. Accumulating evidence emphasises that active parental engagement in children's chronic pain treatment reduces parental distress and improves both CYP's and parental functioning (Kemani et al. 2018).

Beyond parental responses, broader family dynamics also influence CYP's chronic pain experiences.

- Families of a CYP with chronic pain report worse functioning compared to those without a CYP with chronic pain. However, it is unclear if the stresses of the CYP's pain negatively impact family function or if disrupted family functioning decreases coping in the presence of pain (Lewandowski et al. 2010).
- CYP of parents with chronic pain are at increased risk of developing chronic pain (Higgins et al. 2015).

Consequently, a family's chronic pain history should be included in routine pain assessment and management approaches.

During adolescence the influence of peers, particularly close friends, may affect chronic pain experience. Having chronic pain may impact friendships (Forgeron et al. 2011, 2013):

- negatively, e.g. loss of friendships, feelings of loneliness, increases in pain intensity and distress
- positively, e.g. increases in social support leading to increases in school attendance and activities.

Teachers are key social figures in the lives of CYP and can also play a significant role in pain management among CYP with chronic pain (Vervoort et al. 2014). Research is starting to identify that teachers are key in the return to school for young people who experience nociceptive surgical pain (Dagg et al. 2020).

ADDITIONAL INFORMATION

For an overview, see Palermo, T.M., Valrie, C.R. and Karlson, C.W. (2014) Family and parent influences on pediatric chronic pain: a developmental perspective. *American Psychologist* 69(2), 142–152.

Summary

- Pain is a biopsychosocial phenomenon, with a wide range of biological, psychological and social factors interacting in shaping CYP's experiences of pain.
- It is often difficult to separate biological, psychological and social factors as they typically interact to impact CYP's pain experiences.
- Most evidence has studied factors increasing pain experiences (e.g. fear, catastrophic thinking); more recent research explores factors reducing pain experiences (e.g. optimism).
- Numerous factors affecting CYP's perceptions of pain can help to explain why individuals behave differently in similar painful situations.
- Health professionals must consider biological, psychological and social factors when assessing and managing pain in CYP.

Multiple Choice Questions

1. Which one of the following is the main difference between sex and gender?
   a. Sex refers to the biological differences between boys and girls, while gender refers to the psychosocial differences between boys and girls.
   b. Sex influences pain experiences, but gender does not.
   c. Sex has a clear impact on pain experiences, with boys experiencing less pain than girls, while there is mixed evidence for the impact of gender on pain experiences.
   d. There is no difference between sex and gender, and both terms can be used interchangeably.

2. Which of the following statements is *incorrect*?
   a. Research into the role of psychological factors in influencing childhood pain experiences has mostly focused on factors negatively influencing pain.
   b. Taking into account country alone is not sufficient to understand the impact of culture on childhood pain experiences.
   c. There is a clear distinction between the influence of biological, psychological and social factors that influence childhood pain experiences.
   d. Parental responses and family dynamics have a strong influence on childhood pain experiences.

3. Adolescence is a particularly challenging time in the context of pain management. Why is this the case?
   a. Adolescence is a sensitive period for the development of executive functioning skills.
   b. During adolescence the influence of peers can impact their pain experiences.
   c. The onset of puberty during adolescence can impact pain perceptions and experiences.
   d. All of the above reasons.

4. What is the conclusion of a systematic review evaluating the role of temperament in CYP's pain experiences?

   a. CYP's activity and mood are the most consistent temperament factors influencing pain experiences.
   b. CYP's temperament shows no consistent relationship with CYP's pain perception and experiences.
   c. While CYP's temperament shows a clear relationship with CYP's pain perceptions, it does not moderate the impact of pain management interventions.
   d. There is a very limited amount of research available exploring the impact of temperament on CYP's pain experiences.

References

Bandura, A. (1977) *Social Learning Theory*. Prentice-Hall, Hoboken, NJ.

Blakemore, S.J. and Choudhury, S. (2006) Development of the adolescent brain: implications for executive function and social cognition. *Journal of Child Psychology and Psychiatry* 47(3–4), 296–312.

Boerner, K.E., Birnie, K.A., Caes, L., Schinkel, M. and Chambers, C.T. (2014) Sex differences in experimental pain among healthy children: a systematic review and meta-analysis. *Pain* 155(5), 983–993.

Boerner, K.E., Schinkel, M. and Chambers, C.T. (2015) It is not as simple as boys versus girls: the role of sex differences in pain across the lifespan. *Pain Management* 5(1), 1–4.

Boerner, K.E., Chambers, C.T., Gahagan, J., Keogh, E., Fillingim, R.B. and Mogil, J.S. (2018) Conceptual complexity of gender and its relevance to pain. *Pain* 159(11), 2137–2141.

Bournaki, M.-C. (1997) Correlates of pain-related responses to venipuncture in school-age children. *Nursing Research* 46(3), 147–154.

Bouwmeester, N.J., Hop, W.C.J., van Dijk, M., Anand, K.J.S., van den Anker, J.N. and Tibboel, D. (2003) Postoperative pain in the neonate: age-related differences in morphine requirements and metabolism. *Intensive Care Medicine* 29, 2009–2015.

Brown, E.A., De Young, A., Kimble, R., et al. (2018) Review of a parent's influence on pediatric procedural distress and Recovery. *Clinical Child and Family Psychology Review* 21(2), 224–245.

Chan, J.Y.C. and von Baeyer, C.L. (2016) Cognitive developmental influences on the ability of preschool-aged children to self-report their pain intensity. *Pain* 157(5), 997–1001.

Chen, E., Zeltzer, L.K., Craske, M.G. and Katz, E.R. (2000) Children's memories for painful cancer treatment procedures: implications for distress. *Child Development* 71, 933–947.

Chess, S. and Thomas, A. (1986) *Temperament in Clinical Practice*. Guildford Press, New York.

Conte, P.M., Walco, G.A. and Kimura, Y. (2003) Temperament and stress response in children with juvenile primary fibromyalgia syndrome. *Arthritis and Rheumatism* 48, 2923–2930.

Cousins, L.A., Cohen, L.L. and Venable, C. (2015) Risk and resilience in pediatric chronic pain: exploring the protective role of optimism. *Journal of Pediatric Psychology* 40(9), 934–942.

Cousins, L.A., Tomlinson, R.M., Cohen, L.L. and McMurtry, C.M. (2016) The power of optimism: applying a positive psychology framework to pediatric pain. *Pediatric Pain Letter* 18(1), 1–5.

Craig, K. (1986) Social modelling influences. In *The Psychology of Pain* (ed. R.A. Strenbach), pp. 67–95. Raven Press, New York.

Crandall, M., Lammers, C., Senders, C. and Braun, J.V. (2009) Children's tonsillectomy experiences: influencing factors. *Journal of Child Health Care* 13, 308–321.

Dagg, W., Forgeron, P., Macartney, G. and Chartrand, J. (2020) Adolescent patients' management of post-operative pain after discharge: a qualitative study. *Pain Management Nursing* 21(6), 565–571.

Eccleston, C., Fisher, E.A., Vervoort, T. and Crombez, G. (2012) Worry and catastrophizing about pain in youth: a re-appraisal. *Pain* 153(8), 1560–1562.

Forgeron, P.A., McGrath, P.J., Stevens, B., et al. (2011) Social information processing in adolescents with chronic pain: my friends don't really understand me. *Pain* 152(12), 2771–2780.

Forgeron, P.A., Evans, J., McGrath, P.J., Stevens, B. and Finley, G.A. (2013) Living with difference: exploring the social self and friendships of adolescents with chronic pain. *Pain Research and Management* 18(6), e115–e123.

Finley, G.A., Kristjansdottir, O. and Forgeron, P.A. (2009) Cultural influences on the assessment of children's pain. *Pain Research and Management* 14, 33–37.

Fitzgerald, M. (2009) Development of nociception. In *Encyclopedia of Neuroscience* (eds M.D. Binder, N. Hirokawa and U. Windhorst), pp. 953–956. Springer, Berlin, Heidelberg.

Gaffney, A. (1993) Cognitive development aspects of pain in school-age children. In *Pain in Infants, Children and Adolescents* (eds N.L. Schechter, C.B. Berde and M. Yaster), pp. 75–86. Williams and Wilkins, Baltimore, MD.

Gidron, Y., McGrath, P.J. and Goodday, R. (1995) The physical and psychosocial predictors of adolescents' recovery from oral surgery. *Journal of Behavioral Medicine* 18, 385–399.

Goubert, L. and Simons, L.E. (2013) Cognitive styles and processes in paediatric pain. In *Oxford Textbook of Pediatric Pain* (eds P.J.McGrath, B.J. Stevens, S.M. Walker and W.T. Zempsky), pp. 95–101. Oxford University Press, Oxford.

Higgins, K.S., Birnie, K.A., Chambers, C.T., et al. (2015) Offspring of parents with chronic pain: a systematic review and meta-analysis of pain, health, psychological, and family outcomes. *Pain* 156(11), 2256–2266.

Huguet, A., McGrath, P.J. and Pardos, J. (2011) Development and preliminary testing of a scale to assess pain-related fear in children and adolescents. *Journal of Pain* 12(8), 840–848.

Hurley, A. and Whelan, E.G. (1988) Cognitive development and children's perception of pain. *Pediatric Nursing* 14(1), 21–24.

Jongudomkarn, D., Aungsupakorn, N. and Camfield, L. (2006) The meanings of pain: a qualitative study of the perspectives of children living with pain in north-eastern Thailand. *Nursing and Health Sciences* 8, 156–163.

Kemani, M.K., Kanstrup, M., Jordan, A., Caes, L. and Gauntlett-Gilbert, J. (2018) Acceptance and commitment therapy for adolescents with chronic pain and their parents: evaluation of parent and adolescent outcomes and the relation between parent psychological flexibility and adolescent pain acceptance. *Journal of Pediatric Psychology* 43(9), 981–994.

King, S., Chambers, C.T., Huguet, A., et al. (2011) The epidemiology of chronic pain in children and adolescents revisited: a systematic review. *Pain* 152, 2729–2738.

Kleiber, C., Schutte, D.L., McCarthy, A.M., Floria-Santos, M., Murray, J.C. and Hanrahan, K. (2007) Predictors of topical anesthetic effectiveness in children. *Journal of Pain* 8(2), 168–174.

Kotzer, A.M. (2000) Factors predicting postoperative pain in children and adolescents following spine fusion. *Issues in Comprehensive Pediatric Nursing* 23, 83–102.

Kristjansdottir, O., Unruh, A.M., McAlpine, L. and McGrath, P.J. (2012) A systematic review of cross-cultural comparison studies of child, parent, and health professional outcomes associated with pediatric medical procedures. *Journal of Pain* 12(3), 207–219.

Kristjansdottir, O., McGrath, P.J., Finley, G.A., et al. (2018) Cultural influences on parental responses to children's pain. *Pain* 159, 2035–2049.

Kuba, T. and Quinones-Jenab, V. (2005) The role of female gonadal hormones in behavioral sex differences in persistent and chronic pain: clinical versus preclinical studies. *Brain Research Bulletin* 66(3), 179–188.

Lewandowski, A.S., Palermo, T.M., Stinson, J., Handley, S. and Chambers, C.T. (2010) Systematic review of family functioning in families of children and adolescents with chronic pain. *Journal of Pain* 11(11), 1027–1038.

Lynch, A.M., Kashikar-Zuck, S., Goldschneider, K.R. and Jones, B.A. (2007) Sex and age differences in coping styles among children with chronic pain. *Journal of Pain and Symptom Management* 33(2), 208–216.

McCarthy, A.M., and Kleiber, C. (2006) A conceptual model of factors influencing children's responses to a painful procedure when parents are distraction coaches. *Journal of Pediatric Nursing* 21(2), 88–98.

McCarthy, A., Kleiber, C., Hanrahan, K., Zimmerman, M.B., Westhus, N. and Allen, S. (2010) Factors explaining children's responses to intravenous needle insertions. *Nursing Research* 59(6), 407–416.

McGrath, P.A. and Hillier, L.M. (2003) Modifying the psychologic factors that intensify children's pain and prolong disability. In *Pain in Infants, Children and Adolescents*, 2nd edn (eds N.L. Schechter, C.B. Berde and M. Yaster), pp. 85–127. Lippincott, Williams and Wilkins, Baltimore, MD.

McGrath, P.J. and McAlpine, L. (1993) Psychologic perspectives on pediatric pain. *Journal of Pediatrics* 122, S2–S8.

McMurtry, C.M., Noel, M., Chambers, C.T. and McGrath, P.J. (2011) Children's fear during procedural pain: preliminary investigation of the Children's Fear Scale. *Health Psychology* 30(6), 780–788.

McMurtry, C.M., Riddell, R.P., Taddio, A., et al. (2015) Far from 'just a poke': common painful needle procedures and the development of needle fear. *Clinical Journal of Pain* 31(10 Suppl.), S3–S11.

Martin, A.L., McGrath, P.A., Brown, S.C. and Katz, J. (2007) Children with chronic pain: impact of sex and age on long-term conditions. *Pain* 128, 13–19.

Mironenko, I.A. and Sorokin, P.S. (2018) Seeking for the definition of 'culture': current concerns and their implications. A comment on Gustav Jahoda's article 'Critical reflections on some recent definitions of "Culture"'. *Integrative Psychological and Behavioral Science* 52, 331–340.

Mogil, J.S., Yu, L. and Basbaum, A.I. (2000) Pain genes? Natural variation and transgenic mutants. *Annual Review of Neuroscience*, 23, 777–811.

Noel, M., Chambers, C.T., Petter, M., McGrath, P.J., Klein, R.M. and Stewart, S.H. (2012) Pain is not over when the needle ends: a review and preliminary model of acute pain memory development in childhood. *Pain Management* 2, 487–497.

Noel, M., Palermo, T.M., Chambers, C.T., et al. (2015) Remembering the pain of childhood: applying a developmental perspective to the study of pain memories. *Pain* 156(1), 31–34.

Palermo, T.M., Valrie, C.R. and Karlson, C.W. (2014) Family and parent influences on pediatric chronic pain: a developmental perspective. *American Psychologist* 69(2), 142–152.

Patanwala, A.E., Norwood, C., Steiner, H., et al. (2019) Psychological and genetic predictors of pain tolerance. *Clinical and Translational Science* 12, 189–195.

Ranger, M. and Campbell-Yeo, M. (2008) Temperament and pain response: a review of the literature. *Pain Management Nursing* 9(1), 2–9.

Rocha, E.M. and Prkachin, K.M. (2007) Temperament and pain reactivity predict health behavior seven years later. *Journal of Pediatric Psychology* 32(4), 393–399.

Rocha, E.M., Prkachin, K.M., Beaumont, S.L., Hardy, C.L. and Zumbo, B.D. (2003) Pain reactivity and somatization in kindergarten-age children. *Journal of Pediatric Psychology* 28, 47–57.

Sheldon, L.K. and Foust, J.B. (2014) *Communication for Nurses: Talking with Patients*, 3rd edn. Jones & Bartlett Learning, Burlington, MA.

Simons, L.E., Sieberg, C.B., Carpino, E., Logan, D. and Berde, C. (2011) The Fear of Pain Questionnaire (FOPQ): assessment of pain-related fear among children and adolescents with chronic pain. *Journal of Pain* 12(6), 677–686.

Simons, L.E., Smith, A., Kaczynski, K. and Basch, M. (2015) Living in fear of your child's pain: the parent fear of pain questionnaire. *Pain* 156(4), 694–702.

Slater, R., Cantarella, A., Gallella, S., et al. (2006) Cortical pain responses in human infants. *Journal of Neuroscience* 26(14), 3661–3666.

Sullivan, M.J.L., Bishop, S.R. and Pivik, J. (1995) The Pain Catastrophizing Scale: development and validation. *Psychological Assessment* 7, 524–532.

Vervoort, T., Goubert, L., Eccleston, C., Bijttebier, P. and Crombez, G. (2006) Catastrophic thinking about pain is independently associated with pain severity, disability, and somatic complaints in school children and children with chronic pain. *Journal of Pediatric Psychology* 31, 674–683.

Vervoort, T., Logan, D.E., Goubert, L., De Clercq, B. and Hublet, A. (2014) Severity of pediatric pain in relation to school-related functioning and teacher support: an epidemiological study among school-aged children and adolescents. *Pain* 155(6), 1118–1127.

Williams, D.G., Patel, A. and Howard, R.F. (2002) Pharmacogenetics of codeine metabolism in an urban population of children and its implications for analgesic reliability. *British Journal of Anaesthesia* 89(6), 839–845.

Wilson, A.C., Lewandowski, A.S. and Palermo, T.M. (2011) Fear-avoidance beliefs and parental responses to pain in adolescents with chronic pain. *Pain Research and Management* 16(3), 178–182.

Wolff, N., Darlington, A.S., Hunfeld, J., et al. (2010) Determinants of somatic complaints in 18-month-old children: the generation R study. *Journal of Pediatric Psychology* 35(3), 306–316.

World Health Organization (2022) Gender and health. https://www.who.int/health-topics/gender#tab=tab_1 (accessed 17 May 2022).

Woolf, C. and Salter, M. (2000) Neuronal plasticity: increasing the gain in pain. *Science* 288(5472), 1765–1769.

Zubieta, J.-K., Heitzeg, M.M., Smith, Y.R., et al. (2003) COMT val158met genotype affects [mu]opioid neurotransmitter responses to a pain stressor. *Science* 299(5610), 1240–1243.

5 Pharmacology of Analgesics

Janice E. Sumpton

This chapter provides an overview of the pharmacology of commonly used analgesics and adjuvant medications. Children and young people (CYP) are unique because of developmental changes that occur from infancy to adulthood which affect drug pharmacology (Eerdekens et al. 2019). Combining analgesics with physical and psychological strategies ensures better pain management outcomes. More information about physical and psychological interventions can be found in other chapters of this book.

In children most analgesic drugs are administered *off-label* (i.e. usage not approved by the official labelled indication(s), including age, disease treated or route of administration) (Benavides and Nahata 2013). There is a lack of paediatric randomised controlled trials (RCTs), leaving clinicians to rely on best practice principles or recommendations from leading children's hospitals (World Health Organization (WHO) 2010, 2020; Kimland and Odlind 2012). The European Union and the USA introduced legislation to improve safety and knowledge of medicines for children, but change is slow (Kimland and Odlind 2012). To optimise pain management, analgesics should be part of a multimodal approach, including rehabilitative, integrative, psychological and interventional strategies (Association of Paediatric Anaesthetists of Great Britain and Ireland (APA) 2012; Friedrichsdorf and Goubert 2020; WHO 2020).

> **PRACTICE POINT**
>
> In assessing the success of a pharmacological intervention, a 50% reduction in pain is considered a 'responder' and a 30% reduction in pain is classified as clinically relevant (Toth and Moulin 2013).

How Drugs Work

A medication is a bioactive molecule that is not normally part of the body. Drug action is the chemical interaction between the medication and body tissue. However, no drug is completely specific in its positive therapeutic action, and it can also have negative effects resulting in adverse drug reactions (ADRs) (Rang et al. 2012). The aim is to give the appropriate dose to achieve a desired effect but not too much to be toxic (Begg 2008). The two key pharmacological actions are pharmacodynamics (drug action or 'what does the drug do to the body?')

Managing Pain in Children and Young People: A Clinical Guide, Third Edition. Edited by Alison Twycross, Jennifer Stinson, William T. Zempsky, and Abbie Jordan.
© 2024 John Wiley & Sons Ltd. Published 2024 by John Wiley & Sons Ltd.

and pharmacokinetics (drug movement or 'what does the body do to the drug?') (Kanneh 2002a,b; Begg 2008). Commonly used pharmacology definitions are outlined in Table 5.1.

Pharmacokinetics

Key pharmacokinetic actions are described in Table 5.2.

Table 5.1 Pharmacology definitions.

Term	Definition
Adjuvants	Drugs that generally have a primary indication other than treating pain but have analgesic properties
Adverse drug reaction (ADR) or side effect	Undesired effect of the drug occurring at common doses
Affinity	The attraction between drug and receptor (described as high or low)
Agonist	A drug that binds to a receptor and activates it (fully or partially)
Antagonist	A drug that binds to a receptor without activating it, but blocks agonist access
Bioavailability	The rate and extent of drug absorbed into the systemic circulation after administration. Bioavailability is 100% after intravenous administration
Ceiling effect	A drug will not produce a greater effect at a higher dose
Clearance	The rate at which a drug is eliminated from the body over time
Dose interval	Time needed between drug doses to keep the drug within the therapeutic index
Drug–drug interaction	When the effects of one drug are altered, increased or decreased by another drug
Duration of action	Time the drug action lasts at an effective concentration
Enzymes	Proteins that regulate the rate of chemical reactions in the body
First-pass metabolism	Drugs taken orally enter the portal (hepatic) circulation and are partly metabolised before entering the systemic circulation
Half-life ($t_{1/2}$)	Time taken for the drug concentration in blood to fall by half its original value
Ion channels	Pores in the cell membrane that allow passage of ions into and out of the cell
Loading dose	A drug administered at a higher dose to achieve early therapeutic plasma levels
Maintenance dose	Dose required to maintain plasma drug levels at a steady state
Onset of action	Time it takes for the drug to begin working
Prodrug	A drug that is metabolised in the body to another form before it becomes active
Receptors	Protein molecules activated by transmitters or hormones
Steady state	The drug at a uniform level in the body, where administration rate equals elimination rate. Time to steady state is generally five half-lives
Therapeutic index (or 'therapeutic window')	The variance between the therapeutic dose and the toxic dose of a drug: ■ Narrow or low therapeutic index drugs have a high risk of toxicity ■ Wide or high therapeutic index drugs have a low risk of toxicity
Volume of distribution	How and where the drug is distributed in the body

Sources: Kanneh (2002a,b); Begg (2008); Kraemer (2010); Neal (2012).

Table 5.2 Pharmacokinetics definitions.

Term	Definition
Absorption	■ Involves entrance of the drug into the circulatory system ■ Dependent on factors including drug formulation, route of administration, blood flow at the site of administration and surface area exposed to the drug (Kanneh 2002b) ■ Topically applied drugs in infants can have significant systemic absorption because of their larger surface area per unit of mass and a thinner stratum corneum compared to adults (Benavides and Nahata 2013)
Distribution	■ Occurs once the drug enters the circulatory system and reaches the target tissue ■ Drugs are mostly bound to plasma proteins and piggy-back on them to get to their destination ■ Drug distribution is affected by cardiac output, total amount of body water and concentration of plasma proteins (Kanneh 2002b) ■ The increased percentage of body water in infants causes a decrease in drug concentration for highly water-soluble drugs (decreased effect) ■ The decreased proteins for drug binding lead to a greater percentage of unbound (active) drug for highly bound drugs (increased effect) (Berde and Sethna 2002; Benavides and Nahata 2013)
Metabolism	■ The process of breaking down drugs into active and/or inactive components (metabolites) prior to elimination ■ Mostly carried out by enzymes and occurs predominantly in the liver ■ The major enzyme group involved in metabolism of 70–80% of drugs is cytochrome P450 (CYP) (Begg 2008; Bryant and Knights 2010) ■ Is slower in infants secondary to immature CYP enzymes, whereas two- to six-year-old children have increased liver metabolism compared to adults (Berde and Sethna 2002)
Elimination	■ The removal of drug from the body ■ Renal excretion is most common ■ Lesser amounts are removed via the gastrointestinal system, saliva, sweat and tears ■ Renal function changes from birth onwards, reaching adult function by one year of age. This significantly impacts the ability to clear drugs in young infants, requiring dose adjustment to avoid toxicity (Berde and Sethna 2002)

PRACTICE POINT

The capacity for cytochrome P450 enzymes to metabolise drugs has a genetic basis. Individuals can be poor metabolisers, intermediate metabolisers, extensive metabolisers or ultrametabolisers. Individual variations can range from no drug effect to serious ADRs (e.g. respiratory depression, death).

Screening to determine cytochrome P450 phenotypes (pharmacogenetics) may allow for tailoring of analgesia specific to the individual's genetic composition, reducing ADRs and allowing the smallest dose for the greatest effect.

■ If patients have liver dysfunction, they will have decreased rates of drug metabolism, and therefore increased drug levels and increased risk of toxicity for drugs metabolised by the liver.

■ If patients have renal dysfunction, they will have decreased drug elimination, and therefore increased drug levels and increased risk of toxicity for drugs renally excreted.

Routes of Drug Administration

The route of drug administration (Table 5.3) affects the speed of onset and therapeutic response (Bryant and Knights 2010). If a rapid effect is desired, then the parenteral, inhaled or oral transmucosal route is best. Oral administration is most common. The physical and chemical characteristics of the drug and the rate of gastric emptying affect its bioavailability (Benavides and Nahata 2013; Lam et al. 2014). The advantages and disadvantages of using different routes in CYP are outlined in Table 5.4.

PRACTICE POINT

- Intravenous administration delivers the most rapid analgesia.
- Liquid preparations are absorbed faster than tablet or capsule formulations.
- Rectal administration can lead to erratic drug absorption due to drug placement issues, rectal blood flow and faecal loading.

Medication Challenges in Infants, Children and Young People

One of the biggest challenges is the quest for a suitable dosage form. For CYP who cannot or will not swallow tablets, some immediate-release tablets can be crushed, or capsules opened and contents sprinkled on soft food (apple sauce, pudding, yoghurt, ice cream) just before administration (Benavides and Nahata 2013). A small amount of food may be mixed in to ensure the entire dose is given. A pharmacist should be consulted before manipulating the marketed drug to ensure the drug will remain active. Chocolate syrup is ideal for masking bitter-tasting medicines and hazelnut spreads can mask bad-tasting medicines (avoid if nut allergy).

Table 5.3 Main routes of drug administration.

Route	Example
Enteral (via the gastrointestinal system)	Oral (PO), nasogastric (NG), nasojejunal (NJ), percutaneous endoscopic gastrostomy/gastric tube (PEG or G), rectal (PR)
Parenteral (via injection)	Intravenous (IV), subcutaneous (SC), intramuscular (IM), intra-articular, intrathecal (spinal) (IT), epidural, intraosseous (IO)
Inhalation (via the respiratory system)	Gas, mist/aerosol, nebuliser/inhaler
Topical/transmucosal (via the skin or mucous membranes)	Skin, eyes, ears, transdermal (TD), intranasal (IN), oral transmucosal (sublingual [SL], buccal)

Sources: Bryant and Knights (2010); Lam et al. (2014).

Caregivers must be made aware of the importance of knowing the milligram (mg) or microgram (mcg or μg) dose in addition to the volume of liquid they administer (what they generally know from repetition). Errors occur when only one number is remembered and stated incorrectly during medication history. Caregivers knowing the concentration of non-prescription analgesic liquids such as paracetamol (acetaminophen) and ibuprofen is key since multiple strengths are available. This will avoid inadvertent dosing errors with product selection. Correct administration of over-the-counter drugs by caregivers only occurs approximately 30% of the time (Kozer et al. 2006).

PRACTICE POINT

It is important to give an adequate trial of one analgesic before abandoning that drug or adding another analgesic.

Table 5.4 Advantages and disadvantages of routes of analgesic administration.

Route	Advantages	Disadvantages
Oral	■ Painless, least invasive ■ Many marketed choices ■ Preferred by children	■ Slow-acting, reliant on gut function, first-pass metabolism ■ Problem if child is nauseated/vomiting or unable to swallow ■ Analgesics with unpleasant taste/texture ■ If no marketed dosage form suitable for children
Nasogastric	■ Many marketed choices ■ Useful for high-volume/unpleasant tasting medication	■ Slow-acting, reliant on gut function, first-pass metabolism ■ Invasive/painful to insert NG tube ■ Additional nursing care required ■ Disliked by some children
Rectal	■ Useful if CYP is nauseated/vomiting ■ Less first-pass metabolism ■ Not reliant on gut function ■ Useful if no IV, avoids IM injections	■ Unreliable bioavailability ■ Slowest acting ■ Limited marketed choices ■ Disliked by some children
Intravenous	■ Fast-acting, allows rapid analgesia ■ Avoids first-pass metabolism ■ Useful for intermittent bolus, infusion and patient-controlled analgesia (PCA)	■ Invasive/painful to insert IV ■ Additional nursing care required ■ More ADR due to high drug bio-availability
Intramuscular (obsolete): painful and not recommended in patients under 18 years		■ Painful ■ Disliked by infants and children ■ Slower onset ■ Variability in absorption
Subcutaneous	■ Avoids need for IV ■ Useful in community settings ■ Useful for intermittent bolus or infusion	■ Invasive/painful to insert ■ Slower onset
Epidural	■ Fast-acting ■ Extremely effective, allows complete analgesia	■ Invasive, needs highly skilled clinicians ■ Inserted under sedation/anaesthesia ■ Additional nursing care required ■ Risks/adverse effects of procedure
Intranasal	■ Fast-acting ■ Minimal discomfort	■ Limited choices available
Oral transmucosal	■ Avoids first-pass metabolism ■ Not reliant on gut function ■ Fast-acting and short-acting ■ Less invasive	■ Variable acceptability by children ■ Needs adhesive properties to remain in the oral cavity ■ Limited marketed choices
Topical	■ Least invasive route ■ Painless	■ Limited marketed choices

For definition of abbreviations, see Table 5.3.
Sources: WHO (2010, 2012); Batchelor et al. (2014); Frey et al. (2019).

Doses are calculated as mg/kg (or mcg/kg) in infants and children. Some doses are listed as mg/kg per dose *or* mg/kg per day, requiring careful reading to prescribe appropriately. Infants need recalculation of their doses as they grow (Benavides and Nahata 2013). In older children, if mg/kg dosing is used then the dose can be too high. Doses are capped at 50 kg, which generally are the adult doses. In other words, a 75-kg 13 year old would *not* receive a mg/kg dose (e.g. oral morphine 0.3 mg/kg × 75 kg = 22.5 mg which exceeds 0.3 mg × 50 kg = 15 mg). Do *not* exceed the adult starting dose. Opioids may then be titrated higher to effect.

To increase adherence, involve the CYP in their care. Education includes reason for drug use, dosing regimen and proper measurement, possible side effects, duration and goals of treatment, and safe storage (Benavides and Nahata 2013).

PRACTICE POINT

Health professionals should educate caregivers

- Always measure liquid doses with an accurate measuring device (oral syringe with necessary volume markings). Never use a kitchen tea-spoon/tablespoon because they are very inaccurate, leading to under- or over-dosing.
- Caregivers should keep a detailed list of medications with mg or mcg doses to avoid errors.
- Doses per kilogram body weight are capped at 50 kg. Children weighing 50 kg and greater should be prescribed the adult dose and *not* the mg/kg dose.

Selection of analgesics

For optimal analgesic selection assess the type and severity of pain (see Chapter 6 for information about assessing pain in CYP). Assess the benefits and risks of the drug and select the most appropriate analgesic. Administer for the shortest duration. For optimal analgesia, combinations of analgesics with different mechanisms of action can be given. Analgesic regimens are selected based on the specific needs of the CYP, including patient/caregiver preferences and costs of the medications.

The WHO (2012) guidelines were updated in 2020 to provide evidence-based recommendations for pain management in children experiencing chronic pain (lasting at least three months). The WHO (2020) guidelines are based on the most current evidence in accordance with the highest recognised standards in methodology, but there are considerable gaps in research regarding the effectiveness and safety of medication use in children with chronic pain.

Non-opioid Analgesics

Paracetamol

Paracetamol is the most commonly used analgesic in CYP, with antipyretic activity and minimal anti-inflammatory effects. It is highly effective as a sole analgesic for mild pain with an excellent safety profile (Southey et al. 2009; Pierce and Voss 2010). Paracetamol enhances analgesia when used in combination with nonsteroidal anti-inflammatory drugs (NSAIDs) or tramadol (Remy et al. 2006). Paracetamol has opioid-sparing effects of up to 20% in adults and CYP when given in combination with opioids (Remy et al. 2006; Hong et al. 2010).

Action The mechanism of action is not fully understood. Involvement of the cyclooxygenase, serotoninergic, endocannabinoid, opioidergic, adrenergic and cholinergic systems have all been postulated (Beaulieu et al. 2010).

Metabolism/Elimination Paracetamol is metabolised in the liver primarily to glucuronide and sulphate metabolites, which are excreted via the kidneys. Another metabolite, *N*-acetyl-*p*-benzo-quinone imine (NAPQI), is responsible for the toxic effects. NAPQI is metabolised by glutathione and when levels are excessive glutathione is unable to metabolise NAPQI rapidly enough, leading to liver toxicity (Beaulieu et al. 2010).

Adverse Drug Reactions Minor ADRs are uncommon but include gastrointestinal upset and skin reactions. Early symptoms of paracetamol poisoning are non-specific (nausea/vomiting, anorexia, abdominal pain). Liver toxicity and subsequent fulminant liver failure present a few days after an overdose (see Appendix for dosing information).

PRACTICE POINT

- With long-term use in children and adolescents the maximum daily dose is 2–3 g (McCrae et al. 2018).
- Suppositories deliver inconsistent drug dosages. If dividing a suppository, cut it length-wise (tip to end) rather than cross-wise for most accurate dosing.

Non-steroidal Anti-inflammatory Drugs

NSAIDs are used for the treatment of mild to moderate pain and have antipyretic and anti-inflammatory effects (APA 2012). NSAIDs have a high safety and efficacy profile, with a significant opioid-sparing effect (Southey et al. 2009; Pierce and Voss 2010; APA 2012). Ibuprofen is the most studied NSAID in children, with more evidence of safety and efficacy than other NSAIDs (Kraemer 2010; APA 2012; WHO 2012). Non-opioid analgesic drugs have a ceiling effect.

Action NSAIDs inhibit the synthesis of prostaglandins by inhibiting the production of cyclo-oxygenase (COX)-1 and COX-2 enzymes. COX-1 is present in most body tissues and is involved in cell homeostasis, including maintenance of the protective mucous lining in the gastrointestinal tract, renal blood flow, platelet function and bronchodilation. COX-2 is present during inflammation, pain or cancer. It is responsible for multiple mediators that lead to vasodilation, oedema, hyperalgesia and fever.

Non-selective NSAIDs (e.g. ibuprofen, ketorolac, naproxen, acetylsalicylic acid [ASA]) block both COX-1 and COX-2. COX-2 inhibitors (e.g. celecoxib) block COX-2 much more than COX-1 (Conaghan 2012; Friedrichsdorf and Goubert 2020). Current recommendations suggest that both coxibs and non-selective NSAIDs should be used at their lowest effective dose and long-term use be avoided where possible (Conaghan 2012).

Metabolism/Elimination Most NSAIDs undergo metabolism in the liver, with metabolites excreted via the kidneys and in the faeces (Kokki 2003).

Adverse Drug Reactions Less serious ADRs include skin reactions, diarrhoea, and nausea and vomiting (minimise by taking with food). NSAIDs are *not* recommended as analgesics for infants under the age of six months due to risk of renal toxicity, and they may interfere with cerebral and pulmonary blood flow (APA 2012).

PRACTICE POINT

Reye's syndrome

- Use of ASA (aspirin) in children with viral illnesses is associated with an increased risk of developing Reye's syndrome (acute encephalopathy with liver damage), although the degree of causality is questioned.
- Do not use ASA in children unless on the advice of a physician (Schror 2007).

Non-selective NSAIDs have the potential for bleeding, gastric irritation and renal impairment. The risk of bleeding after surgery (mainly tonsillectomy) is present (Kokki 2003; Anderson and Palmer 2006; APA 2012). NSAIDs may induce asthma in ASA/NSAID-sensitive asthmatics, particularly those with multiple allergies, severe eczema or nasal polyp disease (Anderson and Palmer 2006; APA 2012). Renal failure occurs particularly in children with pre-existing renal impairment, hypovolaemia or dehydration (APA 2012).

Celecoxib is an alternative to non-selective NSAIDs if a side effect (e.g. increased bleeding risk or gastric ulcer) is a concern (Friedrichsdorf and Goubert 2020). See Appendix for NSAID dosing information.

PRACTICE POINT

If unable to swallow a celecoxib capsule, then just before administration:

- the capsule can be opened and the contents sprinkled on apple sauce (Lexicomp 2019a) *or*
- a liquid can be compounded by pharmacy *or*
- capsule contents can be mixed in 10 mL of water to give a milky suspension and administered orally or via a ≥8 Fr nasogastric tube (White and Bradnam 2015).

Are Paracetamol and Ibuprofen Equally Efficacious and Safe for Nociceptive (Acute) Pain Management?

A review by Pierce and Voss (2010) of 18 studies comparing ibuprofen and paracetamol in postoperative settings, with musculoskeletal trauma, headaches and febrile discomfort showed the following results:

- Ibuprofen showed superior analgesia in one-third of the studies, better on day of surgery but not thereafter in one study.
- Of 18 studies, 11 showed no significant difference in efficacy between ibuprofen and paracetamol.
- All but one study showed no statistical difference between paracetamol and ibuprofen and their adverse events.
- One study reported that paracetamol was better tolerated than ibuprofen.

A more recent systematic review and meta-analysis compared paracetamol with ibuprofen in children less than two years old. Ibuprofen resulted in less pain at 4–24 hours compared with paracetamol. Side effects were uncommon, with similar serious side-effect profiles (Tan et al. 2020).

Are Paracetamol and Ibuprofen Equally Efficacious and Safe for Chronic Pain Management?

A Cochrane review found no evidence (RCTs) to support or refute paracetamol for chronic non-cancer pain (CNCP) in children and adolescents (Cooper et al. 2017a). A Cochrane review of NSAIDs for CNCP in children and adolescents found only a few studies to review, which led to insufficient data for analysis on efficacy or safety of NSAIDs used chronically (Eccleston et al. 2017).

Should Paracetamol and Ibuprofen be Used Together or Alternately?

Minimal evidence exists about whether paracetamol and ibuprofen should be used together or alternately. A study of nociceptive pain in the emergency department setting compared paracetamol alone, ibuprofen alone and both drugs used together. Pain score reductions were similar in all three groups (Motov et al.

2020). The National Institute for Health and Care Excellence (NICE) in England and Wales (NICE 2019a) and the American Academy of Pediatrics (Sullivan and Farrar 2011) advise against using ibuprofen and paracetamol simultaneously or in alternating doses.

However, alternating paracetamol and ibuprofen is still recommended by health professionals and practised by caregivers. Alternating may have the advantage of improved analgesia if inadequate response is seen with either drug alone. Theoretically, when used together there is:

- potential for additive or synergistic antinociceptive activity;
- an increased risk of renal and hepatic toxicity.

Best practice should ensure that a single drug be given in the correct dose first, and reserve alternating drugs for pain that is unresponsive to monotherapy (Smith and Goldman 2012). Paediatric studies have shown that pain is often undertreated (Barbagallo and Sacerdote 2019; Friedrichsdorf and Goubert 2020; Beal 2021). In addition, more than half of caregivers give incorrect doses (Li et al. 2000; Goldman and Scolnik 2004). Therefore, it is critical that very explicit instructions are given to caregivers.

PRACTICE POINT

Dosing regimen for paracetamol alternating with ibuprofen when an inpatient

For analgesia every three hours:

- six-hourly paracetamol, at 6 a.m., noon, 6 p.m. and midnight *and*
- six-hourly ibuprofen, at 9 a.m., 3 p.m., 9 p.m. (and at 3 a.m. if night-time pain).

However, for a family at home it cannot be reasonably expected for a caregiver and the child to wake up every three hours to administer medications. As such, we recommend administering ibuprofen and paracetamol every six to eight hours together.

Opioid Analgesics

Opioids are used for treating moderate to severe pain. Table 5.5 lists the definitions used in opioid terminology. *Weak opioids* include

Table 5.5 Definitions of opioid terminology.

Term	Definition
Tolerance (pharmacological)	Decreased effectiveness of a drug over time, so that a higher dose of the drug is needed to achieve the same effect. Tolerance develops to desired and undesired effects of opioids at different rates
Physical dependence	A physiological response to the abrupt discontinuation (or dose reduction or reversal) of a drug that leads to a withdrawal (abstinence) syndrome
Substance use disorder	A cluster of cognitive, psychological and behavioural symptoms indicating that the person continues using the substance despite significant substance-related problems
Withdrawal syndrome	A cluster of physiological signs and symptoms that occur after the abrupt discontinuation of an opioid
Pseudoaddiction	Behaviours that may seem inappropriately drug seeking but which are a result of undertreatment of pain and resolve when pain relief is adequate
Opioid-induced hyperalgesia	Opioid use or increased opioid dose causing hyperalgesia in response to the opioid itself (Colvin et al. 2019)

Source: Schug et al. (2020).

Pharmacology of Analgesics

Pharmacology of Analgesics **59**

codeine, hydrocodone and tramadol (see section Mixed Opioids for the non-opioid effects of tramadol). *Strong opioids* include morphine, hydromorphone and fentanyl. Strong opioids (unlike weak opioids) do not have a ceiling effect (Benavides and Nahata 2013; Friedrichsdorf and Goubert 2020). Morphine is the preferred opioid in children (Kraemer 2010; Friedrichsdorf and Goubert 2020). A Cochrane review found no evidence to support or refute the use of opioids for management of CNCP in CYP (Cooper et al. 2017b). WHO (2020) recommends that morphine may be given when tailored to specific indications under the principles of opioid stewardship and in the setting of end-of-life care. Opioids should only be prescribed by trained providers having weighed the risk–benefit ratio. Once prescribed, the CYP should be continuously monitored. This includes a plan for ongoing assessment for potential dose tapering and discontinuation of the opioid where appropriate (WHO 2020).

Action Opioids bind to opioid receptors located in the peripheral and central nervous systems and spinal cord. The mu (μ) receptor and, for some, also kappa (κ) receptor are the main sites of action. Doses are titrated based on analgesia and ability to tolerate adverse effects (Kraemer 2010; Benavides and Nahata 2013).

Metabolism/Elimination Opioids are converted into metabolites (active and inactive) in the liver and then excreted mostly by the kidneys. Morphine and hydromorphone are metabolised by glucuronidation (Smith 2009). Codeine, tramadol, hydrocodone and oxycodone are metabolised by cytochrome P450 (CYP)2D6 to form biologically active metabolites. Differences in CYP2D6 activity result in unpredictable clinical effects due to genetic variants. Pharmacogenetic differences can lead to opioid overdoses in individuals who are

ultra-metabolisers, or inadequate analgesia in individuals who are poor metabolisers (Chidambaran et al. 2017). Oxycodone, tramadol and fentanyl are metabolised by CYP3A4, which may lead to drug interactions with drugs that are CYP3A4 substrates, inhibitors or inducers. These interactions may result in altered drug effects (Smith 2009).

Both morphine and hydromorphone are metabolised into 'bad' metabolites (morphine-3-glucuronide and hydromorphone-3-glucuronide, respectively), which increase neuroexcitability and are renally cleared. Fentanyl and methadone do not have active metabolites and are less affected than other opioids in renal and hepatic impairment (Smith 2009).

PRACTICE POINT

- Codeine should *not* be used in children (Schug et al. 2020).
- The American Academy of Pediatrics states 'Codeine: time to say "No" ' (Tobias et al. 2016).
- Hydrocodone (metabolised to hydromorphone by CYP 2D6) cannot be recommended in paediatrics for the same reason that codeine has become obsolete.

Adverse Drug Reactions Most adverse reactions of opioids are dose-related and include respiratory depression, sedation, nausea and vomiting, constipation, miosis, euphoria, dysphoria, urinary retention and pruritis (Rang et al. 2012). Tolerance develops to most side effects except for miosis and constipation. The central nervous system (CNS) effects of opioids (sedation, euphoria or dysphoria) are generally short-lived and resolve within several days of starting opioids or increasing the dose. Switching to another opioid that is better tolerated may decrease adverse effects (Benavides and Nahata 2013). Pethidine (meperidine) should *not* be used as an analgesic in children because of the risk of norpethidine toxicity (Kraemer 2010; Benavides and Nahata 2013). See Appendix for opioid dosing information.

Opioid Misuse and Substance Use Disorder

We are in the midst of two opioid crises in one world. While there is opioid over-prescribing for patients with chronic pain in the USA, 2.5 million children in low- to middle-income countries die without analgesia (Knaul et al. 2018). Prescribers need mitigation strategies to minimise opioid misuse, substance use disorder (SUD) and opioid use disorder (OUD). These strategies include prescribing opioids in the lowest effective dose for the shortest duration necessary, using short-acting opioids and avoiding concomitant benzodiazepines (Volkow and McLellan 2016; Chua et al. 2020).

The fear of SUD must be balanced with adequate pain control. A 2017 study in two paediatric emergency departments showed only half of the caregivers accepting opioids for moderate pain, despite their child continuing to experience pain after receiving non-opioid analgesics. Reasons given were fears of side effects, masking the diagnosis, addiction and overdose (Jun et al. 2019).

PRACTICE POINT

- Ensure effective analgesia.
- Be aware that some patients may have or develop opioid-induced hyperalgesia.
- *Do not* withhold opioids (this places the patient at risk of acute opioid withdrawal).
- Be alert for signs of opioid withdrawal (sweating, nausea and/or vomiting, agitation, diarrhoea, yawning, dilated pupils, anxiety, insomnia, tachycardia, hypertension and cramping abdominal pain) (Schug et al. 2010).

Opioid Tapering

Most hospitalised children in high-income countries receive opioids (often concurrently with benzodiazepines and alpha-agonists) to provide sedation while being intubated on intensive care units. Treatment of nociceptive pain is the second most common reason for paediatric opioid administration. The practice of the Department of Pain Medicine, Palliative Care and Integrative Medicine at Children's Minnesota in Minneapolis/St Paul, USA is to taper opioids after five or more days of scheduled administration to avoid withdrawal. The following guidelines (which need to be adjusted to the individual clinical case) have been shown to be effective for several thousand paediatric patients for morphine, oxycodone, fentanyl, hydromorphone and methadone:

- The duration of the taper should not generally be longer than the duration of the opioid administration; for example, for a child who has been on opioids for 12 days we plan for a 12-day (or shorter) taper.
- Wean by 10% per day of current dose (or more to not exceed above rule).
- Measure withdrawal with validated tools, such as the Withdrawal Assessment Tool (WAT)-1 (Franck et al. 2012).
- When 50% of a normal starting dose of the opioid is reached (see Appendix), change from scheduled to as-needed dosing for 24 hours and then stop.
- If children seem particularly sensitive, the taper may have to be decreased (e.g. less than 10% or weaning morphine and lorazepam on alternating days by 10% respectively, rather than on the same day).

Mixed Opioids

Tramadol

Tramadol is used for mild to moderate pain, having an effect on nociceptive and neuropathic pain.

Action   Tramadol is a partial agonist at the mu-opioid receptor, with no affinity for the delta or kappa opioid receptors (Bozkurt 2005). Its main action occurs centrally where it inhibits reuptake of the neurotransmitters noradrenaline and serotonin at the nerve synapse.

Adverse Drug Reactions   Tramadol causes nausea and vomiting at similar or reduced rates to other opioids (Bozkurt 2005). Respiratory depression and sedation occur less frequently (Kraemer 2010). Tramadol can lower the seizure threshold and should be used with caution or avoided in patients with seizures. Use caution when combined with other drugs that increase serotonin levels and monitor for serotonin syndrome (Benavides and Nahata 2013).

In 2017, the Food and Drug Administration (FDA) warned against the use of tramadol in children under 12 years of age (Food and Drug Administration 2017). See Appendix for dosing information.

Buprenorphine

Buprenorphine is available as a transdermal patch for chronic pain and and as a sublingual preparation (combined with naloxone) labelled for use in OUD (Borodovsky et al. 2018; Haupt et al. 2019).

Action   Buprenorphine is a partial agonist at the mu receptor and an antagonist at the kappa receptor (Beaulieu et al. 2010). There is a ceiling effect to the opioid agonist effects that may decrease its potential for misuse (Borodovsky et al. 2018).

Metabolism/Elimination   Buprenorphine patches applied topically avoid first-pass metabolism through the liver, allowing lower doses to be utilised (Haupt et al. 2019). Buprenorphine is metabolised in the liver by CYP3A4 and CYP2C8 and extensive glucuronidation. The glucuronidated metabolites are then eliminated by the biliary and renal systems (Davis et al. 2018).

Adverse Drug Reactions   Some patients report mild side effects with transdermal use (nausea/vomiting, constipation, headaches and local skin irritation) (Haupt et al. 2019). A review of three RCTs using buprenorphine in adolescents and young adults with OUD found buprenorphine well tolerated (Borodovsky et al. 2018). The American Academy of Pediatrics Committee on Substance Use Prevention (2016) found no age-related safety concerns with buprenorphine for OUD.

PRACTICE POINT

Patch safety

- Store patches safely away from children, preferably in a locked box.
- Apply to upper back where the child cannot reach it.
- Patches should be returned to the pharmacy for proper disposal, as a significant amount of drug remains at end of the dose interval.
- Avoid exposure to a heat source (e.g. fever) as this increases the release of opioid, leading to potential toxicity.

Partial Patches for Dose Titration

- Do *not* cut patches.

Applicable to patches where drug release is proportional to the size of the patch

- Round patches many be subdivided like pieces of a pie, whereas square patches can be subdivided into halves or thirds (draw a line on the writing side of the patch).
- Apply an occlusive dressing (e.g. Tegaderm) to the skin first, then affix the opioid patch on top of the Tegaderm with the remaining portion of the opioid patch (part to deliver drug) directly on the patient's skin (Mitchell and Smith 2010).

Opioid Antagonists

Naloxone

Naloxone is a pure opioid antagonist that occupies and displaces opioids from all opioid receptors, with greatest affinity for the mu-opioid receptor. It is used to manage opioid-induced ADRs and may be combined with opioids to reduce gastrointestinal adverse effects of opioids without loss of analgesia (Power 2011). See Appendix for naloxone dosing information.

Anaesthetics

Local Anaesthetics

Local anaesthetics (LAs) are drugs that *reversibly* block transmission of pain along nerve fibres (Neal 2012).

Action   Local anaesthetics can be used topically (for skin anaesthesia), by subcutaneous infiltration (for wound infiltration), by intravenous infusion (lidocaine) for neuropathic pain conditions (Nathan et al. 2005; Moulin et al. 2007), by direct injection to a peripheral nerve (for ring block or femoral nerve block) or injected adjacent to the spinal cord (e.g. caudal, epidural or intrathecal). Smaller diameter nerve fibres (pain and autonomic) are more sensitive to LAs than larger diameter (motor and proprioceptive) nerve fibres.

Mixing vasoconstrictors (most often adrenaline) with LAs prolongs the effect by slowing the rate of absorption and metabolism, particularly in single-shot regional anaesthesia techniques, such as caudal and limb blocks. Other drugs may be added to LAs for regional anaesthesia (e.g. epidural) to enhance analgesic effect (e.g. ketamine or opioids).

Longer-acting LAs (e.g. bupivacaine, ropivacaine or levobupivacaine) provide more effective analgesia for regional anaesthesia than short-acting LAs (e.g. lidocaine) (APA 2012). When used in regional anaesthesia, they offer a range of benefits including decreased surgical stress response, reduced use of general anaesthesia, reduced need for postoperative ventilatory support, enhanced analgesia, reduced haemodynamic instability and earlier return of gut function (APA 2012; Bosenberg 2012).

The two main types of local anaesthetics are *amides* and *esters*. The amides (e.g. lidocaine, prilocaine, bupivacaine, ropivacaine, levobupivacaine) are the most common *injected* anaesthetics, have a longer duration of action, are metabolised by the liver, have a low incidence of allergy and are more stable in solution. The esters (e.g. amethocaine (tetracaine), cocaine, procaine, benzocaine) are the most common *topical* anaesthetics, have a shorter duration of action, are metabolised by tissue esterases and have a high incidence of allergy (including anaphylaxis).

Adverse Drug Reactions   Most of the adverse reactions of LAs are due to high plasma concentrations, which mainly affect the cardiac system and CNS. This may occur with accidental injection of the LA into the general circulation. To avoid ADRs, maximum safe doses for age and weight are recommended and should be strictly adhered to (APA 2012).

Topical Local Anaesthetics

Topical LAs are extremely effective for the management of procedure-related pain in children, particularly venepuncture and intravenous cannulation (Murat et al. 2003; Zempsky 2008; Curtis et al. 2012). LA gels or sprays are used for surface anaesthesia before nasogastric tube or urinary catheter insertion, or for painful conditions of the nose, mouth or throat (APA 2012). Various drug combinations have been developed for surface anaesthesia, including mixtures of lidocaine, adrenaline and amethocaine in liquid or gel. These are commonly used for repair of face and scalp lacerations (Murat et al. 2003; APA 2012). Protocols and guidelines should be implemented to optimise topical LA utilisation.

The most common topical LAs used for children are:

- 4% liposomal lidocaine (ELA-Max, Maxilene or LMX4);
- lidocaine/prilocaine (EMLA);
- amethocaine (Ametop, Pontocaine, Dicaine or AnGel);
- 1% buffered lidocaine via needleless applicator (J-Tip);
- lidocaine/amethocaine topical patch (Synera).

PRACTICE POINT

- LA combinations cannot be used for end-arterial supplied areas (e.g. digits, genitalia, nose or ears) as adrenaline (epinephrine) can cause excessive vasoconstriction and tissue necrosis (APA 2012).
- Cocaine-containing LA preparations are not recommended for use in children (Murat et al. 2003).

Ketamine

Ketamine is an anaesthetic with powerful analgesic properties, even at very low doses. It is used in anaesthesia, procedural sedation and analgesia (Roelofse 2010). It reduces opioid-induced tolerance and hyperalgesia and is probably most efficacious for escalating pain or for opioid-resistant pain (Schug et al. 2020). For analgesia ketamine is used primarily in severe acute pain episodes as a low-dose continuous infusion (e.g. sickle cell vaso-occlusive pain, severe postoperative pain) or in end-of-life care (Lubega et al. 2018; Anghelescu and Tesney 2019; Cote and Wilson 2019; Alshahrani and Alghamdi 2020).

Action   Ketamine is an *N*-methyl-D-aspartate (NMDA) receptor channel inhibitor that blocks pain wind-up (sensitisation) (Schug et al. 2020).

Single doses of ketamine are less effective than an infusion because it has a very short half-life (Roelofse 2010).

Metabolism/Elimination   Ketamine is metabolised in the liver with minimal drug remaining for renal excretion. It is useful for patients with renal or liver dysfunction.

Adverse Drug Reactions   The main ketamine ADR at standard dosing is dysphoria, particularly vivid dreams and hallucinations (Schug et al. 2020). This occurs in 10% of patients and may be similar to the rates of dysphoric effects of opioids (Anderson and Palmer 2006). In contrast to opioids, respiratory depression and cardiovascular changes are minimal. At higher doses for procedural sedation, increased salivation, agitation and emergence reactions (imagery, hallucinations, delirium) have been reported. See Appendix for dosing information.

Adjuvant Drugs

Adjuvant drugs work in a variety of ways to enhance analgesia (Knotkova and Pappagallo 2007; Khan et al. 2011). Adjuvants include gabapentinoids, tricyclic antidepressants and α_2-adrenergic agonists (Friedrichsdorf and Goubert 2020). Many drug treatments are extrapolated from adult studies with insufficient evidence other than consensus to guide practice in CYP.

Gabapentinoids

Gabapentin and pregabalin are gabapentinoids used in complex pain. They are first-line agents for neuropathic pain in adults (Smith et al. 2013; Moulin et al. 2014; Finnerup et al. 2015). Management of neuropathic pain in adults focuses on diabetic neuropathy and post-herpetic neuralgia, which are not seen in children. However, Anghelescu and Tesney (2019) have published a summary of recommendations for treating neuropathic pain in children. An RCT using pregabalin in young people with fibromyalgia did not significantly improve pain scores but did find significant improvement in secondary pain measures and global impression of change. Safety was consistent with adult use (Arnold et al. 2016). Case series in children found gabapentin the most frequently used anticonvulsant (Scottish Government 2018). This guideline recommends gabapentin be tried first and pregabalin second, if gabapentin is ineffective or has intolerable side effects (Scottish Government 2018). Using gabapentin first because of increased use in children for seizures is reasonable (Hauer and Houtrow 2017).

Pharmacokinetics   Gabapentin may require dosing every six hours in infants younger than 12 months, as opposed to every eight hours in older children, because of its shorter half-life (Friedrichsdorf and Goubert 2020). In comparison, pregabalin can be given twice daily (Attal and Finnerup 2010). Gabapentin has non-linear bioavailability: as the dose is increased, the percentage absorbed decreases (Toth and Moulin 2013). Pregabalin exhibits linear kinetics, resulting in plasma concentrations that increase proportionally as the dose is increased (Bockbrader et al 2010). Onset of analgesia may be quicker with pregabalin than gabapentin because the dose can be titrated more quickly (Toth and Moulin 2013). Gabapentin is suspected to have poor rectal absorption (due to a missing active transporter), whereas pregabalin is absorbed when given rectally (Kriel et al. 1997; Doddrell and Tripathi 2015; Kram et al. 2020). Gabapentin and pregabalin are excreted unchanged in the urine, so dose reduction is necessary in renal impairment (Bockbrader et al. 2010; Toth and Moulin 2013).

Action   Gabapentin and pregabalin are calcium channel modulators. They bind to the $\alpha_2\delta$ ligand of the voltage-gated calcium channel in the excited neuron, which decreases the release of neurotransmitters (e.g. glutamate and substance P) (Toth and Moulin 2013; Moulin et al. 2014). Pregabalin may also have anxiolytic properties and a beneficial effect on sleep (Toth and Moulin 2013).

Adverse Drug Reactions   The most common adverse effect is sedation. This is best handled by starting with a low dose and increasing slowly (Beaulieu et al. 2010). Start with a bedtime dose for a few days before introducing the morning dose (and a few more days before starting the midday dose if using gabapentin). When increasing the daily dose, consider increasing the bedtime dose first. Other side effects include dizziness, dry mouth and, with pregabalin, peripheral oedema and weight gain (Toth and Moulin 2013).

Switching Between Gabapentin and Pregabalin   To provide equal analgesia, milligram for milligram pregabalin is about six times more potent than gabapentin (Ifuku et al. 2011), so that 1 mg pregabalin is equivalent to 6 mg gabapentin.

Switching between the two drugs is performed as follows.

1. Calculate the total *daily* dose the patient is currently taking.
2. Give the last dose of the first drug at bedtime and then the next day start the second drug with first dose at breakfast.
3. Round down the dose if it is not equally divisible and/or the patient is experiencing side effects.
4. *Example*: current dose is gabapentin 100 mg three times daily = 300 mg per day. To switch to pregabalin: 300 mg ÷ 6 = 50 mg per day, so start pregabalin 25 mg twice daily.

PRACTICE POINT

If a pregabalin liquid is required:

- Liquid is commercially available in the USA and other countries.
- Alternatively:
  - The capsule can be opened and contents mixed in water; pregabalin is water soluble so a partial dose may be given (discard unused portion).
  - Mix the contents of one 25-mg capsule in 5 mL of water to give 5 mg/mL concentration.
  - Give orally or via ≥ 8 Fr nasogastric tube (White and Bradnam 2015).

Tricyclic Antidepressants

A Cochrane review examining antidepressants for CNCP in children and adolescents found a small number of studies with insufficient data for analysis (Cooper et al. 2017c). A review published in 2019 looking at CNCP and cancer-related pain reinforced the paucity of data in children (Eccleston et al. 2019). Despite the lack of trials tricyclics are used in CYP with chronic pain.

Action   Tricyclics modulate pain by affecting the descending inhibitory pathway through inhibition of the reuptake of noradrenaline and serotonin (Kraemer 2010). They also block sodium channels and inhibit NMDA-induced sensitisation (Toth and Moulin 2013). The onset of analgesia is a few weeks as opposed to the four- to eight-week onset needed for the antidepressant effect (Lexicomp 2019b). The inhibition of noradrenaline appears necessary for analgesia since selective serotonin inhibitors do not provide effective analgesia (Kraemer 2010). Amitriptyline and nortriptyline are the most commonly used tricyclics in children.

Metabolism/Elimination
Amitriptyline is metabolised in the liver to the active metabolite nortriptyline (Taketomo et al. 2008, pp. 110–112). Nortriptyline undergoes first-pass metabolism in the liver via hydroxylation and glucuronide conjugation. The metabolites and unchanged nortriptyline are eliminated in the urine with small amounts eliminated in the bile (Taketomo et al. 2008, pp 1276–1278).

PRACTICE POINT

- Despite the name, tricyclic antidepressants are *not* effective for treating anxiety and/or depression in children (Hazell and Mirzaie 2013; Wang et al. 2017).
- Take amitriptyline after supper (7 p.m.) to maximise sedation. Taking at bedtime is too late in the day since peak effects are two to five hours after administration (Lexicomp 2019b).

Adverse Drug Reactions   Obtain a baseline ECG before starting a tricyclic because of their ability to cause cardiac conduction abnormalities (Chambliss et al. 2002; Anghelescu and Tesney 2019). Additional QT interval monitoring may be necessary (Benavides and Nahata 2013). Common side effects include sedation and anticholinergic effects (dry mouth, constipation, urinary retention, tachycardia, orthostatic hypotension and blurred vision) (Chambliss et al. 2002; Attal and Finnerup 2010). Nortriptyline is an alternative drug that exhibits fewer anticholinergic side effects (Friedrichsdorf and Kang 2007). See Appendix for adjuvant drug dosing information.

Cannabinoids

Challenges exist in assessing the efficacy and safety of cannabis given the variation in products, route of administration (oral, vaped, smoked), source of cannabinoid (plant or synthetic), variation of formulation (cannabidiol to THC ratios) and calculation of the exact dose delivered (Campbell et al. 2019). A meta-analysis of 91 publications of cannabis used in CNCP reported that to achieve a decrease in pain by 30% in one patient required treatment of 24 patients (number needed to treat = 24), and treatment in only six patients was required for one patient to experience harm (number needed to harm = 6) (Stockings et al. 2018). The NICE guideline does not recommend using cannabis to manage chronic pain, to use cannabidiol in adults only if part of a clinical trial, and to weigh carefully the additional risks before using in children (NICE 2019b).

Cannabis use and legalisation in some countries has led to many questions about its use in CYP (Ali and Parker 2020). Clinical evidence of cannabis use in children is sparse and mainly comprises case reports (Rieder 2016).

Action   Cannabis comprises Δ^9-tetrahydrocannabinol (THC), which has psychoactive properties, and cannabidiol (CBD), which has behavioural and other CNS effects but no psychoactive properties (Rieder 2016). Cannabis affects the endocannabinoid system via CBD1 receptors primarily in the central and peripheral nervous systems and CBD2 receptors mainly in the immune system (Crawley et al. 2018). THC stimulates the cannabinoid receptors that modulate secretion of GABA and glutamate in the CNS, producing significant neurodevelopmental effects on the brain (Grant and Belanger 2017).

Adverse Drug Reactions   The frontal cortex is responsible for higher-order cognitive processes and undergoes rapid changes up to 25 years of age (Grant and Belanger 2017). Cannabis should not be used in CYP under 25 years of age since it is toxic to cortical neuronal networks and there is an increase in health harms with intensity of use (Kelsall 2017).

In 2017 the Canadian Paediatric Society position statement cautioned that there is a strong link in CYP between cannabis use and increased presence of mental illness (depression, anxiety, psychosis), impaired neurological development and cognitive decline, decreased school performance and lifetime achievement, initiation and maintenance of tobacco smoking, and cannabis dependence and other substance use disorders (Grant and Belanger 2017).

Cannabis impairs short-term memory, complex mental tasks, attention and judgement. Motor skills and reaction times are compromised (Grant and Belanger 2017). Cannabis hyperemesis syndrome presents as cyclic vomiting in chronic high-dose users. Its mechanism of action is not well understood but vomiting is relieved by taking hot baths/showers (Crawley et al. 2018). Cannabis withdrawal symptoms include headaches, sleep disruption, irritability and anxiety (Rieder 2016).

In 2021 the International Association for the Study of Pain (IASP) issued a position statement on the use of cannabis and cannabinoids for analgesia, stating that it did not endorse general use of cannabis and cannabinoids for relief of pain because there is a lack of high-quality evidence to support its use (IASP Presidential Task Force on Cannabis and Cannabinoid Analgesia 2021).

PRACTICE POINT

Cannabinoids (including THC and CBD preparations) have not been shown to be an efficacious analgesic and are *not* safe in children. They cannot be recommended as an analgesic.

Summary

- Many analgesic drugs have not been tested in children or are administered off-label.
- Misconceptions about analgesic drugs, particularly opioids, contribute to the undertreatment of pain in children.
- Confusion about opioid terminology leads to anxiety in families and health professionals and suboptimal pain management practice.
- Combining analgesics with physical and psychological strategies ensures better pain management outcomes.
- Health professionals need to be aware of the patient's liver and renal function and the need for reduced doses of analgesics if these are impaired.
- The route of administration affects the onset and efficacy of a drug. There are advantages and disadvantages with different administration routes, which should be considered before analgesic selection.
- Analgesics should be selected using a stepwise approach based on the type and severity of pain, onset and peak effect of the drug, and benefits and risks.
- Keep all drugs stored away from children and dispose of at the pharmacy.

Multiple Choice Questions

1. Until what age is dose adjustment of renally excreted drugs required, when renal function equals adult function?
   a. 1 month
   b. 3 months
   c. 6 months
   d. 12 months
2. What is the correct order of speed of onset of analgesia, from fastest to slowest?
   a. Oral solid dosage form > oral liquid > intravenous > subcutaneous
   b. Intravenous > subcutaneous > oral solid dosage form > oral liquid
   c. Intravenous > subcutaneous > oral liquid > oral solid dosage form
   d. Subcutaneous > intravenous > oral liquid > oral solid dosage form
3. Which of the following opioids does not require metabolism by CYP2D6?
   a. Tramadol
   b. Hydromorphone
   c. Hydrocodone
   d. Oxycodone
   e. Codeine
4. Which of the following statements is *false*?
   a. Gabapentin and pregabalin cause sedation
   b. Pregabalin can be titrated faster than gabapentin
   c. Pregabalin has linear kinetics whereas gabapentin has saturable absorption
   d. 1 mg gabapentin = 6 mg pregabalin
5. Why should cannabis be used with caution in CYP?
   a. Cannabis use is linked with mental illness
   b. Cannabis use is linked with decrease in school performance
   c. Cannabis use is linked with increased use of tobacco and other substance use disorders
   d. All of the above

Acknowledgements

The author thanks Dr Stefan Friedrichsdorf for writing the section on opioid tapering and for supplying the dosing tables. We'd like to acknowledge the original contributions of Stephanie Dowden to this Chapter in the Second Edition of this book

Useful Web Resources

UK
British Pain Society, www.britishpainsociety.org/
Anaesthesia UK, www.frca.co.uk/

USA
American Academy of Pain Medicine (AAPM), www.painmed.org
American Academy of Pediatrics, www.aap.org/
Medline Plus information about pain management, www.nlm.nih.gov/medlineplus/pain.html
Children's Hospital of Minnesota, www.childrensmn.org/

Canada
Hospital for Sick Children, www.sickkids.ca/HealthcareProfessionalsandStudents/index.html

International
Special Interest Group on Pain in Childhood (IASP), http://childpain.org/

Opioid Information
https://healthsci.mcmaster.ca/npc
Michael G. DeGroote, National Pain Centre
http://www.sickkids.ca/clinical-practice-guidelines/clinical-practice-guidelines/Export/CLINH303/Main%20Document.pdf

Cannabis Patient Information
www.edcan.ca/articles/cannabis-what-are-the-risks-for-students/
www.ccsa.ca/help-your-teen-understand-whats-fact-and-fiction-about-marijuana-infographic
www.camh.ca/en/search?query=cannabis

References

Ali, S. and Parker, A.P.J. (2020) Medicinal use of cannabis-based products: a practical guide for paediatricians *Paediatrics and Child Health* 30(2), 79–83.

Alshahrani, M.S. and Alghamdi, M.A. (2020) Ketamine for sickle cell vaso-occlusive crises: a systematic review. *Saudi Journal of Medicine and Medical Sciences* 9(1), 3–9.

American Academy of Pediatrics, Committee on Substance Use and Prevention, Policy Statement (2016) Medication-assisted treatment of adolescents with opioid use disorders. *Pediatrics* 138(3), e20161893.

Anderson, B.J. and Palmer, G.M. (2006) Recent developments in the pharmacological management of pain in children. *Current Opinion in Anaesthesiology* 19, 285–292.

Anghelescu, D.L. and Tesney, J.M. (2019) Neuropathic pain in pediatric oncology: a clinical decision algorithm. *Pediatric Drugs* 21, 59–70.

Arnold, L.M., Schikler, K.N., Bateman, L., et al. (2016) Safety and efficacy of pregabalin in adolescents with fibromyalgia: a randomized, double-blind, placebo-controlled trial and a 6-month open-label extension study. *Pediatric Rheumatology Online Journal* 14(1), 46.

Association of Paediatric Anaesthetists of Great Britain and Ireland (APA) (2012) *Good Practice in Postoperative and Procedural Pain Management*, 2nd edn. *Pediatric Anesthesia* 22(Suppl. 1), 1–79. Available at http://onlinelibrary.wiley.com/doi/10.1111/j.1460-9592.2012.03838.x/pdf (accessed 5 September 2022).

Attal, N. and Finnerup, N.B. (2010) Pharmacological management of neuropathic pain. *Pain Clinical Updates* 18(9), 1–7. Available at http://www.wps.ac.nz/Portals/9/Documents/Neuropathic-pain.pdf

Barbagallo, M. and Sacerdote, P. (2019) Ibuprofen in the treatment of children's inflammatory pain: a clinical and pharmacological overview. *Minerva Pediatrica* 71(1), 82–99.

Batchelor, H.K., Fotaki, N. and Klein, S. (2014) Paediatric oral biopharmaceutics: key considerations and current challenges. *Advanced Drug Delivery Reviews* 73, 102–126.

Beal, J.A. (2021) Pediatric pain remains undertreated. *MCN American Journal of Maternal/Child Nursing* 46(5), 300.

Beaulieu, P., Lussier, D., Porreca, F. and Dickenson, A.H. (eds) (2010) *Pharmacology of Pain*, pp. 45–46, 68–76, 537, 557. IASP Press, Seattle, WA.

Begg, E.J. (2008) *Instant Clinical Pharmacology*, 2nd edn. John Wiley & Sons, Chichester.

Benavides, S. and Nahata, M.C. (eds) (2013) *Pediatric Pharmacotherapy*, pp. 10, 12–13, 18–33, 844–850. American College of Clinical Pharmacy, Lenexa, KS.

Berde, C.B. and Sethna, N.F. (2002) Analgesics for the treatment of pain in children. *New England Journal of Medicine* 347(14), 1094–1103.

Bockbrader, H.N., Wesche, D., Miller, R., Chapel, S., Janiczek, N. and Burgeret, P. (2010) A comparison of the pharmacokinetics and pharmacodynamics of pregabalin and gabapentin. *Clinical Pharmacokinetics* 49(10), 661–669.

Borodovsky, J.T., Levy, S., Fishman, M., Marsch, L.A. (2018) Buprenorphine treatment for adolescents and young adults with opioid use disorders: a narrative review. *Journal of Addiction Medicine* 12(3), 170–183.

Bosenberg, A. (2012) Benefits of regional anesthesia in children. *Pediatric Anesthesia* 22, 10–18.

Bozkurt, P. (2005) Use of tramadol in children. *Pediatric Anesthesia* 15, 1041–1047.

Bryant, B. and Knights, K. (2010) *Pharmacology for Health Professionals*, 3rd edn. Elsevier Australia, Melbourne.

Campbell, G., Stockings, E. and Nielsen, S. (2019) Understanding the evidence for medical cannabis and cannabis-based medicines for the treatment of chronic non-cancer pain. *European Archives of Psychiatry and Clinical Neuroscience* 269, 135–144.

Chambliss, C.R., Heggen, J., Copelan, D.N. and Pettignano, R. (2002) The assessment and management of chronic pain in children. *Pediatric Drugs* 4(11), 737–746.

Chidambaran, V., Sadhasivam, S. and Mahmoud, M. (2017) Codeine and opioid metabolism: implications and alternatives for pediatric pain management. *Current Opinion in Anesthesiology* 30, 349–356.

Chua, K.-P., Brummett, C.M., Conti, R.M. and Bohnert, A. (2020) Association of opioid prescribing patterns with prescription opioid overdose in adolescents and young adults. *JAMA Pediatrics* 174(2), 141–148.

Colvin, L.A., Bull, F. and Hales, T.G. (2019) Perioperative opioid analgesia: when is enough too much? A review of opioid-induced tolerance and hyperalgesia. *Lancet* 393, 1558–1568.

Conaghan, P.G. (2012) A turbulent decade for NSAIDs: update on current concepts of classification, epidemiology, comparative efficacy, and toxicity. *Rheumatology International* 32(6), 1491–1502.

Cooper, T.E., Fisher, E., Anderson, B., Wilkinson, N.M.R., Williams, D.G. and Eccleston, C. (2017a) Paracetamol (acetaminophen) for chronic non-cancer pain in children and adolescents. *Cochrane Database of Systematic Reviews* (8), CD012539.

Cooper, T.E., Fisher, E., Gray, A.L., et al. (2017b) Opioids for chronic non-cancer pain in children and adolescents. *Cochrane Database of Systematic Reviews* (7), CD012538.

Cooper, T.E., Heathcote, L.C., Clinch, J., et al. (2017c) Antidepressants for chronic non-cancer pain in children and adolescents. *Cochrane Database of Systematic Reviews* (8), CD012535.

Cote, C.J. and Wilson, S. (2019) Guidelines for monitoring and management of pediatric patients before, during, and after sedation for diagnostic and therapeutic procedures. *Pediatrics* 143(6), e20191000.

Crawley, A., LeBras, M. and Regier, L. (2018) Cannabinoids overview. RxFiles© https://www.rxfiles.ca/rxfiles/uploads/documents/pain-qanda-cannabinoids.pdf (accessed 22 August 2022).

Curtis, S., Wingert, A. and Ali, S. (2012) The Cochrane Library and procedural pain in children:

an overview of the reviews. *Evidence-Based Child Health* 7, 1363–1399.

Davis, M.P., Pasternak, G. and Behm, B. (2018) Treating chronic pain: an overview of clinical studies centered on the buprenorphine option. *Drugs* 78(12), 1211–1228.

Doddrell, C. and Tripathi, S.S. (2015) Successful use of pregabalin by the rectal route to treat chronic neuropathic pain in a patient with complete intestinal failure. *BMJ Case Reports* 2015, bcr2015211511.

Eccleston, C., Cooper, T.E., Fisher, E., Anderson, B. and Wilkinson, N.M.R. (2017) Non-steroidal anti-inflammatory drugs (NSAIDs) for chronic non-cancer pain in children and adolescents. *Cochrane Database of SysematicReviews* (8), CD012537.

Eccleston, C., Fisher, E., Cooper, T.E., et al. (2019) Pharmacological interventions for chronic pain in children: an overview of systematic reviews. *Pain* 160, 1698–1707.

Eerdekens, M., Beuter C., Lefeber C. and van den Anker, J. (2019) The challenge of developing pain medications for children: therapeutic needs and future perspectives. *Journal of Pain Research* 12, 1649–1664.

Finnerup, N.B., Attal, N., Haroutounian, S. et al. (2015) Pharmacotherapy for neuropathic pain in adults: a systematic review and meta-analysis. *Lancet Neurology* 14, 162–173.

Food and Drug Administration (2017) FDA Drug Safety Communication: FDA restricts use of prescription codeine pain and cough medicines and tramadol pain medicines in children; recommends against use in breastfeeding women. `www.fda.gov/drugs/drug-safety-and-availability/fda-drug-safety-communication-fda-restricts-use-prescription-codeine-pain-and-cough-medicines-and` (accessed 27 January 2020).

Franck, L.S., Scoppettuolo, L.A., Wypij, D. and Curley, M.A.Q. (2012) Validity and generalizability of the Withdrawal Assessment Tool-1 (WAT-1) for monitoring iatrogenic withdrawal syndrome in pediatric patients. *Pain* 153(1), 142–148.

Frey, T.M., Florin, T.A., Caruso, M., Zhang, N., Zhang, Y. and Mittiga, M.R. (2019) Effect of intranasal ketamine vs fentanyl on pain reduction for extremity injuries in children. The PRIME randomized clinical trial. *JAMA Pediatrics* 173(2), 140–146.

Friedrichsdorf, S.J. and Goubert, L. (2020) Pediatric pain treatment and prevention for hospitalized children *Pain Reports* 5(1), e804.

Friedrichsdorf, S.J. and Kang, T.I. (2007) The management of pain in children with life-limiting illnesses. *Pediatric Clinics of North America* 54, 645–672.

Goldman, R.D. and Scolnik, D. (2004) Underdosing of acetaminophen by parents and emergency department utilization. *Pediatric Emergency Care* 20(2), 89–93.

Grant, C.N. and Belanger, R.E. (2017) Canadian Paediatric Society Position Statement: Cannabis and Canada's children and youth. *Paediatrics and Child Health* 22(2), 98–102.

Hauer, J. and Houtrow, A.J. (2017) Pain assessment and treatment in children with significant impairment of the central nervous system. *Pediatrics* 139(6), e20171002.

Haupt, T.S., Smyth, M. and Gregoire, M.-C. (2019) A scoping review of transdermal buprenorphine use for non-surgical pain in the pediatric population. *Cureus* 11(10), e9594.

Hazell, P. and Mirzaie, M. (2013) Tricyclic drugs for depression in children and adolescents. *Cochrane Database of Systematic Reviews*, (6), CD002317.

Hong, J.Y., Kim, W.O., Koo, B.N., Cho, J.S., Suk, E.H. and Kil, H.K. (2010) Fentanyl-sparing effect of acetaminophen as a mixture of fentanyl in intravenous parent-/nurse-controlled analgesia after pediatric ureteroneocystostomy. *Anesthesiology* 113(3), 672–677.

IASP Presidential Task Force on Cannabis and Cannabinoid Analgesia (2021) International Association for the study of Pain Presidential Task Force on cannabis and cannabinoid analgesia position statement. *Pain* 162(Suppl.), S1–S2.

Ifuku, M., Iseki, M., Hidaka, I., Morita, Y., Komatus, S. and Inada, E. (2011) Replacement of gabapentin with pregabalin in postherpetic neuralgia therapy. *Pain Medicine* 12, 1112–1116.

Jun, E., Ali, S., Yaskina, M., et al. (2021) A two-centre survey of caregiver perspectives on opioid use for children's acute pain management. *Paediatrics and Child Health* 26, 19–26.

Kanneh, A. (2002a) Paediatric pharmacological principles: an update Part 1: Drug development and pharmacodynamics. *Paediatric Nursing* 14(8), 36–42.

Kanneh, A. (2002b) Paediatric pharmacological principles: an update Part 2: Pharmacokinetics: absorption and distribution. *Paediatric Nursing* 14(9), 39–43.

Kelsall, D. (2017) Cannabis legislation fails to protect Canada's youth. *Canadian Medical Association Journal* 189(21), e737–e738.

Khan, M.I., Walsh, D. and Brito-Dellan, N. (2011) Opioid and adjuvant analgesics: compared and contrasted. *American Journal of Hospice and Palliative Care* 28(5), 378–383.

Kimland, E. and Odlind, V. (2012) Off-label drug use in pediatric patients. *Clinical Pharmacology and Therapeutics* 91(5), 796–801.

Knaul, F.M., Farmer, P.E., Krakauer, E.L. et al. (2018) Alleviating the access abyss in palliative care and pain relief: an imperative of universal health coverage. The Lancet Commission report. *Lancet* 391, 1391–1454.

Knotkova, H. and Pappagallo, M. (2007) Adjuvant analgesics. *Medical Clinics of North America* 91, 113–124.

Kokki, H. (2003) Nonsteroidal anti-inflammatory drugs for postoperative pain: a focus on children. *Pediatric Drugs* 5(2), 103–123.

Kozer, E., Greenberg, R., Zimmerman, D.R. and Berkovitch, M. (2006) Repeated supratherapeutic doses of paracetamol in children: a literature review and suggested clinical approach. *Acta Paediatrica* 95, 1165–1171.

Kraemer, F.W. (2010) Treatment of acute pediatric pain. *Seminars in Pediatric Neurology* 17, 268–274.

Kram, S., Tatum, M., Iboaya, E. and Klapper, J. (2020) Nonenteral administration of pregabalin for withdrawal in a surgical critically ill patient. *Critical Care Medicine* 48(Suppl. 1), 420.

Kriel, R.L., Birnbaum, A.K., Cloyd, J.C., Ricker, B.J., Jones Saete, C. and Caruso, K.J. (1997) Failure of absorption of gabapentin after rectal administration. *Epilepsia* 38(11), 1242–1244.

Lam, J.K.W., Xu, Y., Worsley, A. and Wong, I.C.K. (2014) Oral transmucosal drug delivery for pediatric use. *Advanced Drug Delivery Reviews* 73, 50–62.

Lexicomp (2019a) Celecoxib monograph. Lexi-Comp Online, Pediatric and Neonatal Lexi-Drugs Online. https://online.lexi.com (accessed 23 December 2019).

Lexicomp (2019b) Amitriptyline monograph. Lexi-Comp Online, Pediatric and Neonatal Lexi-Drugs Online. https://online.lexi.com (accessed 23 December 2019).

Li, S.F., Lacher, B. and Crain, E.F. (2000) Acetaminophen and ibuprofen dosing by parents. *Pediatric Emergency Care* 16(6), 394–397.

Lubega, F.A., DeSilva, M.S., Munube, D., et al. (2018) Low dose ketamine versus morphine for acute severe vaso occlusive pain in children: a randomized controlled trial. *Scandinavian Journal of Pain* 18(1), 19–27.

McCrae, J.C., Morrison, E.E., MacIntyre, I.M., Dear, J.W. and Webb, D.J. (2018) Long-term adverse effects of paracetamol: a review. *British Journal of Clinical Pharmacology* 84, 2218–2230.

Mitchell, A. and Smith, H.S. (2010) Applying partially occluded fentanyl transdermal patches to manage pain in pediatric patients. *Journal of Opioid Management* 6(4), 290–294.

Motov, S., Butt, M., Masoudi, A., et al. (2020) Comparison of oral ibuprofen and acetaminophen with either analgesic alone for pediatric emergency department patients with acute pain. *Journal of Emergency Medicine* 58(5), 725–732.

Moulin, D.E., Clark, A.J., Gilron, I., et al (2007) Pharmacological management of chronic neuropathic pain: consensus statement and guidelines from the Canadian Pain Society. *Pain Research and Management* 12(1), 13–21.

Moulin, D.E., Boulanger, A., Clark, A.J., et al. (2014) Pharmacological management of chronic neuropathic pain: revised consensus statement from the Canadian Pain Society. *Pain and Research and Management* 19(6), 328–335.

Murat, I., Gall, O. and Tourniaire, B. (2003) Procedural pain in children, evidence-based best practice and guidelines. *Regional Anesthesia and Pain Medicine* 28, 561–572.

Nathan, A., Rose, J.B., Guite, J.W., Hehir, D. and Milovcich, K. (2005) Primary erythromelalgia in a child responding to intravenous lidocaine and oral mexiletine treatment. *Pediatrics* 115(4), e504–e507.

National Institute for Health and Care Excellence (NICE) (2019a) Fever in under 5s: assessment and initial management. NICE Guideline NG143. Available at www.nice.org.uk/guidance/ng143 (accessed 22 August 2022).

National Institute for Health and Care Excellence (NICE) (2019b) Cannabis-based medicinal products. NICE Guideline NG144. Available at www.nice.org.uk/guidance/ng144 (accessed 23 December 2019).

Neal, M.J. (2012) *Medical Pharmacology at a Glance*, 7th edn. John Wiley & Sons, Chichester.

Pierce, C.A. and Voss, B. (2010) Efficacy and safety of ibuprofen and acetaminophen in children and adults: a meta-analysis and qualitative review. *Annals of Pharmacotherapy* 44(3), 489–506.

Power, I. (2011) An update on analgesics. *British Journal of Anaesthesia* 107(1), 19–24.

Rang, H.P., Dale, M.M., Ritter, J.M., Flower, R.J. and Henderson, G. (2012) *Pharmacology*, 7th edn. Elsevier/Churchill Livingstone, Edinburgh.

Remy, C., Marret, E. and Bonnet, F. (2006) State of the art of paracetamol in acute pain therapy. *Current Opinion in Anesthesiology* 19, 562–565.

Rieder, M.J. (2016) Canadian Paediatric Society Drug Therapy and Hazardous Substances Committee Position Statement: Is the medical use of cannabis a therapeutic option for children? *Paediatrics and Child Health* 21(1), 31–34.

Roelofse, J.A. (2010) The evolution of ketamine applications in children. *Paediatric Anaesthesia* 20(3), 240–245.

Schror, K. (2007) Aspirin and Reye syndrome: a review of the evidence. *Pediatric Drugs* 9(3), 191–200.

Schug, S.A., Palmer, G.M., Scott, D.A., Alcock, M., Halliwell, R. and Mott, J.F. (eds) (2020) *Acute Pain Management: Scientific Evidence*, 5th edn. Australian and New Zealand College of Anaesthetists and Faculty of Pain Medicine, Melbourne. Available at https://www.anzca.edu.au/resources/college-publications/acute-pain-management/apmse5.pdf (accessed 22 August 2022).

Scottish Government (2018) *Management of Chronic Pain in Children and Young People. A National Clinical Guideline*. Available at https://sign.ac.uk/media/1538/chronic_pain_in_childrenpdf.pdf (accessed 22 August 2022).

Smith, B.H., Lee, J. and Baranowski, A.P. (2013) Neuropathic pain: a pathway for care developed by the British Pain Society. *British Journal of Anaesthesia* 111(1), 73–79.

Smith, C. and Goldman, R.D. (2012) Alternating acetaminophen and ibuprofen for pain in children. *Canadian Family Physician* 58, 645–647.

Smith, H.S. (2009) Opioid metabolism. *Mayo Clinic Proceedings* 84(7), 613–624.

Southey, E.R., Soares-Weiser, K. and Kleijnen, J. (2009) Systematic review and meta-analysis of the clinical safety and tolerability of ibuprofen compared with paracetamol in paediatric pain and fever. *Current Medical Research and Opinion* 25(9), 2207–2222.

Stockings, E., Campbell, G., Hall, W.D., et al. (2018) Cannabis and cannabinoids for the treatment of people with chronic noncancer pain conditions: a systematic review and meta-analysis of controlled and observational studies. *Pain* 159, 1932–1954.

Sullivan, J.E. and Farrar, H.C. (2011) Fever and antipyretic use in children. *Pediatrics* 127(3), 580–587.

Taketomo, C.K., Hodding, J.H., Kraus, D.M. (eds) (2008) *Pediatric Dosage Handbook*. American Pharmacists Association, Washington, DC.

Tan, E., Braithwaite, I., McKinlay, C.J.D. and Dalziel, S.R. (2020) Comparison of acetaminophen (paracetamol) with ibuprofen for treatment of fever or pain in children younger than 2 years: a systematic review and meta-analysis. *JAMA Network Open* 3(10), e2022398.

Tobias, J.D., Green, T.P. and Cote, C.J. (2016) Codeine: Time to say 'no'. *Pediatrics* 138(4), e20162396.

Toth, C. and Moulin, D.E. (eds) (2013) *Neuropathic Pain: Causes, Management and Understanding*, pp. 226–229. Cambridge University Press, Cambridge.

Volkow, N.D. and McLellan, A.T. (2016) Opioid abuse in chronic pain: misconceptions and mitigation strategies. *New England Journal of Medicine* 374, 1253–1263.

Wang, Z., Whiteside, S.P.H., Sim, L., et al. (2017) Comparative effectiveness and safety of cognitive behavioral therapy and pharmacotherapy for childhood anxiety disorders: a systematic review and meta-analysis. *JAMA Pediatrics* 171(11), 1049–1056.

White, R. and Bradnam, V. (eds) (2015) *Handbook of Drug Administration via Enteral Feeding Tubes*, 3rd edn, pp. 169, 568–569. Pharmaceutical Press, London.

World Health Organization (2010) *Model Formulary for Children*. WHO, Geneva.

World Health Organization (2012) *Persisting Pain in Children: WHO Guidelines on the Pharmacological Treatment of Persisting Pain in Children with Medical Illnesses*. WHO, Geneva.

World Health Organization (2020) *Guidelines on the Management of Chronic Pain in Children*. WHO, Geneva.

Zempsky, W.T. (2008) Pharmacologic approaches for reducing venous access pain in children. *Pediatrics* 122(Suppl. 3), S140–S153.

6

Pain Assessment

Lindsay Jibb and Jennifer Stinson

Many health professionals are involved, either directly or indirectly, in assessing pain in children and young people (CYP). Health professionals have a key role in identifying CYP who are experiencing pain: appropriately assessing the pain and its impact on each CYP and their family, relieving pain using available resources, and evaluating the effectiveness of those actions. This chapter provides the theoretical knowledge required by health professionals to enable them to successfully assess pain in CYP.

Pain Measurement and Pain Assessment

Most pain assessment tools focus on *measuring* pain intensity. However, a wider and more holistic *assessment* provides information such as the location of pain, the frequency of pain, and how much pain impacts on well-being. In the context of assessment, seminal research (Melzack 1975) established the importance of recognising pain as a multidimensional experience comprising sensory, affective and evaluative components:

- Sensory: the quality (what pain feels like), intensity (how much pain hurts), location (spatial distribution of pain) and duration (how long pain lasts) of pain.
- Affective: the emotional impact of pain (e.g. the extent to which pain is perceived as unpleasant or distressing).
- Evaluative: the degree to which pain is perceived to interfere with physical (activity, sleep), psychological, role and social functioning.

Assessing Pain in Children and Young People

Pain assessment is the first step in the management of pain. To treat pain effectively, ongoing assessment of the presence and severity of pain and the CYP's response to treatment are essential. When assessing pain in CYP there are three key steps (Box 6.1).

Managing Pain in Children and Young People: A Clinical Guide, Third Edition. Edited by Alison Twycross, Jennifer Stinson, William T. Zempsky, and Abbie Jordan.

Parents and other significant family members know the CYP best and can recognise subtle changes in manner or behaviour. These individuals have a particularly important role in pain assessment and should be involved in all three steps.

Taking a Pain History

Conducting a thorough history of the CYP's prior pain experiences and current pain issue is the first step in pain assessment. Standardised pain history forms are available to structure conversations with CYP and parents about pain.

For CYP in (acute) nociceptive pain, the questions outlined in Table 6.1 generally provide the health professional with sufficient pain history information. For CYP with chronic pain, a more detailed pain history as outlined in Table 6.2 should be taken (see also Figure 6.1).

Assessing CYP's Pain Using a Developmentally Appropriate Pain Assessment Tool

The three approaches to measuring pain are:

- self-report (what CYP say)
- behavioural indicators (how CYP behave)
- physiological indicators (how the CYP's body reacts).

These three approaches may be used separately but have also been combined in several pain assessment tools available for use in practice.

Self-report tools should be used with CYP who are old enough to understand and use the scales and who are not overly distressed. Chronological age is the best predictor of whether a child is able

Table 6.1 Pain history for CYP with nociceptive pain.

Questions for children and young people	Questions for parents/carers
■ Can you tell me what pain is? ■ Can you tell me about the hurt you have had before? ■ Do you tell others when you hurt? If yes, who? ■ What do you want to do for yourself when you are hurting? ■ What do you want others to do for you when you are hurt? ■ What don't you want others to do for you when you hurt? ■ What helps the most to take your hurt away? ■ Is there anything special that you want me to know about when you hurt? (If yes, have CYP describe).	■ What word(s) does your CYP use in regard to pain? ■ Describe the pain experiences your CYP has had before. ■ Does your CYP tell you or others when they are hurting? ■ How do you know when your CYP is in pain? ■ How does your CYP generally react to pain? ■ What do you and your CYP do when they are hurting? ■ What works best to decrease or take away your CYP's pain? ■ Is there anything special that you would like me to know about your CYP and pain? (If yes, describe).

Source: Adapted from Hester et al. (1998).

Table 6.2 Pain history questions for CYP with chronic pain and their parents/carers.

Description of pain	**Type of pain**
	▪ *Is the pain nociceptive* (e.g. medical procedures, postoperative pain, accidental injury), *recurrent* (e.g. headaches) *or chronic* (e.g. juvenile idiopathic arthritis)?
	Onset of pain
	▪ *When did the pain begin? What were you doing before the pain began? Was there any initiating injury, trauma or stressors?*
	Duration
	▪ *How long has the pain been present?* (e.g. hours/days/ weeks/months)
	Frequency
	▪ *How often is pain present? How long does the pain last?*
	Location
	▪ *Where is the pain located? Can you point to the part of the body that hurts? Does the pain go anywhere else?* (Body outlines such as in Figure 6.1 can be used to help children over three to four years of age indicate where they hurt and pain radiation)
	Intensity
	▪ *What is your pain intensity at rest? What is your pain intensity with activity?* (Use a developmentally appropriate intensity assessment tool)
	▪ *Over the past week what is the least pain you have had? What is the worst pain you have had? What is your usual level of pain?*
	Unpleasantness
	▪ *How unpleasant/bothersome is the pain right now?* (Use a developmentally appropriate unpleasantness assessment tool)
	▪ *Over the past week what is the least unpleasant/bothersome your pain has been? What is most unpleasant/bothersome your pain has been? How unpleasant/bothersome is it generally?*
	Quality of pain
	▪ *Describe the quality of your pain* (e.g. word descriptors such as sharp, dull, achy, stabbing, burning, shooting or throbbing). School-age children can communicate about pain in more abstract terms. Word descriptors can provide information on whether the pain is nociceptive or neuropathic in nature or a combination of both
Associated symptoms	▪ *Are there any other symptoms that go along with or occur just before or immediately after the pain?* (e.g. nausea, vomiting, light-headedness, tiredness, diarrhoea or difficulty walking)
	▪ *Are there any changes in the colour or temperature of the affected extremity or painful area?* (These changes most often occur in CYP with conditions such as complex regional pain syndrome)
Temporal or seasonal variations	▪ *Is the pain affected by changes in seasons or weather?*
	▪ *Does the pain occur at certain times of the day?* (e.g. after eating or going to the toilet)

(Continued)

Table 6.2 (Continued)

Impact on daily living	▪ *Has the pain led to changes in daily activities and/or behaviours?* (e.g. sleep disturbances, change in appetite, physical activity, mood, social interactions or school attendance) ▪ *What level would the pain need to be so that you could do all your normal activities?* (i.e. tolerability) ▪ *What level would the pain need to be so that you won't be bothered by it?* (Rated on same developmentally appropriate scale as pain intensity)
Pain relief measures	▪ *What has helped to make the pain better?* ▪ *Have you taken medication to relieve your pain? If so, what was the medication and did it help? Were there any side effects?* ▪ It is important to also ask about the use of physical, psychological and complementary and alternative treatments, if tried, and how effective these methods are in relieving pain. The degree of pain relief (or change in pain intensity) after a pain-relieving treatment/intervention should be determined

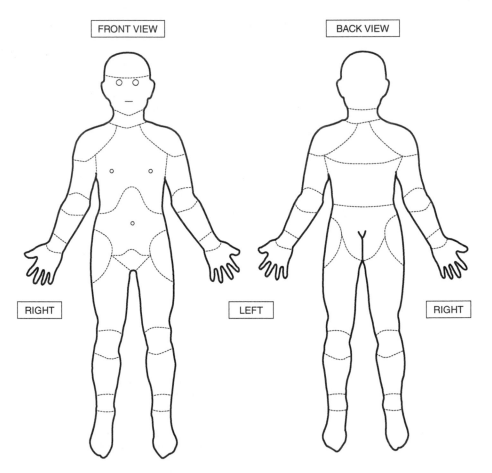

Figure 6.1 Body map from the Standardized Universal Pain Evaluation for Pediatric Rheumatology Providers (SUPER-KIDZ) tool.

Source: Reproduced with permission from Luca et al. (2017). © Journal of Orthopaedic and Sports Physical Therapy.

to accurately self-report pain (von Baeyer et al. 2011). Most CYP aged five to six years and older are able to self-report their current pain when provided with a developmentally appropriate tool (von Baeyer et al. 2017). With CYP who are sedated or have learning disabilities, behavioural pain assessment tools should be used (Beltramini et al. 2017). If CYP are overtly distressed (e.g. due to pain, anxiety or some other stressor), no meaningful self-report can be obtained at that time. Instead, pain should be estimated using a behavioural pain assessment tool until the CYP is less distressed (e.g. after the administration of analgesic drugs).

Self-report Tools

Verbal Rating Scales

- A verbal rating scale (VRS) consists of a list of simple word descriptors or phrases to indicate varying degrees or intensities of pain.
- One example of a VRS is using word descriptors of 'None' = 0, 'Very mild' = 1, 'Mild' = 2, 'Moderate' = 3, 'Severe' = 4, 'Very severe' = 5 (Miró et al. 2019).
- CYP are asked to select the word or phrase that best represents their level of pain intensity, and the score is the number associated with the chosen word.
- Interpretive caution is required in the use of these scales as VRS scores may reflect CYP's perceptions of other constructs in addition to pain intensity, including the ways pain interferes with a CYP's activities of daily living (Miró et al. 2019).

Graphic Rating Scales

- The most commonly used graphic rating scale is the Pieces of Hurt Tool (Hester 1979), also known as the Poker Chip Tool.
- This tool consists of four tokens (i.e. poker chips), with one token representing 'a little hurt' and four tokens representing 'the most hurt you could ever have', and was designed to be applicable to the cognitive abilities of a child around four years old.
- The Pieces of Hurt Tool has been studied in the context of hospital- and community-based CYP with nociceptive procedural pain and is easy to use and score. Instructions have been translated into several languages (Birnie et al. 2019).
- Limitations associated with its use include the need to clean the chips after each patient, the potential to lose chips, and evidence of insufficient measurement properties in younger children and CYP experiencing postoperative pain (Birnie et al. 2019).

Faces Pain Scales

- Faces pain scales present CYP with drawings or photographs of facial expressions representing different levels of pain intensity, in rank order. Examples of drawings include the Faces Pain Scale–Revised (Hicks et al. 2001; Figure 6.2) and the Wong-Baker FACES Pain Scale (Wong and Baker 1988); an example of photographs includes The Oucher (Beyer et al. 2009).
- CYP are asked to select the face that best represents their pain intensity, and their score is the number of the expression chosen.
- Faces scales have been validated for use in CYP aged 5–18 years across several ethnic and cultural groups (Birnie et al. 2019). No or only weak evidence indicates that children of three to four years of age can use faces scales in a reliable or valid way (von Baeyer et al. 2017).
- Smiling 'no pain' and crying 'most pain possible' anchor faces of the Wong-Baker FACES Pain Scale (viewable at www.wongbakerfaces.org) may confound ratings of pain with affect (Tomlinson et al. 2010). Faces pain scales with neutral expressions

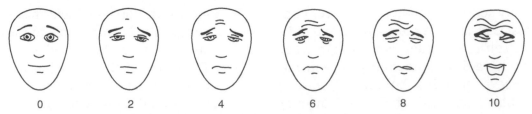

Figure 6.2 Faces Pain Scale–Revised.

Source: Reproduced with permission from Hicks et al. (2001) / Elsevier.

for 'no pain' (Figure 6.2) are therefore generally recommended.

- The more commonly used and well-validated faces pain scales are outlined in Table 6.3.

Numerical Pain Scales

- Numerical rating scales (NRS) comprise a range of numbers (e.g. 0–10 or 0–100) that can be represented in verbal or graphical format (Figure 6.3).
- CYP are told that the lowest number represents 'no pain' and the highest number represents a construct such as 'the most pain possible'. CYP are instructed to circle, record or state the number that best represents their pain intensity.
- Verbal NRS tend to be the most frequently used pain intensity tool with CYP over eight years of age in clinical practice because of the ease of implementation.
- NRS are strongly recommended for use in nociceptive pain and weak recommendations are made for its use in chronic pain (Birnie et al. 2019). However, it is not recommended for use in children aged six years and under.

Visual Analogue Scales

- Visual analogue scales (VAS) require CYP to select a point on a vertical or horizontal line to represent pain, where the ends of the line are defined as the extreme limits of pain intensity. The line is typically 100 mm in length and corresponds to a 0–10 or 0–100 scale.
- Strategies have been employed to improve reliability, validity and accessibility, including by using graphic or other methods to enhance CYP's understanding of the tool (e.g. Colour Analogue Scale; McGrath et al. 1996).
- VAS are supported by evidence of reliability, validity and responsiveness, and have received a weak recommendation for CYP aged six years and older with nociceptive and chronic pain (Birnie et al. 2019).
- While VAS are easy to reproduce, photocopying may alter the line length and VAS pain assessment also requires the extra step of measuring the line, which increases the burden and probability of errors in assessment.

Multidimensional Pain Tools

Although pain intensity is the most commonly assessed aspect of pain, a more comprehensive pain assessment is often necessary. Table 6.4 presents a sample of multidimensional self-report pain tools that have been shown to be reliable and valid.

Validated measures to assess the cognitive–affective impact of chronic pain (e.g. pain

Table 6.3 A sample of validated faces pain tools.

Tool	Characteristics	Considerations
Faces Pain Scale–Revised (FPS-R) (Hicks et al. 2001)	■ Six gender-neutral faces (Figure 6.2) ■ Faces range from *no pain* to *as much pain as possible* ■ Scored 0–10	■ Intended for use in CYP aged 5–12 years; used in CYP aged 3–18 years ■ Well-established evidence of reliability, validity and responsiveness (Birnie et al. 2019) ■ High clinical utility (quick and easy to use) ■ Translated into >35 languages ■ Disadvantages: limited evidence regarding inter-pretability of scores and mixed evidence about the acceptability of the scale to CYP
Oucher, photo-graphic scale (Beyer et al. 2009)	■ Composed of two scales presented together: a 0–10 point numerical rating scale presented alongside a six photograph scale ■ Available as Caucasian, African-American, Hispanic, Canadian First Nations, and Asian faces scales with instructions available in English, Chinese and Spanish ■ A numerical competency screening (i.e. counting to 100 by ones or tens, and identifying which of any two numbers is larger) or preference assessment may be used to determine which of the two scales to use ■ Scored 0–10	■ Intended for use in children aged 3–7 years; used in CYP aged 3–18 years ■ Evidence of reliability, validity and ability to detect change (Birnie et al. 2019). However, further test-ing in children aged 3–4 years needed (von Baeyer et al. 2017) ■ Moderate clinical utility ■ Mixed acceptability compared to other faces scales ■ Disadvantages: photos are not gender or ethnically neutral and are of CYP with nociceptive rather than chronic pain, limiting the clinical contexts in which it can be used
Wong-Baker FACES Pain Scale (Wong and Baker 1988)	■ Six hand-drawn faces ranging from smiling to cry-ing (viewable at www.wongbakerfaces.org) ■ Face 0, 'no hurt'; face 1, 'hurts a little bit'; face 2, 'hurts a little more'; face 3, 'hurts even more'; face 4, 'hurts a whole lot'; face 5, 'hurts worst' ■ Scored 0–5 or 0–10	■ Intended for use in those 3 years and over ■ Evidence of validity and responsiveness (Birnie et al. 2019) ■ High clinical utility (quick and simple to use) ■ High acceptability ■ Translated into more than 60 languages ■ Readily available (can be obtained free of charge) ■ Wearable water-resistant badges are available for purchase ■ Disadvantages: confounding of pain intensity with affect caused by use of smiling and crying anchor faces (Tomlinson et al. 2010)

No pain	0	1	2	3	4	5	6	7	8	9	10	Most pain

Figure 6.3 Numerical rating scale (NRS).

Table 6.4 A sample of validated multidimensional self-report pain tools.

Tool	Components	Considerations
Bath Adolescent Pain Questionnaire (BAPQ) (Eccleston et al. 2005)	▪ 61 items assessing the impact of pain on social and physical functioning, depression, anxiety, family functioning, and development	▪ Well-established evidence of validity and reliablity in 11–18 year olds with chronic pain ▪ Usable and feasible computerised version developed (BAPQ-C) (Jordan et al. 2020) ▪ Length of instrument decreases clinical utility ▪ Viewable at www.bath.ac.uk/publications/bath-adolescent-pain-questionnaire-bapq/
Pediatric Pain Questionnaire (PPQ) (Varni et al. 1987)	▪ Pain intensity measured using a 0–10 cm VAS anchored with happy and sad faces for present and worst pain ▪ Gender-neutral body outline to describe location of pain ▪ 46 word descriptors to assess the sensory, affective and evaluative qualities of pain	▪ Originally developed for CYP with chronic pain (e.g. arthritis) ▪ Intended for use in CYP 5–16 years; used in CYP 4–18 years ▪ Child, young person and parent versions ▪ Children younger than 7 years may need to be read the instructions to complete the VAS and body outline ▪ Well-established evidence of reliability and validity and some evidence of ability to detect change ▪ Minimal training and takes 10–15 minutes to complete

anxiety, pain catastrophising and fear of pain) in CYP include the Pain Catastrophizing Scale for Children (PCS-C), Fear of Pain Questionnaire for Children (FOPQ-C) and Child Pain Anxiety Symptoms Scale (CPASS-20) (Fisher et al. 2018). The Patient Reported Outcomes Measurement Information System (PROMIS®), a National Institutes of Health initiative to advance patient-reported outcome assessments, includes pain intensity, pain interference (self-report and parent proxy), pain behaviours (self-report and parent proxy) and pain quality tools. A complete and current list of instruments can be found at www.health-measures.net.

Digital Pain Assessment Tools

Pain diaries represent a means to track pain over time. While paper-based diaries have been used in clinical and research practice for decades, they are prone to recall biases and poor compliance (Jibb et al. 2020). Real-time data collection methods using electronic hand-held devices have been developed for self-report by CYP as young as eight years of age with recurrent and chronic pain (Fortier et al. 2016; Stinson et al. 2015). These measures can be more seamlessly integrated with electronic medical records and pain registries to improve understanding of CYP's pain over time (Lord et al. 2019). Pain-QuILT is an example of such a tool (Lalloo et al.

2014). Patients can choose from a library of pain quality 'icons' to express different types of pain, such as a matchstick for 'burning pain'. Descriptive icons can be assigned a rating of intensity (0–10 NRS) and then dragged-and-dropped onto a detailed virtual body map to show pain location (Figure 6.4). A free version of the tool is available at http://painquilt.com.

ADDITIONAL INFORMATION

For further information about self-report tools see Birnie, K.A., Hundert, A.S., Lalloo, C., et al. (2019) Recommendations for selection of self-report pain intensity measures in children and adolescents: a systematic review and quality assessment of measurement properties. *Pain* 160(1), 5–18.

Behavioural Tools

A wide range of specific expressive behaviours have been identified that are indicative of pain in neonates, infants and young children. Those particularly relevant to newborn infants are shown in Table 6.5.

Tools incorporating these behavioural reactions are indicated for CYP who are (von Baeyer et al. 2011):

- too young to understand and use self-report scales (e.g. less than five to six years old)
- too distressed to use self-report scales
- have learning disabilities
- have verbalisation challenges
- not restricted by bandages, surgical tape, mechanical ventilation or paralysing or sedating drugs

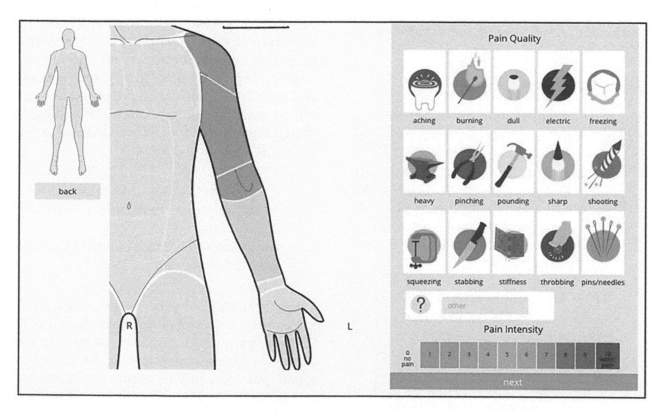

Figure 6.4 Screenshot of Pain-QuILT™.

Table 6.5 Behavioural reactions to pain in newborn infants.

Behavioural indicator	Effect from painful stimuli
Communication	Avoidance of eye contact, locking of gaze, or drifting away
Crying, vocalisations	Longer duration, changes in quality, fussiness, 'silent cry'
Facial expressions, grimacing	Presence and duration of, e.g., brow bulge, eye squeeze, nasolabial furrow, open lips, horizontal mouth stretch, vertical mouth stretch, purse lips, taut tongue and/or chin quiver
Limb movements	Presence and duration of avoiding or more indistinct limb movements, hand movements like fisting or finger spraying
Muscle tone	Increased or decreased
Sleep–wake state	Quality of sleep, hyper-alertness

Source: Reproduced with permission from Eriksson and Campbell-Yeo (2019) / Elsevier.

■ considered to have exaggerated, minimised or unrealistic self-report due to cognitive, emotional or situational factors.

A variety of behavioural pain tools have been developed and validated for use with infants and CYP (Table 6.6).

ADDITIONAL INFORMATION

For further information about behavioural tools that can be used with infants and CYP see:

■ Andersen, R.D., Langius-Eklof, A., Nakstad, B., et al. (2017) The measurement properties of pediatric observational pain scales: a systematic review of reviews. *International Journal of Nursing Studies* 73, 93–101.
■ Beltramini, A., Milojevic, K. and Pateron, D. (2017) Pain assessment in newborns, infants, and children. *Pediatric Annals* 46(10), e387–e395.
■ Giordano, V., Edobor, J., Deindl, P., et al. (2019) Pain and sedation scales for neonatal and pediatric patients in a preverbal stage of development: a systematic review. *JAMA Pediatrics* 173(12), 1186–1197.

Physiological Indicators

Neonates, infants and CYP display physiological and neurophysiological responses to pain, also called biomarkers (Eriksson and Campbell-Yeo 2019). These responses indicate the activation of the sympathetic nervous system, the part of the autonomic nervous system that is responsible for the *fight or flight* response associated with stress. Both an increase and decrease can be seen in many of these physiological changes and they should be recognised as (von Baeyer and Spagrud 2007):

■ generally reflecting stress reactions
■ being only loosely correlated with self-report of pain
■ occurring in response to other states, e.g. exertion, fever and anxiety.

On their own, physiological indicators do not constitute a valid clinical pain measure for CYP. A multidimensional or composite tool that incorporates physiological and behavioural indicators, as well as self-report, is therefore preferred whenever possible (Eriksson and Campbell-Yeo 2019). Physiological parameters that can indicate a CYP is in pain are outlined in Table 6.7. Other physiological indicators of

Table 6.6 A sample of validated behavioural tools.

Tool	Indicators	Considerations
COMFORT Scale (Ambuel et al. 1992); COMFORT-Behavioral Scale (van Dijk et al. 2000); COMFORTneo Scale (van Dijk et al. 2009)	■ Alertness, calmness or agitation, respiratory response, blood pressure, heart rate, muscle tone, physical movement, facial tension ■ Modified to the COMFORT-Behavioural (COMFORT-B) for non-ventilated infants through removal of non-responsive items and addition of crying (van Dijk et al. 2000; Boerlage et al. 2015) ■ COMFORTneo scale validated for use in preterm and term infants and for sedated infants (van Dijk et al. 2009)	■ Original COMFORT scale intended for use in CYP aged 0–17 years; used in CYP aged 0–18 years on ventilator or in critical care ■ Used to rate sedation and pain related to heart surgery, repositioning and mechanical ventilation (Andersen et al. 2017) ■ COMFORT and COMFORT-B have well-established evidence of validity and reliability but inconsistent responsiveness (Andersen et al. 2017) ■ Administration time is about 3 minutes ■ Two hours training needed to use tool
Revised FLACC (r-FLACC) (Malviya et al. 2006)	■ Facial expression, leg movement, activity, cry and consolability	■ Intended for use in children aged 2 months to 8 years; used in CYP aged 0–18 years and those aged 4–21 years with learning disabilities (Malviya et al. 2006) ■ Validated for procedural and postoperative pain (Crellin et al. 2018) ■ Indicators are scored on a 0–2 scale, with a total score from 0 to 10 ■ Evidence of validity and reliability (von Baeyer and Spagrud 2007) ■ High clinical utility due to simplicity of use (Voepel-Lewis et al. 2008) ■ Consolability requires (i) an attempt to console and (ii) a subjective rating of response to that intervention

Table 6.7 Physiological reactions to pain.

Observation	Effect from painful stimuli
Heart rate	Increase or decrease
Respiratory rate	Increase or decrease, apnoea
Blood pressure	Increase or decrease
Oxygen saturation	Decrease
Skin colour	Increase (red) or decrease (pale)

Source: Reproduced with permission from Eriksson and Campbell-Yeo (2019) / Elsevier.

pain include sweating and dilated pupils. Neurophysiological indicators include heart rate variability, skin conductance, cerebral oxygenation, electroencephalography (EEG), intracranial pressure and stress hormone concentrations. However, the measurement of these requires laboratory or technical analyses, making them less useful for clinical practice (Eriksson and Campbell-Yeo 2019).

An emerging area in the field of physiological marker assessment relates to wearable sensor-enabled technologies capable of continuous biometric tracking (e.g. heart rate, respiratory rate, distance walked, sleep) (Davoudi et al. 2020). These devices can provide high-quality health and fitness data to CYP, families and health professionals. Though not clinically well explored in the context of CYP's pain, data gathered by these devices may be useful in providing longitudinal physiological pain assessment data and information on pain's impact on activities of daily living.

Pain Assessment Tools for Neonates

Several pain assessment tools combine behavioural and physiological indicators as well as contextual factors (e.g. gestational age, sleep–wake state) for assessing pain in neonates (Table 6.8). Facial activity is the most comprehensively studied behavioural pain assessment indicator in neonates. The

Table 6.8 A sample of validated multidimensional pain assessment tools for neonates.

Tool	Indicators	Considerations
Neonatal Infant Pain Scale (NIPS) (Lawrence et al. 1993)	Facial expression, cry, breathing patterns, arms, legs, state of arousal	▪ Procedural pain in preterm and term neonates ▪ Indicators are scored on a two-point (0, 1) or three-point (0, 1, 2) scale at 1-minute intervals, before, during and after a procedure ▪ Evidence of validity and reliability (Duhn and Medves 2004) ▪ Cannot be used in intubated or paralysed neonates
Neonatal Pain, Agitation and Sedation Scale (N-PASS) (Hummel et al. 2008)	Cry/irritability, behaviour/state, facial expression, extremities/tone, heart rate, respiratory rate, blood pressure, and/or oxygen saturation	▪ Preterm and term infants ▪ Pain subscale validated for nociceptive (Hummel et al. 2008) and prolonged pain; sedation subscale can reliably detect oversedation, but not adequate sedation and undersedation (Giordano et al. 2019) ▪ Scored by assigning a value of 0, 1 or 2 for pain/agitation and 0, −1 or −2 for sedation for each indicator, total score obtained by adding the scores for each criterion
Premature Infant Pain Profile (PIPP) (Stevens et al. 1996); PIPP-R (Stevens et al. 2014)	▪ Gestational age, behavioural state, heart rate and oxygen saturation, brow bulge, eye squeeze and nasolabial furrow ▪ PIPP-R includes changes to physical layout, detailed instructions for use, and clarification of scoring of indicators for behaviours in preterm and term infants	▪ Procedural pain in preterm and term neonates ▪ Includes contextual indicators (e.g. gestation and behavioural state) ▪ Indicators are scored on a four-point scale (0, 1, 2, 3) for a total score of 0–21 based on the gestation of the neonate ▪ Score of 6 or less generally indicates minimal or no pain, while scores greater than 12 indicate moderate to severe pain ▪ PIPP has evidence of validity, reliability and responsiveness ▪ Pain assessments take 1 minute ▪ PIPP-R has evidence of validity and reliability, and is considered feasible by clinicians

---

BOX 6.2   FACIAL ACTIONS ASSOCIATED WITH PAIN IN NEONATES

- Bulging brow
- Eyes squeezed tightly shut
- Deepening of nasolabial furrow
- Open lips
- Mouth stretched vertically and horizontally
- Taut tongue

Source: Craig (1998)

---

facial actions associated with nociceptive pain in neonates are identified in Box 6.2.

Pain Assessment in Ventilated CYP

Health professionals may find it challenging to assess pain in ventilated infants and CYP because they:

- are intubated
- are generally sedated (with or without pharmacological paralysis)
- may also exhibit distress, anxiety, iatrogenic withdrawal syndrome and delirium, which can be difficult to differentiate from pain
- may have neurological impairment due to trauma, health condition or medications.

In 2016, the European Society of Paediatric and Neonatal Intensive Care (ESPNIC) recommended the use of the well-established and validated COMFORT-B and FLACC scales (for infants and CYP) and the PIPP-R (for neonates) to assess pain in critically ill CYP (Harris et al. 2016).

Pain Assessment in CYP with Learning Disabilities

Emerging evidence suggests that CYP with learning disabilities are equally or more sensitive to pain compared with their typically developing peers (Barney et al. 2020). Infants and CYP with learning disabilities, including those with moderate or severe cerebral palsy, neurodevelopmental disorders, severe developmental delay and autism spectrum disorders, and who are unable to report pain, may be at greater risk for the undertreatment of pain (Box 6.3).

Individualised considerations for this population may provide more meaningful pain assessment and ultimately lead to better pain management (Ely et al. 2016). Although CYP with learning disabilities may have the capacities to provide basic forms of self-report, self-report is best used in conjunction with other methods of assessing their pain (Schiariti and Oberlander 2018). Credible assessment can be obtained from the parent or another person who knows the infant or CYP well (Barney et al. 2020).

BOX 6.3   REASONS FOR INCREASED RISK OF UNDERTREATMENT OF PAIN IN CYP WITH LD

- Multiple medical issues and associated procedures may cause or be a source of pain.
- Idiosyncratic behaviours, such as moaning or laughing, may mask expression of pain or confuse observers.
- Many pain behaviours, such as changes in facial expression and patterns of sleep or play, are already inconsistent and difficult to interpret.

Factors to consider in assessment of pain in CYP with learning disabilities include the following:

- The underlying neurological condition/process (e.g. impact on neurological or musculoskeletal system, progressive or stable, and how this might influence the pain system).
- Developmental level (e.g. cognition, communication, motor function).
- Usual behaviours and health (e.g. baseline condition, pain experiences and everyday function).
- Usual means of communication (e.g. verbal, non-verbal, pain behaviours).
- Caregivers' views and understanding of what is happening.

Behavioural cues used to identify pain in CYP with learning disabilities include (Siden and Oberlander 2008):

- facial expression
- vocalisations (e.g. crying, screaming, moaning)
- movements (both increased and decreased);
- change in muscle tone (increased and decreased)
- guarding/protecting
- change in everyday activities (social interactions, eating and sleeping).

While there are several pain assessment tools for this population, three tools have been found reliable and are well validated.

- Non-Communicating Children's Pain Checklist–Revised (NCCPC-R; Breau et al. 2002).
- Revised Faces, Legs, Activity, Cry, Consolability (r-FLACC; Malviya et al. 2006).
- Paediatric Pain Profile (PPP; Hunt et al. 2004, 2007) (viewable at www.pppprofile.org.uk/).

The NCCPC-R has been used to assess nociceptive, chronic and postoperative pain in CYP with learning disabilities. Postoperative pain has also been assessed with the r-FLACC, and the PPP has been used to assess persistent daily pain. Synthesised data from an evidence-based review, feedback from a family-based hospital advisory board, and a quality improvement study with nurses and parents caring for CYP with learning disabilities have supported the clinical utility of the r-FLACC over the PPP in practice (Chen-Lim et al. 2012). In the absence of gold-standard pain measures, each CYP should be considered as their own control and behaviours and responses to interventions should be compared against previous assessments (Siden and Oberlander 2008).

Ruling Out Delirium, Withdrawal and Other Non-pain Pathologies when Assessing Pain

Untreated anxiety, depression, nausea, sleep disturbance, feeding intolerance, visceral hyperalgesia, fluid overload, constipation, seizure disorder, spasticity/contractures, reflux, medication withdrawal and delirium may significantly contribute to a CYP's pain experience. It is recommended that, along with pain assessment, hyperactive or hypoactive delirium be ruled out. This is particularly important in the case of neonates, infants and CYP under critical care in intensive care units who are receiving opioids, benzodiazepines and/or alpha-agonists. Setting sedation goals on these units (e.g. with the State Behavioral Scale) (Curley et al. 2006) may decrease the amount of analgesia and sedation administered and decrease the delirium risk. The Cornell Assessment of Pediatric Delirium is the only tool validated for non-verbal CYP (Traube et al. 2014). When decreasing doses of opioids, benzodiazepines and/or alpha-agonists, medication withdrawal must be ruled out using tools such as the Withdrawal Assessment Tool 1 (Franck et al. 2008) or producing a modified Finnegan score for infants (Gomez-Pomar and Finnegan 2018).

ADDITIONAL INFORMATION

Additional material, including tools and videos of CYP with and without delirium, can be found at www.icudelirium.org.

Choosing the Right Pain Assessment Tool

There are numerous valid, reliable and clinically useful neonatal, infant and CYP pain assessment tools. However, no easily administered, widely accepted, uniform technique exists for assessing pain in all CYP. Box 6.4 identifies some of the factors to be considered when selecting a pain tool for use in everyday practice.

BOX 6.4   CHOOSING A PAIN ASSESSMENT TOOL FOR EVERYDAY USE

The tool needs to be:

- *valid* (i.e. unequivocally measures a specific dimension of pain)
- *reliable* (i.e. consistent and trustworthy ratings regardless of time, setting or who is administering the tool)
- *responsive* (i.e. able to detect change in pain due to treatment)
- *feasible* to use (i.e. simple to use and not long, short training time, easy to administer and score).

The tool should also be:

- developmentally and culturally appropriate

- easily understood by patients
- well liked by patients, clinicians and researchers
- inexpensive and easy to obtain, reproduce, distribute and disinfect
- available in various languages or easily translatable.

The key points to consider when choosing a pain assessment tool for an individual CYP are outlined in Box 6.5. An example of an algorithm for assessing pain in hospitalised CYP can be seen in Figure 6.5 (Palozzi et al. 2018).

BOX 6.5   KEY POINTS TO CONSIDER WHEN CHOOSING A PAIN ASSESSMENT TOOL FOR AN INDIVIDUAL CHILD OR YOUNG PERSON

- The CYP's age, ethnic background, clinical status and cognitive/developmental level will all impact on the selection of the appropriate tool.
- Careful explanation and appropriate timing of administration are necessary.
- Rehearsal using a tool may be helpful for CYP to understand the task expected of them. Hypothetical painful situations may be used.

ADDITIONAL INFORMATION

- Within the hospital setting it will generally be necessary to have more than one pain assessment tool to cater for all patient groups.
- Each pain assessment tool should, whenever possible, use a common metric (e.g. all rate pain from 0 to 10).
- This means that a pain score of 5 will mean the same whichever pain assessment tool is used and will therefore aid effective communication about CYP's pain.

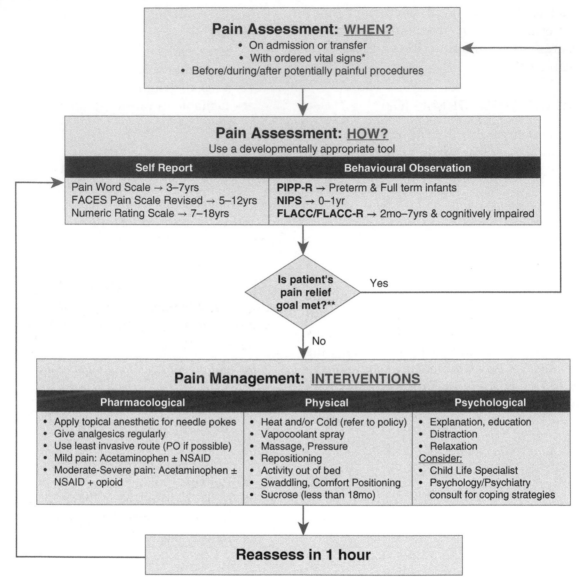

Figure 6.5 Example of an algorithm for assessing pain in hospitalised children and young people. Note that acetaminophen = paracetamol; child life specialist = play therapist.

Source: Reproduced with permission from Palozzi et al. (2018) / The Hospital for Sick Children.

How Often Should Pain be Assessed?

Effective pain management depends on regular assessment of the presence and severity of pain and the patient's response to pain management interventions. Every patient should have their pain assessed:

- when they visit an emergency department or an ambulatory clinic
- on admission to hospital
- at least once per shift (while they are an inpatient)
- before, during and after an invasive procedure.

Pain should be assessed regularly after surgery and/or if the patient has a known painful medical condition. In these cases, pain should be assessed hourly for the first six hours. After this, if the pain is well controlled, it can be assessed less frequently (e.g. every four hours). If the pain is fluctuating, regular assessment should continue for 48–72 hours; after this the pain intensity will generally have peaked and be starting to subside. Chronic pain assessment may be more complex than nociceptive pain assessment and is also likely to benefit from longitudinal measurements (i.e. over a period of days to weeks).

Documentation

The documentation of pain assessment data allows effective treatment and communication among the healthcare team, patient and family. Standardised forms and electronic medical records (e.g. admission assessment forms, vital signs charts) for documentation encourage initial assessment, ongoing reassessments, and enhance the efficacy of pain-relieving interventions. Including pain intensity ratings on the vital signs record reminds staff to consider pain as seriously as the other vital signs they measure.

Summary

- Pain assessment is vital for effective pain management.
- Recording a pain history, assessing a CYP's pain using an appropriate pain assessment tool, and evaluating the effectiveness of the pain-relieving interventions used are all steps to high-quality pain assessment.
- Valid and reliable pain assessment tools are available for CYP of all ages.
- The CYP's self-report of pain is important and should be sought whenever possible.
- Physiological, behavioural and self-report indicators can all be used to assess CYP pain.
- CYP who are non-verbal or who have learning disabilities are vulnerable to having their pain underestimated.
- Pain should be assessed regularly to detect the presence of pain and to evaluate the effectiveness of treatments.
- Documentation of pain facilitates regular reassessment of pain and follow-up.

Acknowledgements

We would like to kindly thank Dr Stefan Friedrichsdorf for his important contribution related to ruling out delirium, withdrawal and other non-pain pathologies when assessing CYP's pain.

Multiple Choice Questions

1. What is the best predictor of whether a child will be able to accurately self-report pain?
   a. Previous familiarity with pain reporting
   b. Relationship with the nurse assessing pain
   c. Chronological age
   d. Literacy level

2. Which of the following is *not* considered a behavioural reaction to pain in newborn infants?
   a. Grimacing
   b. Nausea/vomiting
   c. Finger splaying
   d. Fussiness

3. Which of the following is a graphic rating scale?
   a. Verbal Rating Scale
   b. Wong-Baker Scale
   c. Faces Pain Scale–Revised
   d. Pieces of Hurt Tool

4. Which of the following is *not* an established physiological reaction to pain in young children?
   a. Bradycardia
   b. Increased respiratory rate
   c. Increased oxygen saturation
   d. Increased heart rate

5. Which of the following is *not* a primarily important parameter to consider when choosing a pain assessment tool to use with a child or young person?
   a. The validity, reliability and responsiveness of the tool
   b. The age of the child or young person
   c. The amount of nurse-time a tool will require to administer
   d. The child or young person's sedation status

References

Ambuel, B., Hamlett, K.W., Marx, C.M. and Blumer, J.L. (1992) Assessing distress in pediatric intensive care environments: the COMFORT scale. *Journal of Pediatric Psychology* 17, 95–109.

Andersen, R.D., Langius-Eklof, A., Nakstad, B., Bernklev, T. and Jylli, L. (2017) The measurement properties of pediatric observational pain scales: a systematic review of reviews. *International Journal of Nursing Studies* 73, 93–101.

Barney, C.C., Andersen, R.D., Defrin, R., Genik, L.M., McGuire, B.E. and Symons, F.J. (2020). Challenges in pain assessment and management among individuals with intellectual and developmental disabilities. *Pain Reports* 5(4), e821.

Beltramini, A., Milojevic, K. and Pateron, D. (2017) Pain assessment in newborns, infants, and children. *Pediatric Annals* 46(10), e387–e395.

Beyer, J.E., Villarruel, A.M. and Denyes, M.F. (2009) The Oucher: a user's manual and technical report. www.oucher.org (accessed 5 May 2022).

Birnie, K.A., Hundert, A.S., Lalloo, C., Nguyen, C. and Stinson, J.N. (2019) Recommendations for selection of self-report pain intensity measures in children and adolescents: a systematic review and quality assessment of measurement properties. *Pain* 160(1), 5–18.

Boerlage, A.A., Ista, E., Duivenvoorden, H.J., de Wildt, S.N., Tibboel, D. and van Dijk, M. (2015) The COMFORT behaviour scale detects clinically meaningful effects of analgesic and sedative treatment. *European Journal of Pain* 19(4), 473–479.

Breau, L.M., McGrath, P.J., Camfield, C.S. and Finley, G.A. (2002) Psychometric properties of the non-communicating children's pain checklist-revised. *Pain* 99(1–2), 349–357.

Chen-Lim, M.L., Zarnowsky, C., Green, R., Shaffer, S., Holtzer, B. and Ely, E. (2012) Optimizing the assessment of pain in children who are cognitively impaired through the quality improvement process. *Journal of Pediatric Nursing* 27(6), 750–759.

Craig, K.D. (1998) The facial display of pain in infants and children. In *Measurement of Pain in Infants and Children* (eds G.A. Finley and P.A. McGrath), pp. 103–121. IASP Press, Seattle, WA.

Crellin, D.J., Harrison, D., Santamaria, N., Huque, H. and Babl, F.E. (2018) The psychometric properties of the FLACC Scale used to assess procedural pain. *Pain* 19(8), 862–872.

Curley, M.A.Q., Harris, S.K., Fraser, K.A., Johnson, R.A. and Arnold, J.H. (2006) State Behavioural Scale: a sedation assessment instrument for infants and young children supported on mechanical ventilation. *Pediatric Critical Care Medicine* 7, 107–114.

Davoudi, M., Skokouhyan, S.M., Abedi, M., et al. (2020) A practical sensor-based methodology for the quanititative assessment and classification of chronic non specific low back patients (NSLBP) in clinical settings. *Sensors* 20(10), 2902.

Duhn, L.J. and Medves, J.M. (2004) A systematic integrative review of infant pain assessment tools. *Advances in Neonatal Care* 4(3), 126–140.

Eccleston, C., Jordan, A., McCracken, L.M., Sleed, M., Connell, H. and Clinch, J. (2005) The Bath Adolescent Pain Questionnaire (BAPQ): development and preliminary psychometric evaluation of an instrument to assess the impact of chronic pain on adolescents. *Pain* 118(1–2), 263–270.

Ely, E., Chen-Lim, M.L., Carpenter, K.M., Wallhauser, E. and Friedlaender, E. (2016) Pain assessment of chidren with autism spectrum disorders. *Journal of Developmental and Behavioral Pediatrics* 37(1), 53–61.

Eriksson, M. and Campbell-Yeo, M. (2019) Assessment of pain in newborn infants. *Seminars in Fetal and Neonatal Medicine* 24(4), 101003.

Fisher, E., Heathcote, L.C., Eccleston, C., Simons, L.E. and Palermo, T.M. (2018) Assessment of pain anxiety, pain catastrophizing, and fear of pain in children and adolescents with chronic pain: a systematic review and meta-analysis. *Journal of Pediatric Psychology* 43(3), 3140325.

Fortier, M.A., Chung, W.W., Martinez, A., Gago-Masague, S. and Sender, L. (2016) Pain buddy: a novel use of m-health in the management of children's cancer pain. *Computers in Biology and Medicine* 76, 202–214.

Franck, L.S., Harris, S.K., Soetenga, D.J., Amling, J.K. and Curley, M.A.Q. (2008) The Withdrawal Assessment Tool-1 (WAT-1): an assessment instrument for monitoring opiod and benzodiazepine withdrawal symptoms in pediatric patients. *Pediatric Critical Care Medicine* 9, 573–580.

Giordano, V., Edobor, J., Deindl, P., et al. (2019) Pain and sedation scales for neonatal and pediatric patients in a preverbal stage of development: a systematic review. *JAMA Pediatrics* 173(12), 1186–1197.

Gomez-Pomar, E. and Finnegan, L.P. (2018) The epidemic of neonatal abstinence syndrome, historical references of its' origins, assessment and management. *Frontiers in Pediatrics* 6, 33.

Harris, J., Ramelet, A.S., van Dijk, M., et al. (2016) Clinical recommendations for pain, sedation, withdrawal and delirium assessment in critically ill infants and children: an ESPNIC position statement for healthcare professionals. *Intensive Care Medicine* 42(6), 972–986.

Hester, N.K. (1979) The preoperational child's reaction to immunization. *Nursing Research* 28(4), 250–255.

Hester, N., Foster, R., Jordan-Marsh, M. et al. (1998) Putting pain measurement into clinical practice. In *Measurement of Pain in Infants and Children* (eds G.A. Finley and P.A. McGrath), pp. 179–198. IASP Press, Seattle, WA.

Hicks, C.L., von Baeyer, C.L., Spafford, P.A., van Korlaar, I. and Goodenough, B. (2001) The Faces Pain Scale–Revised: toward a common metric in pediatric pain measurement. *Pain* 93(2), 173–183.

Hummel, P., Puchalski, M., Creech, S. and Weiss, M.G. (2008) Clinical reliability and validity of the N-PASS: neonatal pain, agitation and sedation scale with prolonged pain. *Joural of Perinatology* 28(1), 55–60.

Hunt, A., Goldman, A., Seers, K., et al. (2004) Clinical validation of the paediatric pain profile. *Developmental Medicine and Child Neurology* 46(1), 9–18.

Hunt, A., Wisbeach, A., Seers, K., et al. (2007) Development of the paediatric pain profile: role of video analysis and saliva cortisol in validating a tool to assess pain in children with severe neurological disability. *Journal of Pain and Symptom Management* 33(3), 276–289.

Jibb, L.A., Khan, J.S., Seth, P., et al. (2020) Electronic data capture versus conventional data collection methods in clinical pain studies: systematic review and meta-analysis. *Journal of Medical Internet Research* 22(6), e16480.

Jordan, A., Begen, F.M., Austin, L., Edwards, R.T. and Connell, H. (2020) A usability and feasibility study of a computerized version of the Bath Adolescent Pain Questionnaire: the BAPQC. *BMC Pediatrics* 20(1), 6.

Lalloo, C., Stinson, J.N., Brown, S.C., Campbell, F., Isaac, L. and Henry, J.L. (2014) Pain-QuILT: assessing clinical feasibility of a Web-based tool for the visual self-repot of pain in an interdisciplinary pediatric chronic pain clinic. *Clinical Journal of Pain* 30(11), 934–943.

Lawrence, J., Alcock, D., McGrath, P., Kay, J., MacMurray, S.B. and Dulberg, C. (1993) The development of a tool to assess neonatal pain. *Neonatal Network* 12(6), 59–66.

Lord, S.M., Tardif, H.P., Kepreotes, E.A., Blanchard, M. and Eagar, K. (2019) The Paediatric electronic Persistent Pain Outcomes Collaboration (PaedePPOC): establishment of a binational system for benchmarking children's persistent pain services. *Pain* 160(7), 1572–1585.

Luca, N.J., Stinson, J.N., Feldman, B.M., et al. (2017) Validation of the Standardized Universal Pain Evaluations for Rheumatology Providers for Children and Youth (SUPER-KIDZ). *Journal of Orthopaedic and Sports Physical Therapy* 47, 731–740.

McGrath, P.A., Seifert, C.E., Speechley, K.N., Booth, J.C., Stitt, L. and Gibson, M.C. (1996) A new analogue scale for assessing children's pain: an initial validation study. *Pain* 64(3), 435–443.

Malviya, S., Voepel-Lewis, T., Burke, C., Merkel, S. and Tait, A.R. (2006) The revised FLACC observational pain tool: improved reliability and validity for pain assessment in children with cognitive impairment. *Paediatric Anaesthesia* 16(3), 258–265.

Melzack, R. (1975) The McGill Pain Questionnaire: major properties and scoring methods. *Pain* 1(3), 277–299.

Miró, J., de la Vega, R., Gertz, K.J., Thong, I.S.K., Jensen, M.P. and Engel, J.M. (2019) Do commonly used measures of pain intensity only reflect pain intensity in youths with bothersome pain and a physical disability? *Frontiers in Pediatrics* 7, 229.

Palozzi, L., Campbell, F. and Hurdowar, A. (2018) Pain Management Clinical Practice Guideline, Policies and Procedures Database. Hospital for Sick Children, Toronto, Canada.

Schiariti, V. and Oberlander, T. (2018) Evaluating pain in cerebral palsy: comparing assessment tools using the International Classification of Functioning, Disability and Health. *Disability and Rehabilitation* 41(22), 2622–2629.

Siden, H. and Oberlander, T. (2008) Pain management for children with a developmental disability in a primary care setting. In *Pain in Children: A Practical Guide for Primary Care* (eds K.R. Goldschneider and G.A. Walco), pp. 29–37. Humana Press, New York.

Stevens, B., Johnston, C., Petryshen, P. and Taddio, A. (1996) Premature Infant Pain Profile: development and initial validation. *Clinical Journal of Pain* 12, 13–22.

Stevens, B.J., Gibbins, S., Yamada, J., et al. (2014) The premature infant pain profile-revised (PIPP-r): initial validation and feasibility. *Clinical Journal of Pain* 30(3), 238–243.

Stinson, J.N., Jibb, L.A., Nguyen, C., et al. (2015) Construct validity and reliability of a real-time multidimensional smartphone app to assess pain in children and adolescents with cancer. *Pain* 156(12), 2607–2615.

Tomlinson, D., von Baeyer, C.L., Stinson, J.N. and Sung, L. (2010) A systematic review of faces scales for the self-report of pain intensity in children. *Pediatrics* 26(5), 1168–1198.

Traube, C., Silver, G., Kearney, J., et al. (2014) Cornell Assessment of Pediatric Delirium: a valid, rapid, observational tool for screening delirium in the PICU. *Criticial Care Medicine* 42, 656–663.

van Dijk, N., de Boer, J.B., Koot, H.M., Tibboel, D., Passchier, J. and Duivenvoorden, H.J. (2000) The reliability and validity of the COMFORT scale as a postoperative pain instrument in 0 to 3-year-old infants. *Pain* 84, 367–377.

van Dijk, M., Roofhooft, D.W., Anand, K.J. et al. (2009) Taking up the challenge of measuring prolonged pain in (premature) neonates: the COMFORT neo scale seems promising. *Clinical Journal of Pain* 25(7), 607–616.

Varni, J.W., Thompson, K.L. and Hanson, V. (1987) The Varni/Thompson Pediatric Pain Questionnaire: I. Chronic musculoskeletal pain in juvenile rheumatoid arthritis. *Pain* 28, 27–38.

Voepel-Lewis, T., Malviya, S., Tait, A.R., et al. (2008) A comparison of the clinical utility of pain assessment tools for children with cognitive impairment. *Anesthesia and Analgesia* 106(1), 72–78.

von Baeyer, C.L. and Spagrud, L.J. (2007) Systematic review of observational (behavioral) measures for children and adolescents aged 3 to 18 years. *Pain* 127, 140–150.

von Baeyer, C.L., Uman, L.S., Chambers, C.T. and Gouthro, A. (2011) Can we screen young children for their ability to provide accurate self-reports of pain? *Pain* 152, 1327–1333.

von Baeyer, C.L., Jaaniste, T., Vo, H.L.T., Brunsdon, G., Lao, H.-C. and Champion, G.D. (2017) Systematic review of self-report measures of pain intensity in 3- and 4-year-old children: bridging a period of rapid cognitive development. *Journal of Pain* 18(9), 1017–1026.

Wong, D.L. and Baker, C.M. (1988) Pain in children: comparison of assessment scales. *Pediatric Nursing* 14(1), 9–17.

7 Preventing and Treating Nociceptive Pain

Sueann Penrose and Cate Sinclair

This chapter reviews the causes of nociceptive (acute) pain in children and young people (CYP). Strategies for managing nociceptive pain in hospital and community settings are provided, including a summary of the most appropriate pain assessment tools in this context. The use of analgesic drugs to manage nociceptive pain is outlined, along with the management of specialist analgesic modalities. We also discuss the evidence supporting the use of physical and psychological pain-relieving interventions in nociceptive pain.

What is Nociceptive Pain?

Nociceptive pain, often called acute pain, is short-lived, lasting days to weeks, and generally has a single obvious cause (e.g. tissue damage due to surgery or injury). Nociceptive pain may not be proportionate to the severity of tissue damage. Nociceptive pain is expected to resolve as healing takes place (Franziska and McMahon 2017). Pain lasting over three months is classified as chronic (Schug et al. 2020). Further information about the anatomy and physiology of pain can be found in Chapter 3.

Causes of Nociceptive Pain in Children and Young People

Injury, childhood illnesses and medical conditions, painful procedures and surgery all cause nociceptive pain in CYP (Table 7.1).

Surgical Stress Response

Nociceptive pain induces effects ranging from tissue injury and inflammation to activation of the metabolic, immune and hormone systems. These cause a stress response involving changes in systemic blood flow, blood pressure, heart rate and pulmonary function, leading to complications and negative health outcomes. The magnitude is related to the size and site of injury (enhanced in abdominal and thoracic regions). Different analgesic modalities have varied effects both on pain relief and in reducing the body's stress response; simple analgesics are less effective than opioids, that are in turn less effective than regional anaesthetics (Roberts et al. 2020).

Rosenbloom et al. (2019) report that 20–50% of CYP may develop chronic postoperative pain after major surgery. In this study there

Managing Pain in Children and Young People: A Clinical Guide, Third Edition. Edited by Alison Twycross, Jennifer Stinson, William T. Zempsky, and Abbie Jordan.

Table 7.1 Causes of nociceptive pain in CYP.

Cause of pain	Description
Injury	▪ Unintentional injuries from falls, collisions, burns and cuts are among the most common causes of nociceptive pain and contribute to one-third of emergency department attendances (Arslan and Demir 2022) ▪ With school-aged CYP, injuries most commonly occur at school, during sport and through road traffic accidents (Dorney et al. 2020) ▪ Nociceptive pain from injury is primarily due to tissue damage and inflammation
Illnesses and disease	▪ Illnesses and diseases frequently cause nociceptive pain. Otitis media and pharyngitis are the most frequent diagnoses in CYP attending community-based health services (Glockler et al. 2018) ▪ Pain from tooth decay is prevalent in CYP of low socioeconomic backgrounds with limited access to dental care (Kumar and Joshi 2017) ▪ Nociceptive medical pain may include exacerbation of underlying disease, e.g. acute abdominal pain with Crohn's disease ▪ Medical conditions, e.g. arthritis, cancer, systemic lupus erythematosus, haemophilia, inflammatory bowel disease, sickle cell disease (SCD) and epidermolysis bullosa, have combined nociceptive and chronic pain components due to disease processes, treatment or medical investigations (Rabbitts et al. 2020; World Health Organization (WHO) 2020) ▪ SCD has a nociceptive pain component with vaso-occlusive episodes requiring hospitalisation (Mucalo et al. 2021). Associated nociceptive pain can cause considerable suffering, may be poorly recognised and undertreatment may be compounded by the negative attitudes and inadequate education of clinicians (Hurley-Wallace et al. 2018)
Significant impairment of the nervous system	▪ CYP with significant impairment of the central nervous system (CNS), including those diagnosed with learning disability (intellectual disability), cerebral palsy and autism spectrum disorder, experience nociceptive pain from multiple sources and chronic pain from their underlying condition (Hauer and Houtrow 2017) ▪ Due to cognitive and communication impairments, pain in CYP with significant impairment of the CNS is difficult to identify and often undertreated (Cascella et al. 2019; Carter 2020) ▪ Pain in CYP with significant impairment of the CNS is discussed in more detail in Chapter 14
Pain caused by medical procedures or treatments	▪ Procedural pain and anxiety can be caused by dressing changes, intravenous access, blood tests, injections, vaccinations, lumbar punctures, etc. ▪ The prevention and treatment of procedural pain is discussed in more detail in Chapter 12

was a link between preoperative functional disability, pain and pain-related psychosocial factors. It may therefore be beneficial to implement a preoperative plan to address these issues to reduce the risk of developing chronic postsurgical pain. (Further information about chronic postsurgical pain can be found in Chapter 11.)

A systematic review by Shinnick et al. (2016) showed enhanced recovery after surgery using pathways that aimed to return the patient to previous function as quickly as appropriate, thereby avoiding the complications of prolonged fasting, opioid use and immobility. A study implementing an enhanced recovery pathway for paediatric idiopathic scoliosis

(Temby et al. 2021) delivered improved outcome and decreased length of stay with an early return to normal function.

PRACTICE POINT

Poorly managed nociceptive pain after surgery, burns or injury may result in:

- increased morbidity
- slowed recovery time
- prolonged hospital admission
- delayed return to normal activities
- decreased patient and family satisfaction
- increased risk of chronic pain, including chronic postoperative pain.

The consequences of unrelieved pain are discussed further in Chapter 2.

Managing Nociceptive Pain

Aims of Pain Management

Pain is a biopsychosocial phenomenon (see Chapter 4) and therefore a multimodal approach should include pharmacological, physical and psychological strategies. According to Wright et al. (2021), the aims of managing nociceptive pain in CYP are to:

- rapidly identify pain
- prevent pain when possible
- administer analgesia according to age, weight, pain severity and underlying medical condition
- reassess pain
- reduce surgical stress response
- use multimodal analgesia along with psychological and physical support
- monitor to prevent adverse events
- address emotional components of pain
- continue pain control after discharge from hospital.

Best Practice Guidelines

Current best practice guidelines specific to nociceptive pain management are outlined in Box 7.1.

Pain Assessment

The first step in determining appropriate pain-relieving interventions is assessment of the pain considering the CYP's age, gender, nervous system development, illness, previous pain experiences and sociocultural experiences (Pope et al. 2017). All possible sources of pain and discomfort should be considered including haemorrhage or haematoma, compartment syndrome, urinary retention, bladder spasms, muscle spasms, vomiting, nausea and itching.

In relation to nociceptive pain, children as young as three to four years have the developmental capacity to identify pain cause, location, meaning and quality (Pope et al. 2017). Three

---

BOX 7.1   CURRENT BEST PRACTICE GUIDELINES FOR THE MANAGEMENT OF NOCICEPTIVE PAIN

- Australian and New Zealand College of Anaesthetists and Faculty of Pain Medicine Guidelines on the Management of Acute Pain (2020): https://www.anzca.edu.au/resources/college-publications/acute-pain-management/apmse5.pdf
- American Society of Hematology (2020) Treatment and pain management of sickle cell disease: https://doi.org/10.1182/bloodadvances.2020001851
- European Society for Paediatric Anaesthesiology (ESPA) (2018) Postoperative pain management in children: https://doi.org/10.1111/pan.13373

developmentally appropriate tools have been formulated for the assessment of nociceptive pain in CYP:

- Revised Face, Legs, Activity, Cry, Consolability (rFLACC) for children aged two months to seven years and non-verbal CYP (Malviya et al. 2006a).
- Faces Pain Scale Revised (FPS-r) for CYP who are verbal and aged over five years (Hicks et al. 2001).
- Numerical Rating Scale (NRS) for CYP who are numerate and verbal over the age of six years (Birnie et al. 2019).

Additional information about pain assessment can be found in Chapter 6.

CASE STUDY: PART 1

Jane is a 14 year old with a two-day history of pain in the right upper quadrant. She presents to the emergency department with increased abdominal pain and it is confirmed that she has a ruptured appendix. She does have a past medical history of recurrent abdominal pain secondary to chronic constipation.

Jane has experienced bullying at school with minimal empathy from her extended family. Recently she was referred to mental health specialists due to anxiety related to school.

She has been admitted for an urgent appendectomy. After reviewing the evidence-based approaches to pain assessment:

1. What questions would you ask Jane about her pain?
2. How would you assess her pain?
3. What impact might her anxiety have on her postoperative pain?
4. Why would it be important to know if Jane was taking analgesic drugs at home prior to surgery?

Pain Management in the Hospital Setting

Pain experienced in hospital can vary in intensity. An algorithm to support decision-making can be seen in Figure 7.1. Additional guidance is also available:

- The European Society for Paediatric Anaesthesiology has published a guidance document for the postoperative pain management of children (Vittinghoff et al. 2018).
- Guidance about prescribing opioid analgesic drugs in CYP can be found in Cravero et al. (2019) and Kelley-Quon et al. (2020).
- Australian and New Zealand College of Anaesthetists and Faculty of Pain Medicine Guidelines on the Management of Acute Pain, Section 10 (Palmer et al. 2020).

Pharmacological Pain-relieving Interventions

Multimodal pharmacology is the recommended approach for managing nociceptive pain in hospitalised CYP and helps to reduce the amount of analgesic drugs required (Friedrichsdorf and Goubert 2020). In relation to pharmacological interventions, the WHO analgesic ladder (Anekar et al. 2022), discussed in Chapter 1, offers a two-step strategy for treating pain, recommending that analgesic drugs are given according to pain severity.

Nociceptive pain is short-lived and, once controlled, a step-down rather than a step-up approach should be used, as the pain is expected to diminish. Analgesic drugs should be given regularly (i.e. scheduled) initially, then as needed (PRN) for comfort (Friedrichsdorf and Goubert 2020). If the pain does not lessen as expected, this may indicate complications or an alternative diagnosis.

Step 1: Assess pain

Using a developmentally appropriate pain assessment tool	Consider changes to CYP's behaviour	Ask CYP and parent/carer their opinion

Step 2: Treat pain

Give analgesia according to the WHO ladder taking severity of pain into account	Use physical pain-relieving interventions	Use psychological strategies

Step 3: Reassess pain

Reassess pain 20–30 minutes after the intervention

Step 4: Treat pain

If pain is no better, consider using another analgesic drug (as per the pain ladder)	Consider using other physical or psychological strategies

Step 5: Refer to specialist

Consider referral to an anaesthetist or pain service for advice about additional pain management

Figure 7.1 An algorithm outlining a five-step approach to nociceptive pain management in CYP.

Strategies for optimising the safely of analgesic drugs are discussed below. Following this, the different analgesic drugs are discussed alongside a summary of the research for their use in treating nociceptive pain. Strategies for managing opioid side effects are also outlined, as well as possible routes of administration. The use of specific analgesic delivery techniques is then discussed.

- allows for lower drug doses, thus minimising adverse effects
- allows analgesia to be individualised to the patient or patient group
- targets pain at different points of the pain pathway (see Chapter 3).

Source: Schug et al. (2020)

PRACTICE POINT

Multimodal pharmacology is the combination (by the same or different routes) of two or more analgesic drugs with different mechanisms of action to provide analgesia, which:

- improves pain scores and provides greater pain relief

Optimising the Safety of Analgesic Drugs

Safe administration of analgesic drugs requires education of all involved and careful attention to the organisational aspects in delivering pain relief (Schug et al. 2020). Some of the steps that can be taken are outlined in Box 7.2.

BOX 7.2   OPTIMISING THE SAFETY OF ANALGESIC DRUGS

- Appropriate patient selection considering medical condition, comorbidities, age, surgery/procedure, emotional state and concurrent medications.
- Staff adequately trained and supported, with sufficient staff numbers to safely monitor patients.
- Education about all aspects of analgesics to clinicians, CYP and families.
- Clear guidelines and expectation they will be followed.
- Risk minimisation: labelling, standard drug concentrations, smart pump technology, specific charts, double-checking of pump programming and prescriptions, documentation and appropriate patient monitoring.
- Avoiding co-administration of sedatives and opioids by different routes.
- Regular review of efficacy and adverse effects of analgesia.
- Reportable safety limits individualised to patient type or age groups.
- Emergency protocols to manage adverse events.
- Pain service or pain link nurses to guide/direct staff.
- Regular audit of pain management.

Source: Palmer et al. (2020)

PRACTICE POINT

If a patient on opioids is receiving other medication that can cause sedation (e.g. antihistamines, benzodiazepines or antiepileptics and some antiemetics), there is an increased risk of sedation and respiratory depression.

1. How would you support and prepare Jane for surgery?
2. How would her previous experience of pain affect her response to the surgical pain?
3. How does family reaction to a young person in pain influence pain behaviour?
4. What information and support would you give to her aunt?

CASE STUDY: PART 2

When adopting a multimodal approach to treating pain, it is important to consider the psychological aspects of pain management.

Jane is in the care of her aunt who is concerned about Jane's behaviour and anticipates that she will be in terrible pain after her surgery.

Non-opioids

Non-opioid analgesic drugs are important in nociceptive pain management and may be all that is required for mild pain. For moderate to severe pain, they are key components of multimodal analgesia and are opioid-sparing. Intravenous preparations of paracetamol (acetaminophen) and some non-steroidal anti-inflammatory drugs (NSAIDs) are now widely available and can be used intraoperatively when patients are nil by mouth or when rapid onset of analgesia is required.

Research evidence tells us that:

- combining paracetamol and NSAIDs can be opioid-sparing after myringotomy, minor orthopaedic surgery and multiple dental extractions (Gazal and Al Samadani 2017; Vittinghoff et al. 2018)
- perioperative NSAIDs decrease opioid requirements and postoperative nausea and vomiting (PONV) during the first 24 hours after surgery (Michelet et al. 2012)
- patients who receive perioperative intravenous propacetamol/paracetamol require less opioid immediately postoperatively (Rudikoff et al. 2022)
- low-dose ketamine used preoperatively for tonsillectomy and adenotonsillectomy decreases postoperative analgesic requirements (Persino et al. 2017)
- a ketamine infusion alongside opioids decreases opioid use and nausea and vomiting, and improves pain and patient satisfaction for CYP undergoing scoliosis surgery (Noah and Walters 2019).

Information about dosing for non-opioid analgesics can be found in Appendix 1.

Opioids

Opioids are safe and effective for CYP when titrated to effect and administered for the correct indication (Schug et al. 2020) and are the mainstay for treating severe vaso-occlusive pain in sickle cell disease (Brandow et al. 2020).

We also know that:

- intravenous opioids are an important component of multimodal analgesia for postoperative pain (Palmer et al 2020);

- intranasal fentanyl is equivalent to intravenous morphine for nociceptive pain in the paediatric emergency department setting and improves time to analgesia by up to 50% (Schoolman-Anderson et al. 2018);
- a systematic review of intranasal fentanyl in CYP in acute care showed that time to deliver analgesia was an important factor in managing pain effectively (Setlur and Friedland 2018).

Details of drug dosages can be found in Appendix 1.

Oral Opioids

Oral opioids are used for moderate to severe pain in conjunction with non-opioid analgesics. If the CYP can take medications by mouth, oral opioids may be given instead of parenteral opioids or after infusions have ceased. A small number of CYP require oral opioids for an extended time, e.g. when weaning off opioids or when experiencing continuing tissue injury (e.g. epidermolysis bullosa, osteogenesis imperfecta, metastatic bone cancer). Long-acting (sustained-release, SR) and short-acting (immediate-release, IR) opioids have been shown to be safe and effective after major surgery in CYP (Cravero et al. 2019). However, oral opioids should not be prescribed routinely for postoperative discharge (Farr et al. 2020).

CASE STUDY: PART 3

Jane has had surgery. She is to remain nil by mouth for the next 24–48 hours. She currently weighs 45 kg.

She has a patient-controlled analgesia (PCA) pump delivering morphine. The pump has been programmed for a delivery of 0.9 mg/hour continuous infusion plus 0.9 mg PCA bolus.

She reports her pain to be 4–7 out of 10. She has used 83 mg of morphine in the past 24 hours. Having reviewed the information on postoperative analgesia:

1. What adjuvant drugs would you prescribe?
2. Are there any side effects you would expect and what would you consider to prevent and/or treat these side effects?
3. How might you encourage Jane to participate in her pain management?

PRACTICE POINT

■ Opioids should be for short-term use (ideally days to weeks).
■ If the pain is extended (i.e. lasting over four to six weeks) the patient should be referred to a transitional pain service, pain specialist or chronic pain service for review (Glare et al. 2019).

Intranasal Opioids

Intranasal fentanyl provides safe and effective needle-free analgesia in a variety of clinical settings and is acceptable to CYP (Anderson et al. 2022).

Parenteral Opioids

Intramuscular injections are no longer considered appropriate for use with CYP: they are painful and less effective than other methods of opioid delivery (Schug et al. 2020). Subcutaneous or intravenous methods of administration are preferred.

Intravenous and Subcutaneous Opioids

Intravenous and subcutaneous routes of morphine dose are equally efficacious (Schug et al. 2020). A meta-analysis of paediatric postoperative PCA use showed that the addition of continuous (or background) infusion to the demand (or bolus) dose for intravenous PCA is associated with a higher incidence of respiratory events than PCA bolus alone (Gupta et al. 2018) (see below for more information on PCA).

Intermittent Opioid Boluses

Intermittent opioid boluses are used to manage short-term moderate to severe pain (e.g. fracture reduction or after minor surgery). They are helpful in achieving rapid pain control before starting an infusion or PCA (e.g. with postoperative pain) or as a rescue for severe pain exacerbation.

Continuous Opioid Infusions

Continuous opioid infusions are used for moderate to severe pain expected to last for more than 24 hours, where intermittent bolus dosing provides inadequate analgesia, and PCA or oral analgesia are not suitable. Continuous infusions allow for constant pain relief and decrease staff workload compared to intermittent opioid boluses (Schug et al. 2020).

Initial infusion rates vary according to age and weight and should be titrated to the CYP's response (Schug et al. 2020). Bolus doses may be prescribed for breakthrough pain.

Managing the Adverse Effects of Opioids

Opioids can cause several adverse effects (sedation, nausea, vomiting, urinary retention, pruritus and constipation), but it is important to consider *all* possible causes and not assume the opioid alone is responsible (Schug et al. 2020). Adverse effects are discussed in order of clinical significance.

Sedation/Respiratory Depression Assessing sedation is the key to early identification and treatment of opioid-induced respiratory depression. A lower dose of opioid is required to induce sedation rather than respiratory depression; monitoring of sedation provides effective early detection (Varga et al. 2022).

Sedation should be assessed using a validated sedation scale to ensure consistency between clinicians (Box 7.3). If required, an opioid antagonist (most commonly naloxone) should be administered. All patients receiving opioids should have standing orders (PRN prescriptions) for naloxone to minimise delays. Box 7.4 provides a protocol for managing opioid-induced respiratory depression.

BOX 7.3   UNIVERSITY OF MICHIGAN SEDATION SCALE (UMSS)

0 Awake and alert
1 Minimally sedated: may appear tired/sleepy, responds to verbal conversation and/or sound
2 Moderately sedated: somnolent/sleeping, easily aroused with light tactile stimulation or simple verbal command
3 Deep sedation: deep sleep, arousable only with deep or significant physical simulation
4 Unrousable
S Patient is sleeping

Source: Malviya et al. (2006b)

BOX 7.4   PROTOCOL TO MANAGE OPIOID-INDUCED RESPIRATORY DEPRESSION IN CYP

If opioid-induced respiratory depression is suspected:

- cease the opioid
- stimulate the patient (shake gently, call by name, ask to breathe)
- administer oxygen
- administer naloxone if indicated.

Indications for naloxone

- If patient is significantly sedated (UMSS 3): administer naloxone 2 µg/kg via IV push and repeat every 1–2 minutes as needed (maximum five doses).
- If patient cannot be roused and/or is apnoeic (UMSS 4):
    - Manage airway/resuscitate.
    - Administer naloxone 10 µg/kg via IV push and repeat every 1–2 minutes as needed (maximum five doses).
- Suggested dilution: 0.4 mg naloxone in 20 mL normal saline = 20 µg/mL.

Continue to monitor the patient closely. Naloxone has a shorter duration of action than most opioids, therefore repeated doses may be required. In some situations, a naloxone infusion will be necessary.

Other considerations when managing sedation include the following (Schug et al. 2020):

- If the child is receiving PCA and/or opioid infusion, consider reducing or ceasing the background infusion or reducing the bolus size.
- Optimise doses of non-opioid analgesics, including adjuvant analgesics.
- Check for other contributing factors (e.g. sedatives, dose error, hypoxia, sepsis, hypovolaemia, renal impairment or electrolyte imbalance).

It is important to use valid and reliable tools when assessing pain and sedation (Miller-Hoover 2019).

PRACTICE POINT

Respiratory depression from opioids is caused by:

- decreased responses to hypercapnia and hypoxia
- depression of the cough reflex
- decreased tidal volume (by decreased respiratory rate).

The best clinical indicator of respiratory depression is increasing sedation. Decreased rate of breathing and decreased oxygen saturation are *late* signs (Dunwoody and Jungquist 2018).

Nausea and Vomiting   PONV is caused by complex mechanical and chemical interactions between the brain (vomiting centre or chemoreceptor trigger zone (CTZ)), vestibular apparatus in the middle ear and the gastrointestinal tract. PONV in CYP is multifactorial (i.e. due to type of surgery, anaesthesia, prolonged fasting, opioids, antibiotics, other drugs, ileus, pain, psychological distress, electrolyte imbalance, renal dysfunction), although opioids are generally considered to be the primary cause.

When deciding how best to treat PONV assess for *all* possible causes, as this may influence antiemetic selection. The following need to be considered:

- CYP have a significantly higher rate of PONV than adults, which can be compounded in those with a prior history of PONV or motion sickness.
- Guidelines for managing PONV suggest identifying CYP at high risk for PONV, treating aggressively with prophylactic antiemetic therapy and using a combination of different antiemetic agents from different classes for best results (Gan et al. 2019) (see Appendix 1 for relevant drug dosages).
- Moderate to high risk for PONV will require prophylaxis with two antiemetics (different classes).
- High-risk PONV or failed prophylaxis will require combination therapy with two or three antiemetics (different classes).

PRACTICE POINT

Non-operative nausea and vomiting related to pain or analgesics will generally only require single antiemetic therapy, using drugs acting on the CTZ (e.g. serotonin antagonists), but some CYP require rotation to another opioid or low-dose naloxone infusion.

Source: Schug et al. (2020)

Urinary Retention   Urinary retention after surgery is multifactorial (i.e. due to opioids, pain, bladder spasm, constipation, dehydration, neuraxial blockade or anxiety about using a bedpan or bottle). Even if one cause seems probable, others such as pre-existing neurological deficits or bladder dysfunction may be significant (Schug et al. 2020). Consider:

- conservative management (e.g. observation, reassurance, manual expression of bladder)
- encouragement strategies (e.g. increase privacy, commode by the bed, encourage male patients to stand up if possible, running water)
- intermittent catheterisation or indwelling urinary catheter may be required (De Jong et al. 2021).

If the retention is likely to be opioid induced, consider:

- reducing the opioid dose;
- administering a low-dose opioid antagonist;
- opioid rotation (e.g. switching from one opioid to another to improve analgesia and/or reduce side effects), which may involve a change in drug or route.

Pruritus (Rosen et al. 2022)

- Pruritus (itch) is generally caused by central mechanisms and *not* by opioid-induced histamine release, and usually settles within two or three days of commencing opioids.
- As a result, prescribing antihistamines for this problem is generally ineffective and can cause sedation, constipation and urinary retention.
- A low-dose opioid antagonist is effective.
- If ineffective, rotate the opioid.

Constipation (Schug et al. 2020)

- Constipation is an expected side effect of opioids, caused by delayed gastric emptying and decreased peristaltic activity of the bowel.
- Unlike almost all other adverse opioid effects it does not resolve after a few days and needs management for the duration of the opioid therapy.

- Preventive measures should be implemented *early* after commencement of opioids. Ideally a combination of stool softener and a stimulant laxative should be used.
- Ensuring adequate fluids and a high-fibre diet will assist in constipation management.
- Peripherally acting opioid antagonists may offer alternative management.

Local Anaesthetics

- Local anaesthetic (LA) infiltration before tonsillectomy has been found to reduce pain and analgesic use postoperatively in CYP (Bangera 2017).
- Intraoperative LA reduces postoperative pain after dental extractions (Palmer et al. 2020).
- LAs can be used to provide regional anaesthesia.

Other Analgesic Drugs

Other analgesic drugs (e.g. tramadol or low-dose ketamine) are used for nociceptive pain when full mu-receptor opioids are not indicated and/or adjunct analgesia is required (Friedrichsdorf and Goubert 2020). These may be administered via PCA or intravenous infusion (IV tramadol is not available in the USA). The addition of low-dose ketamine to morphine PCA or infusion improves analgesic efficacy in CYP with mucositis pain with no increase in side effects (Hurrell et al. 2019).

Analgesic Administration Techniques

Patient-controlled Analgesia

PCA uses a programmable infusion pump to allow patients to self-administer analgesia. The aim is optimal pain relief and improved patient and parent/carer satisfaction. Use of small frequent boluses allows the patient to titrate the analgesia to their pain, thus receiving only what they need (Cravero et al. 2019).

- PCA is used for the management of moderate to severe pain in CYP aged over five or six years (Schug et al. 2020).
- It is used for postoperative pain, trauma and burns, cancer pain and during palliative care.
- PCA is safe, effective and viewed as a highly satisfactory method of analgesia by staff, patients and families.
- Adverse effects are rare and can be reduced by the addition of opioid-sparing analgesics (Schug et al. 2020).

Other advantages of PCA include improved analgesia during sleep–wake cycles and movement as well as providing increased autonomy for CYP (Cravero et al. 2019).

When using PCA:

- the CYP's parents/carers must understand the PCA system, so they can support their CYP in its use
- the PCA button should *only* be used by the patient in order to reduce the risk of opioid-induced adverse effects (Schug et al. 2020).

CYP who are unwilling or unable to use PCA should have an opioid infusion or PCA-by-proxy (e.g. nurse-administered PCA) instead.

PRACTICE POINT

To use PCA the child must:

- have the cognitive ability to associate pressing the PCA button with receiving pain relief
- be physically able and willing to press the button to control their pain.

The terminology used for PCA administration is outlined in Box 7.5.

Observations necessary during intravenous opioid infusions and PCA are shown in Table 7.2 and Box 7.6.

BOX 7.5   PCA TERMINOLOGY

Bolus dose	When the patient presses the remote button, the PCA delivers the programmed bolus dose of analgesia.
Lockout time	The PCA will not deliver a dose during lockout time. This allows each bolus to reach peak effect before another bolus, therefore reducing the risk of overdose. The lockout time is generally set at 5–10 minutes.
Dose duration	Ranges from 30 to 120 seconds, depending on the PCA pump. The dose duration can be increased to prevent problems, such as light-headedness or nausea associated with a rapid peak of onset of analgesia.
Background	A *continuous* infusion that may be added to improve analgesia.
Maximum limit	This setting may be used to limit the amount of medication the patient may request in a certain period (e.g. one hour or four hours, depending on pump type and settings).

Note that terminology varies slightly in different countries and with different PCA pumps.

Sources: San Diego Patient Safety Council (2014); Ocay et al. (2018)

Table 7.2 Suggested observations for CYP receiving opioid infusion or patient-controlled analgesia (PCA).

Parameter	Suggested frequency	Comments
Sedation score	1-hourly for the duration of the opioid infusion/PCA	Use a validated paediatric sedation scale, e.g. University of Michigan Sedation Scale (see Box 7.3)
Respiratory rate and heart rate	1-hourly for the duration of the opioid infusion/PCA	
Pain score	1-hourly while awake	Use a developmentally appropriate pain assessment scale (see Chapter 6)
Nausea/vomiting assessment	1-hourly for the first 12 hours, then 4-hourly as indicated	
Pulse oximetry	As indicated (see Box 7.6)	Strongly recommended. Most leading children's hospitals in North America have implemented a policy of pulse oximetry while CYP are receiving PCA (exceptions may include when awake and in play room. etc.)

Note: observation requirements vary between organisations and countries. Readers are advised to follow their own institution's guidelines.

BOX 7.6   INDICATIONS FOR PULSE OXIMETRY, WHEN NOT AVAILABLE FOR ALL PATIENTS WITH PCA

Pulse oximetry must be used *continuously* in high-risk patients with:

- UMSS sedation score >2 (see Box 7.3)
- age under six months
- significant cardiorespiratory impairment
- sleep apnoea, snoring or airway obstruction
- spot oximetry less than 94% SaO_2.

Or in patients receiving:

- supplementary oxygen
- concurrent sedative agents.

Clinical indicators for 'spot' pulse oximetry are:

- tachypnoea or bradypnoea
- respiratory distress
- pallor, cyanosis or impaired oxygenation
- confusion or agitation
- hypotension
- nurse concern.

Note: observation requirements vary between organisations and countries. Readers are advised to follow their own institution's guidelines.

PCA-by-proxy

PCA-by-proxy is the delivery of medication from a PCA device by someone other than the patient, typically either a parent or nurse. It is sometimes called *parent-controlled* or *nurse-controlled* analgesia. PCA-by-proxy is used when the CYP is too young, physically unable, cognitively impaired or during end-of-life care. When the designated proxy is carefully chosen and educated, PCA-by-proxy is safe and effective (Cravero et al. 2019).

PRACTICE POINT

When commencing an opioid infusion or PCA, or if the rate is to be increased:

- a loading dose may be required to ensure therapeutic plasma levels are reached quickly
- it takes approximately four half-lives (approximately eight hours for morphine/hydromorphone; approximately 1.5 hours for fentanyl) for opioids to reach steady-state plasma concentrations.

Source: Palmer et al. (2020)

PRACTICE POINT

- Any adverse effects relating to specialist analgesia techniques should be reported urgently to the pain service or anaesthetist.
- Any observations outside reportable limits or outside normal values for age should be reported.
- The effectiveness of the analgesia should be documented in the CYP's healthcare record.

Weaning PCA

Most CYP self-wean from PCA as the pain improves, making a natural progression to simple analgesics and oral opioids if needed.

PRACTICE POINT

CYP who have required high doses or prolonged periods on opioids risk developing opioid abstinence syndrome (*withdrawal*) if opioids are decreased too rapidly. Instead, a careful weaning regimen should be implemented (see Chapter 5).

CASE STUDY: PART 4

After two days Jane is tolerating clear fluids and able to increase her oral intake. It is important to discuss options for pain management when transitioning to oral analgesia to ensure Jane and her family are well informed. Oral opioids will replace her PCA. Jane has continued to report high pain scores on IR oxycodone and is reluctant to increase her oral intake, only drinking smoothies. She is prescribed SR oxycodone twice per day and encouraged to mobilise.

1. What physical and psychological interventions might you want to include in Jane's pain management plan?
2. Which members of the multidisciplinary team might you want to involve?
3. What other concerns would you have?

CASE STUDY: PART 5

Jane has progressed from surgery three days ago with no physical complications, her mobilisation has slightly improved, but she is still refusing solid food. There is a plan for her to be discharged on simple analgesia and oxycodone IR for two more days.

Her analgesia requirement has decreased, and she has reported her pain to have improved. However, her aunt reports that Jane has more pain and does not want to take her home. She is angry and unsatisfied with the information given to her. Jane's oral intake has further decreased.

1. What questions might you ask Jane in order to explore any spiritual dimensions to her pain?
2. How do you think the family and previous pain experiences influence Jane's pain?
3. How would you plan Jane's discharge?

Regional Anaesthesia

Regional anaesthesia (RA) or *neuraxial analgesia* is the administration of LAs into the epidural space (caudal or epidural), around a peripheral nerve plexus or into the intrathecal space (spinal) to block pain transmission. RA provides excellent analgesia, reduces the surgical stress response and can significantly diminish the need for opioids and other analgesics (Schug et al. 2020; Heydinger et al. 2021). RA is used in CYP of all ages. It needs to be managed by competently trained staff to minimise complications (Schug et al. 2020).

- In paediatric caudal epidurals, levobupivacaine, bupivacaine and ropivacaine are equivalent in efficacy, but bupivacaine produces a longer-acting motor block (Kumar et al. 2019).
- Addition of clonidine or ketamine to paediatric caudal epidurals may improve analgesia compared to using LA alone.
- Adding ketamine to caudal anaesthesia has been found to be effective in a randomised controlled trial in managing postoperative pain, and reduced the use of opioids (Khoshfetrat et al. 2018).
- The addition of opioids to epidural or caudal provides equivalent or improved analgesia to LA alone but increases side effects, particularly itch, respiratory depression and PONV (Berger and Goldschneider 2019).

Central Blocks

- The most frequently used central RA technique in CYP is the caudal block, which is used for surgical procedures below the umbilical region. It is generally a single-dose technique (Adler et al. 2020).
- Epidurals are used for major surgery of the spine, chest and abdomen (thoracic epidural) or lower limbs (lumbar epidural).

They are delivered by patient-controlled epidural anaesthesia (PCEA) or continuous infusion. It can be the sole technique or used in conjunction with general anaesthesia (Marcelino et al. 2019).

- In neonates, epidurals are inserted into the caudal epidural space, then threaded to the lumbar or thoracic levels as needed (Palmer et al. 2020).
- Intrathecal analgesia is administered as a single dose or by infusion and provides an alternative to general anaesthesia (Heydinger et al. 2021).

Peripheral Blocks

- The use of peripheral nerve (*perineural*) blocks is increasing and, in some cases, replacing central RA techniques as the analgesia is comparable with fewer adverse effects. They are most useful for site-specific analgesia (e.g. limb surgery) and are administered as a single dose or by infusion (Palmer et al. 2020).
- Continuous peripheral nerve blocks (CPNB) enable prolonged analgesia and can be delivered via a portable pump, allowing early discharge from hospital (Schlechter et al. 2022).
- Depending on the LA used, analgesia can last for 6–24 hours with a single-dose technique or longer with infusion. Bupivacaine, levobupivacaine and ropivacaine are the LA drugs most often used. Opioids, clonidine or ketamine may be added to the LA solution (Palmer et al. 2020). Information about drug doses is provided in Appendix 1.

Optimising the Safety of Regional Anaesthesia

The practices to optimise safety suggested in Box 7.6 also apply to RA techniques. Suggested observations required while receiving RA infusions are outlined in Table 7.3.

Table 7.3 Suggested observations for CYP receiving regional anaesthesia.

Parameter	Suggested frequency	Comments
Sedation score	1-hourly for the duration of the epidural infusion	Use a validated paediatric sedation scale (see Box 7.3)
Respiratory rate and heart rate	1-hourly for the duration of the epidural infusion	
Temperature and blood pressure	1-hourly for the *first 4 hours* then 4-hourly until epidural ceased	
Pain score	1-hourly while awake	Use a developmentally appropriate pain assessment scale (see Chapter 6)
Nausea/vomiting score	1-hourly for the first 12 hours, then 4-hourly as indicated	
Pulse oximetry	As indicated (see Box 7.6)	
Sensory and motor assessment	4-hourly	See Boxes 7.7 and 7.8

Note: observation requirements vary between organisations and countries. Readers are advised to follow their own institution's guidelines.

Assessment of Sensory and Motor Block

Assessment of sensory and motor block enables early detection of complications and ensures analgesia can be optimised. The method for assessment of sensory block is outlined in Box 7.7. Figure 7.2 demonstrates the dermatome distribution in CYP.

BOX 7.7   ASSESSMENT OF SENSORY BLOCK

Rationale

Sensory nerve fibres respond to pain, temperature, touch and pressure. As pain and temperature nerve fibres are similarly affected by local anaesthetic drugs, changes in temperature perception indicate the anaesthetised area.

At each vertebra, nerve roots exit from the spinal cord bilaterally. Dermatomes are areas of skin that are primarily innervated by a single spinal nerve.

It is important to assess sensory block:

- to ensure effective pain relief
- to ensure the block is not too extensive, which may increase the risk of complications.

Procedure

1. Explain procedure to patient/parent/carer.
2. Wrap an ice cube in tissue/paper towel leaving part exposed.

3. Place ice on an area well away from the affected dermatomes (e.g. face) and ask the patient to tell you how cold it feels to them.
4. Apply the ice to an area likely to be numb on the same side of the body and ask the patient 'Does this feel the same cold as your face/arm or different?' Patients may report the ice feeling colder, warmer or the same.
5. Apply the ice to areas above and below this point until you can determine the upper and lower margins of the block.
6. Repeat the procedure on the opposite side of the body (blocks may be uneven or unilateral).
7. Document the blocked dermatomes on the observation chart. Record both the upper and lower margins of the block, e.g. T7–L1, L = R *or* R: T7–L1, L: T10–L2.
8. It is possible to assess dermatome levels on infants or non-verbal/cognitively impaired CYP by observing flinching and facial expression in response to ice on presumed blocked and unblocked dermatomes. Another way is by observing the patient's response to movement and response to very gentle palpation of the operative site.

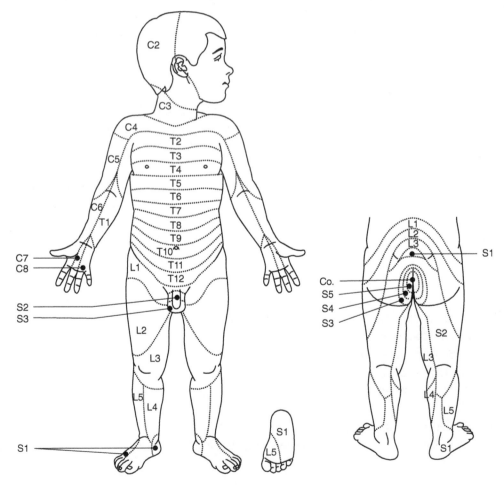

Figure 7.2 Distribution of dermatomes in CYP.

Source: Used with permission from Royal Children's Hospital, Melbourne (2021a).

Sensory block should be assessed *every four hours* and at the following times:

- in the recovery room on waking from anaesthetic
- on return to the ward/unit from the recovery room
- if the patient complains of pain
- one hour after a bolus or rate change.

The patient should be reviewed by the pain service or anaesthetist if:

- the block is higher than T3 dermatome
- there is no block
- the block is insufficient to relieve pain
- any major change in motor function (particularly any sudden change)

- almost complete or complete motor block in legs (Bromage score 2–3)
- reduced motor function in hands or fingers with thoracic epidural.

The method for assessment of motor block is outlined in Box 7.8. Figure 7.3 demonstrates the Bromage scale to assess motor function in CYP.

Motor block should be assessed *every four hours* and at the following times:

- in the recovery room on waking from anaesthetic
- on return to the ward/unit from the recovery room
- before ambulation
- one hour after a bolus or rate change.

BOX 7.8 ASSESSMENT OF MOTOR BLOCK

Rationale

Motor nerves (as well as sensory nerves) may be affected by local anaesthetics. It is important to assess motor block:

- to prevent pressure areas
- to ensure the patient is safe to walk (if permitted)
- to detect the onset of complications (e.g. epidural haematoma or abscess).

The degree of motor block in both legs should be assessed using the *Bromage scale*, the standard method of assessing motor function, scored as shown below:

Score 0 (none)	Full flexion of knees and feet
Score 1 (partial)	Just able to move knees and feet
Score 2 (almost complete)	Able to move feet only
Score 3 (complete)	Unable to move feet or knees

Procedure

1. Explain procedure to patient/parent/carer.
2. Ask the patient to flex their knees and ankles. Rate their movement according to the Bromage scale.
3. Document the score on the observation chart. If motor function is different in each leg, document this accordingly, e.g. Bromage L = 2, R = 0.

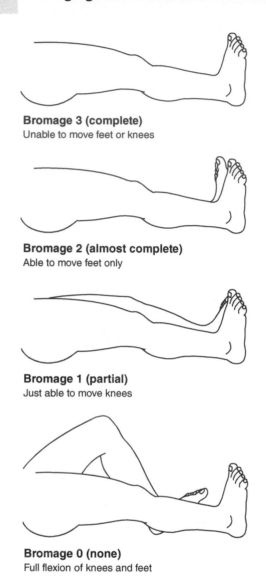

Bromage 3 (complete)
Unable to move feet or knees

Bromage 2 (almost complete)
Able to move feet only

Bromage 1 (partial)
Just able to move knees

Bromage 0 (none)
Full flexion of knees and feet

Figure 7.3 The Bromage scale to assess motor function in CYP.

Source: Used with permission from Royal Children's Hospital, Melbourne (2021b).

PRACTICE POINT

Assessing sensory and motor block can assist in ensuring optimal efficacy of continuous peripheral nerve blocks. As the nerve block affects a single limb, a modified assessment is required. The type and frequency of assessment should be guided by the region being blocked and specific institutional protocols.

Catheter Position and Insertion Site

- The catheter insertion site should be inspected at least eight-hourly for redness, tenderness, leaking and dressing integrity.
- The catheter markings should be checked to ensure the catheter has not migrated (moved).

Pressure Area Care

- The decreased sensation and motor blockade produced by epidural and perineural analgesia can cause pressure sores and nerve compression.
- Generally, the heels, medial and lateral malleoli and sacrum are involved but *all* pressure points are at risk.
- Superficial nerves (e.g. common peroneal nerve) are vulnerable to damage from unrecognised pressure due to decreased sensation.
- The use of pressure-relief devices (e.g. air mattresses, pressure pads) and meticulous nursing care minimises the risk.

Anticoagulant Medication

If a patient is prescribed anticoagulant medications while receiving RA, the timing for catheter removal must be considered to minimise bleeding risk (Schug et al. 2020).

Urinary Retention

- Patients with lumbar or caudal epidural infusions are at increased risk of urinary retention. Risk is higher in patients receiving epidural opioids.
- Patients may require a urinary catheter, which should remain in situ until the epidural infusion is ceased.

Regional Anaesthesia: Problem-solving

Inadequate Analgesia   If the patient complains of pain or appears to be in pain:

- assess sensory block
- check catheter position, insertion site and connections for leakage/dislodgement
- assess severity and location of pain
- contact the pain service or anaesthetist for advice and report findings.

Manage as per institutional epidural guidelines:

- the infusion rate may be increased, or a bolus administered
- a review may be required if at risk of surgical complications (e.g. compartment syndrome or haemorrhage).

Reportable Observations   Contact the pain service or anaesthetist *urgently* if any of the following occur:

- high block >T3
- back pain
- dense motor block (Bromage score 2–3)

- UMSS sedation score ≥3 with or without respiratory depression
- fever >38.5°C
- hypotension
- signs of local anaesthetic toxicity
- signs of infection at catheter entry site
- oedema or swelling at catheter entry site.

Complications of Regional Anaesthesia   The incidence of RA complications is 1 in 2000 for serious complications and 1 in 10 000 for persisting complications (Ecoffey et al. 2022).

Epidural complications and suggested treatments are presented in Tables 7.4 and 7.5.

CASE STUDY: PART 6

Jane is being discharged home. Her surgery and expected progress were discussed with Jane and her aunt. She is going home with a small number of oxycodone tablets for pain.

1. What information would you give her family regarding oxycodone?
2. Who would you refer Jane to in the community?
3. Why do you think follow-up and support is important?

Table 7.4 Complications related to insertion of epidural catheter.

Problem	Comments	Treatment
Headache	<ul><li>May be due to dural tap (incidence 1–2%)</li><li>May not present until patient mobilises</li></ul>	<ul><li>Analgesia</li><li>Bed rest</li><li>Fluids</li><li>Epidural blood patch if prolonged, typical postural headache</li></ul>
Back pain	<ul><li>Generally at insertion site</li><li>Mild back pain is common and usually transient</li><li>Moderate or severe back pain must be thoroughly investigated</li></ul>	<ul><li>Simple analgesics and reassurance for mild back pain with regular check-ups until resolved</li><li>If moderate to severe pain and/or fever, needs *urgent* review to rule out epidural abscess or haematoma (see below)</li></ul>
Sympathetic blockade	<ul><li>May cause hypotension (generally in children aged >8 years).</li></ul>	<ul><li>Posture (lie flat, *not* head down)</li><li>IV fluid bolus</li></ul>

Table 7.4 (Continued)

Problem	Comments	Treatment
High blockade	■ Dermatome block higher than T3: numbness or tingling in fingers or arms ■ Horner's syndrome: miosis, ptosis, dry/warm skin on face (unilateral) ■ Respiratory distress (intercostal block) ■ Bradycardia (high thoracic block) ■ Unconsciousness (total spinal block)	■ Resuscitation ■ Cease epidural infusion ■ The infusion might be recommenced at a lower rate if epidural position is confirmed
Dense motor block (see Box 7.8)	■ Usual immediately after surgery due to higher concentrations of solution used intraoperatively ■ Prolonged dense motor block >6 hours after surgery must be investigated to rule out epidural abscess or haematoma	■ Regularly assess amount of motor block (using Bromage scale) ■ Report Bromage score 2–3 ■ Investigate if indicated
Nerve damage	■ Very rare ■ May present with weakness or numbness that is generally transient	■ Neurology referral ■ Investigate if indicated
Epidural abscess	■ Very rare ■ Presents with moderate to severe back pain, fever, sensory or motor deficits, malaise	■ Urgent investigation: full blood examination, inflammatory markers, blood culture, MRI ■ Urgent neurology or neurosurgical review
Epidural haematoma	■ Very rare ■ Presents with moderate to severe back pain, sensory or motor deficits	■ Urgent investigation: full blood examination, coagulation studies, MRI ■ Urgent neurology or neurosurgical review

Table 7.5 Drug-related problems with regional anaesthesia (RA).

Problem	Comments	Treatment
Local anaesthetic drugs		
Overdose/ toxicity	Signs of LA toxicity: dizziness, blurred vision, decreased hearing, restlessness, tremor, hypotension, bradycardia, arrhythmia, seizures, sudden loss of consciousness	■ Resuscitation ■ Management of cardiac, neurological and respiratory side effects ■ Cease RA infusion
Allergy	Extremely rare. Signs of anaphylaxis or allergic reaction may be present	■ Resuscitation with IV fluids, adrenaline, antihistamines and steroids ■ Cease RA infusion
Clonidine		
Sedation	Clonidine increases sedation	■ May need dose decreased or removed
Hypotension/ bradycardia	Clonidine increases hypotension	■ Consider IV fluid bolus ■ Monitor urine output and blood pressure ■ May need dose decreased or removed

Stopping Regional Anaesthesia Infusions

To minimise adverse effects, RA infusions are generally limited to three or four days (Schug et al. 2020). Oral analgesia should be administered as soon as the RA infusion has ended rather than waiting until sensation has returned. If the patient cannot receive oral analgesia, PCA or intravenous administration will be required. Analgesia needs to be given regularly for 12–24 hours, with doses available for pain escalation. After this period, analgesia should be given on a PRN basis, depending on the surgery and expected pain.

Pain Problem-solving: What to Do if the Pain Management Plan Is Not Working

An important component of pain management is problem-solving why analgesia is inadequate or why the CYP is not responding as expected. It is useful to consider all possibilities. Distress may not be due to pain; it can be due to hunger, parental separation or being in an unfamiliar place. Sometimes the prescribed analgesic drugs are adequate for rest but inadequate for activity.

PRACTICE POINT

When assessing for efficacy of analgesia, ensure it is sufficient:

- for rest and sleep
- for movement and turning
- for deep breathing and coughing
- for physiotherapy and nursing care
- to enable mobilising.

Surgical pain usually peaks 24–48 hours after surgery, then decreases rapidly. If there is worsening pain more than 48 hours after surgery, or at any time the pain appears disproportional to the surgery or underlying medical condition, reasons for this should always be considered and thoroughly investigated in addition to administering analgesics (see Table 7.6 for more details).

Transition to Oral Analgesics from Specialist Analgesic Techniques

The transition from specialist analgesia techniques needs to be planned carefully. As the CYP's pain decreases and condition improves, oral medications are generally tolerated, which allows the specialist techniques to be weaned or ceased. If the CYP needs to remain fasting for an extended period, some non-opioid analgesic drugs can be given via the intravenous route. During the transition the assessment of pain and functional activity should continue. It is important to give adequate analgesic drugs to ensure the CYP can mobilise and cough. Ensuring additional rescue doses of analgesic drugs also relieves CYP and parental/carer anxiety.

Pain Medications at Home

Once CYP are ready for discharge from hospital, they and their parents/carers need clear instructions about pain management and safe administration of analgesics, the weaning plan and what to do if the pain is not well controlled (Forster et al. 2021). If CYP need to stay on opioid analgesic drugs for an extended period after discharge from hospital, they may

Table 7.6 Pain problem-solving.

Problem	Possible cause/considerations	Management
Pain escalation	What analgesia has been given and why is it inadequate? Have non-opioid analgesics been given in addition to other analgesics?	Check the doses are correct. Ensure *all* prescribed analgesics are given in a timely manner. If required, administer additional analgesia (titrate to comfort)
	Are the infusion pumps functioning correctly?	Check the infusion delivery device(s) and ensure it is functioning correctly
	Is the IV cannula or RA catheter in place and functioning normally?	Check the device is not leaking, blocked or dislodged
	Is the pain due to a medical or surgical complication (e.g. tight plaster, compartment syndrome, haemorrhage, haematoma, blocked wound drain, ileus)?	Request a medical or surgical review if complications are present or possible. Address the underlying cause of the pain (e.g. split the plaster, adjust the drain(s), insert nasogastric tube)
	Has a *single-dose* RA or perineural block regressed, requiring additional analgesia?	Administer additional analgesia
	Is the RA infusion providing adequate analgesia?	Review rate, consider a bolus. Consider other analgesics
	Is the opioid infusion providing adequate analgesia?	Check rate, consider a bolus. Consider other analgesics
Complaints of pain with PCA	Does the CYP understand how to use the PCA?	Re-educate if necessary
	Is the bolus dose adequate? Is the lockout time appropriate? Is a background infusion required? Is the analgesia adequate for the pain severity?	Consider addition of background infusion or increase bolus size. Consider other analgesics
	Consider other causes: anxiety, confusion, inappropriate use	Address and manage non-pain issues

require telephone follow-up or outpatient review to assist weaning and monitoring for chronic pain.

Most mild nociceptive pain in CYP is managed by parents at home using physical and psychological strategies and (if required) analgesic drugs (Table 7.7). In most situations, moderate pain can be controlled with non-opioid analgesics and low doses of opioid analgesics with the addition of LAs. Severe nociceptive pain is initially managed by parents/carers with the help of community health professionals or emergency responders before referral to hospital for intensive management.

Table 7.7 Treatment of nociceptive pain at home.

Type of pain	Treatment
Otalgia	■ Ibuprofen or paracetamol are equally effective in managing pain associated with otitis media (Schug et al. 2020) ■ Topical local anaesthesia to the ear canal is effective for managing pain from acute otitis media
Acute pharyngitis	■ Although glucocorticoids have been associated with faster reduction of pain compared with placebo (Schug et al. 2020), they offer no significant benefit over simple analgesics (paracetamol and NSAIDs) in CYP ■ Medicated topical therapies (sprays or lozenges) offer no advantage over saltwater gargling or sucking hard candy (Drutz and Correa 2021)
Dental pain	■ NSAIDs alone provide adequate analgesia after dental extractions. Local anaesthesia reduces pain after dental extraction (Palmer et al. 2020)
Tonsillectomy	■ Paracetamol and NSAIDS may not be enough for postoperative pain in some CYP ■ Tramadol was seen to be more effective (Palmer et al. 2020)

Psychological Pain-relieving Interventions

A recent systematic review supports the provision of distraction, hypnosis, combined cognitive behavioural therapy and breathing exercises as psychological interventions for nociceptive pain in CYP (Birnie et al. 2018). Other research shows that:

- creating a calm child-friendly environment, with adequate parent/carer information and training, assists in reducing distress and nociceptive pain (Pancekauskaite and Jankauskaite 2018)
- environments with ambient lighting have been found to decrease both pain ratings and rates of pain medication (Robinson and Green 2015)
- digital distraction produces a modest reduction in pain and distress, while the effectiveness of these strategies over non-digital distractors is yet to be established (Gates et al. 2020).

We also know that anxiety, catastrophising and depression impact the perception of pain, and affect CYP experiencing nociceptive pain. The Pain Catastrophizing Scale has been validated in nociceptive pain populations (Durand et al. 2017), and is recommended as a screening tool in acute settings to target appropriate pain management. The screening tool may be offered to patients who are attending pre-assessment clinics before orthopaedic surgery.

In high-catastrophising CYP, distraction has not been found to be an effective technique to reduce pain, and can intensify pain experiences (Verhoeven et al. 2012). Psychological acceptance-based therapies have also been found to reduce nociceptive pain for CYP with cancer (Cederberg et al. 2017). Acceptance and cognitive therapies, rather than distraction, may assist CYP and parents with higher levels of catastrophising to reduce nociceptive pain and distress.

Further information about psychological pain-relieving interventions can be found in Chapter 1.

Physical Pain-relieving Interventions

Physical interventions for nociceptive pain have less clear evidence than psychological interventions.

- In pre-hospital and emergency department settings, use of RICE (rest, ice, compression/splinting and elevation) for soft-tissue and musculoskeletal injuries and haemophilia bleeds appears effective (Gourde and Damian 2012).
- Massage has not been shown to effectively reduce nociceptive pain or anxiety in CYP after cardiac surgery (Staveski et al. 2018).
- For babies experiencing nociceptive pain, evidence supports non-nutritive sucking, swaddling, and comfort positioning using skin-to-skin contact (Taddio et al. 2019; Lisanti et al. 2020). More information about the management of neonatal pain can be found in Chapter 13.

Spirituality and Nociceptive Pain in Children and Young People

Spiritual aspects of nociceptive pain in CYP have received minimal consideration in the literature. Illness and pain can disrupt a person's biological, interpersonal and spiritual relationships, while spiritual practice can potentially decrease a person's pain experience (Dedeli and Kaptan 2013), and is associated with positive psychological adjustment in adults (Ferreira-Valente et al. 2019). Prayer is a universal practice, with varied cultural forms. Creating a respectful place for spiritual practice in hospital and community settings may empower parents/carers and CYP to access psychological strengths that can assist in alleviating nociceptive pain.

Summary

- Nociceptive pain is a common experience for CYP, and is generally of short duration and usually resolves completely.
- There are multiple causes of nociceptive pain, including illnesses, injury, surgery or pre-existing medical conditions.
- CYP with developmental disabilities experience significant pain in their daily life.
- Opioids are important for the management of severe nociceptive pain but should be combined with simple analgesics as these have an opioid-sparing effect.
- Multimodal analgesia allows for optimal pain management, while minimising adverse effects by using combinations of analgesics at lower doses.

- Regional anaesthesia offers superior pain relief compared with most other analgesic techniques, as it can completely block pain.
- Close monitoring is key in preventing serious adverse events related to opioid and regional analgesia techniques.
- Problem-solving can assist clinicians in improving the pain management of patients.
- Any pain disproportional to the surgery or condition should always be investigated as it may indicate medical or surgical complications.
- Transition to oral analgesia following specialist analgesia techniques requires planning to ensure optimal pain management.

- Physical and psychological interventions combined with multimodal pharmacological pain management provides the best outcomes.

- Parents should be given clear instructions about managing pain at home after their CYP's discharge from hospital, and CYP should ideally be reviewed by their medical practitioner or pain specialist.

Acknowledgements

We'd like to acknowledge the original contributions of Stephanie Dowden to this Chapter in the Second Edition of this book.

Key to Case Study

Part 1

1. It is important to understand Jane's pain experience and response to pain in the past, as this will help make decisions to support her through the postsurgical pain. A pain history documenting where Jane experiences pain, what triggers it or makes it worse and also what helps to make it better is important. Pain is subjective and each patient should be believed when reporting their pain.

2. An appropriate pain assessment tool would be the Wong–Baker FACES Pain Rating Scale, as using this would reduce the need for verbal communication. A comprehensive explanation of the tool will help Jane use the tool to identify her level of pain.

3. Jane has experienced chronic constipation and anxiety due to situational stress at school, which will mean her expressions of pain and responses to varying stimuli will be individual and potentially more heightened.

4. If Jane has been taking analgesia prior to surgery, this will need to be taken into consideration for potential tolerance. Surgical pain is often severe in the first 24 hours postoperatively, and for Jane it will be important to ensure adequate analgesic drugs are given and assure her that she can be given additional medication to help manage the pain if needed.

Part 2

1. Given Jane's previous experience of school-based anxiety and recurrent pain, she would meet with a member of the acute pain team prior to the surgery to discuss how her pain would be managed. Jane would benefit from a psychologist and play therapist (child life therapist) to give her some strategies for helping manage the postoperative pain and address her past pain experience.

2. Presurgical pain, anxiety and parental/ guardian catastrophising influences pain behaviour and the risk of developing persistent pain after surgery.

3. Anxiety and fear may limit Jane's progress and coping skills, and be influenced by her aunt's anxiety.

4. It is important to provide education to Jane and her aunt on what to expect after the surgery and ways to help cope with pain based on a biopsychosocial framework.

Part 3

1. Jane has a PCA which she can use at her discretion. It would benefit her to have adjuvant analgesic drugs to decrease opioid use, for example clonidine which would not only have an analgesic effect but would help her anxiety and sleep. Jane needs to be provided education about medication to feel confident that other drugs can help alleviate her pain.
2. Side effects from opioids such as constipation should be explained and managed with a combination of a stool softener and a stimulant laxative until opioids are stopped. Opioids may cause pruritis but this should resolve. If nausea persists, antiemetics may be required for a short period.
3. Jane can participate in her pain management through communication with clinicians, managing the PCA and practising psychological and physical pain-relieving strategies. An explanation for a multimodal approach to analgesia to decrease opioid use and side effects may help with compliance.

Part 4

1. Pharmacological pain management should always be supported by physical and psychological pain-relieving interventions such as light movement, relaxation, imagery and possibly hypnosis. Distraction techniques such as music and craft may help Jane cope with her pain better.
2. Physiotherapists and occupational therapists may be able to give Jane strategies to manage her postoperative recovery and pain.
3. It is important to ensure analgesia is adequate for mobilising and any physiotherapy.

Part 5

1. Jane's ongoing experience of pain may be complex and feel overwhelming. She will require an opportunity to meet again with members of the pain team, such as the psychologist or play therapist, to understand the emotional, spiritual and physical aspects of her pain, and practice physical and psychological pain-relieving strategies.
2. In the past, Jane's family gave her little empathy and were dismissive of her physical and psychological experiences. They lacked understanding of the complexity of pain for young people with anxiety. Jane's aunt appears angry, frustrated and concerned about Jane's pain. It is important to recognise that an adult's pain experience impacts the pain experience of young people. Family members would benefit from meeting with a member of the acute pain team to explore their own pain experience, build an understanding of the relationship between stress and Jane's pain behaviour, and build skills in communicating effectively with Jane about her pain.
3. Discharge planning should involve referrals to local specialists including a dietitian for guidance on high-fibre foods, and a psychologist to ensure Jane has appropriate support going forward related to school anxiety. This support will enable Jane to develop strategies to reach her potential socially, culturally and spiritually.

Part 6

1. As Jane will be discharged on oxycodone, her aunt should be given information about the safe use and disposal of opioids.

2. As well as referrals to dietitians and psychologists, a letter could be sent to her general practitioner (GP) and possibly her school through a social worker or psychologist, to address the bullying Jane has experienced. Her surgical procedure is only one aspect of her pain journey.

3. Young people who experience anxiety and presurgical pain are at risk of developing persistent postsurgical pain and require follow-up and potential referral to a chronic pain management team for ongoing support.

Multiple Choice Questions

1. A three-year-old boy has returned from having orthopaedic surgery and is on a morphine infusion for pain. What clinical observation is the most important to determine opioid toxicity?
   a. Blood pressure
   b. Respiratory rate
   c. Oxygen saturation
   d. Sedation score

2. A 14-year-old girl has had a large laparotomy for inflammatory bowel disease 24 hours ago. She has a thoracic epidural at T7 with levobupivacaine 0.125%. She is comfortable, but you are concerned she cannot move her legs. What would you be most concerned about?
   a. She is unable to get out of bed
   b. She may have an epidural haematoma
   c. The epidural catheter may have migrated out
   d. She may have nerve damage

3. You are caring for a two-year-old girl who has had a laparotomy and stoma formed after a bowel obstruction. What pain assessment tool would you use?
   a. Numerical pain scale
   b. Behavioural assessment tools

   c. Self-report
   d. Faces Pain Scale Revised

4. Your patient has arrived from theatre after a hip reduction spica for hip dysplasia. She is 14 months old and has a morphine infusion attached but not running for pain management. She had local anaesthetic into the caudal space at the start of her surgery. She is crying and unsettled. What do you think is the primary problem?
   a. She is hungry
   b. She is having muscle spasm
   c. Her caudal anaesthetic has worn off
   d. She has an indwelling urinary catheter in situ

5. Why is it important to give your patient alternative analgesia at the same time their regional anaesthetic is ceased?
   a. To help mobilisation
   b. For analgesia to reach effectiveness
   c. To avoid pain when the local anaesthetic has worn off
   d. All of the above

References

Adler, A., Belon, C., Guffey, D., et al. (2020) Real-time ultrasound improves accuracy of caudal block in children. *Anaesthesia and Analgesia* 20(4), 1002–1007.

Anderson, T., Harrell, C., Snider, M. and Kink, R. (2022) The safety of high-dose intranasal fentanyl in the pediatric emergency department. *Pediatric Emergency Care* 38(2), e447–e450.

Anekar, A.A., Hendrix, J.M. and Cascella, M. (2022) WHO analgesic ladder. StatPearls [Internet]. https://www.ncbi.nlm.nih.gov/books/NBK554435/

Arslan, I. and Demir, K. (2022) Evaluation of forensic cases presented to the pediatric emergency department. *Turkish Journal of Emergency Medicine* 22(3), 137–142.

Bangera, A. (2017) Anaesthesia for adenotonsillectomy: an update. *Indian Journal of Anaesthesia* 61(2), 103–109.

Berger, A.S. and Goldschneider, K.R. (2019) The role of neuraxial opioids in pediatric practice. *Clinical Journal of Pain* 35(6), 497–500.

Birnie, K.A., Noel, M., Chambers, C.T., Umen, L.S. and Parker, J.A. (2018) Psychological intervention for needle-related procedural pain in children and adolescents. *Cochrane Database of Systematic Reviews* (10), CD005179.

Birnie, K.A., Hundert, A.S., Lalloo, C., et al. (2019) Recommendations for selection of self-report pain intensity measures in children and adolescents: a systematic review and quality assessment of measurement properties. *Pain* 160(1): 5–18.

Brandow, A., Carroll, P., Creary, S., et al. (2020) American Society of Hematology 2020 guidelines for sickle cell disease: management of acute and chronic pain. *Blood Advances* 4(12), 2657–2701.

Carter, B. (2020) Communicating pain: the challenge of pain assessment in children with profound cognitive impairment. *Comprehensive Child and Adolescent Nursing* 43(1), 10–14.

Cascella, M., Bimonte, S. and Saettini, F. (2019) The challenge of pain assessment in children with cognitive disabilities: features and clinical applicability of different observational tools. *Journal of Paediatrics and Child Health* 55(2), 129–135.

Cederberg, J.T., Dahl, J., von Essen, L. and Ljungman, G. (2017). An acceptance-based intervention for children and adolescents with cancer experiencing acute pain: a single-subject study. *Journal of Pain Research* 10(21), 2195–2203.

Cravero, J.P., Agarwal, R., Berde, C., et al. (2019) The Society for Pediatric Anesthesia recommendations for the use of opioids in children during the perioperative period. *Pediatric Anesthesia* 29(6), 547–571.

Dedeli, O. and Kaptan, G. (2013) Spirituality and religion in pain and pain management. *Health Psychology Research* 1(3), e29.

De Jong, A.C., Maaskant, J.M., Groen, L.A. and van Woensel, J.B.M. (2021) Monitoring of micturition and bladder volumes can replace routine indwelling urinary catheters in children receiving intravenous opioids: a prospective cohort study. *European Journal of Pediatrics* 180, 47–57.

Dorney, K., Dodinton, J.M., James, R., et al. (2020) Preventing injuries must be a priority to prevent disease in the twenty-first century. *Pediatric Research* 87(2), 282–292.

Drutz, J.E. and Correa, A.G. (2021) Acute pharyngitis in children and adolescents: symptomatic treatment. UpToDate. https://www.medilib.ir/uptodate/show/2875 (accessed 2 June 2023).

Dunwoody, D.R. and Jungquist, C.R. (2018) Sedation scales: do they capture the concept of opioid-induced sedation? *Nursing Forum* 53(4), 399–405.

Durand, H., Birnie, K.A., Noel, M., et al. (2017) State versus trait: validating state assessment of child and parental catastrophic thinking about children's acute pain. *Journal of Pain* 18(4), 385–395.

Ecoffey, C., Bosenberg, A., Lonnqvist, P., Suresh, S., Delbos, A. and Ivani, G. (2022) Practice advisory on the prevention and management of complications of pediatric regional anesthesia. *Journal of Clinical Anesthesia* 79, 110725.

Farr, B., Ranstrom, M.S. and Mooney, M.D. (2020) Eliminating opiate prescribing for children after non-perforated appendicectomy. *Journal of the American College of Surgeons* 230(6), 944–946.

Ferreira-Valente, A., Sharma, S., Torres, S., et al. (2019) Does religiosity/spirituality play a role in function, pain-related beliefs, and coping in patients with chronic pain? A systematic review. *Journal of Religion in Health* 61(3), 2331–2385.

Forster, E.M., Kotzur, C., Richards, J. and Gilmour, J. (2021) Paediatric post-discharge pain and parent perceptions of support from an Australian nurse practitioner led pain service. *Journal of Child Health Care* 26(3), 394–406.

Franziska, D. and McMahon, S.B. (2017) Neurological basis for pain vulnerability: why me? *Pain* 158(Suppl. 1), S108–S114.

Friedrichsdorf, S.J. and Goubert, L. (2020) Pediatric pain treatment and prevention for hospitalized children, *Pain Reports* 5(1), e804.

Gan, T., Tong, J., Kumar, B.G., et al. (2019) Fourth consensus guidelines for the management of post-operative nausea and Vomiting. *Anesthesia and Analgesia* 131(2), 411–448.

Gates, M., Hartling, L., Shulhan-Kilroy, J., et al. (2020) Digital technology distraction for acute pain in children: a meta-analysis. *Pediatrics* 145(2), e20191139.

Gazal, G. and Al Samadani, K.H. (2017) Comparison of paracetamol, ibuprofen and diclofenac potassium for pain relief following dental extractions and deep cavity preparations. *Saudi Medical Journal* 38(3), 284–291.

Glare, P., Aubrey, K. and Myles, P. (2019) Transition from acute to chronic pain after surgery. *Lancet* 393, 1537–1546.

Glockler, M., Goebel, W. and Michael, K. (2018) *A Waldorf Guide to Children's Health, Illnesses, Symptoms, Treatments and Therapies*. Floris Books, Edinburgh.

Gourde, J. and Damian, F.J. (2012) ED fracture pain management in children. *Journal of Emergency Nursing* 38(1), 91–97.

Gupta, K., Nagappa, M., Prasad, A., et al. (2018) Risk factors for opioid-induced respiratory depression in surgical patients: a systematic review and meta-analyses. *BMJ Open* 8(12), e024086.

Hauer, J. and Houtrow, A.J. (2017) Pain assessment and treatment in children with significant impairment of the central nervous system. *Pediatrics* 39(6), e1–e27.

Heydinger, G., Tobias, J. and Veneziano, G. (2021) Fundamentals and innovations in regional anaesthesia for infants and children. *Anaesthesia* 76(Suppl. 1), 74–88.

Hicks, C.L., von Baeyer, C.L., Spafford, P.A., van Korlaar, I. and Goodenough, B. (2001) The Faces Pain Scale-Revised: toward a common metric in pediatric pain measurement. *Pain* 93(2), 173–183.

Hurley-Wallace, A., Wood, C., Franck, L.S., Howard, R.F. and Liossi, C. (2018) Paediatric pain education for health care professionals. *Pain Reports* 4(1), e701.

Hurrell, L., Burgoyne, L., Logan, R., Revesz, T. and Gue, S. (2019) The management of pediatric oncology inpatients with oral mucositis. *Journal of Pediatric Hematology/Oncology* 41(8), e510–e516.

Kelley-Quon, L.I., Kirkpatrick, M.G., Ricca, R.L., et al. (2020) Guidelines for opioid prescribing in children and adolescents after surgery: an expert panel opinion. *JAMA Surgery* 156(1), 76–90.

Khoshfetrat, M., Davoodi, R. and Keykha, A. (2018) Comparing the effects of three different doses of ketamine plus bupivacaine on pain control after paediatric surgery. *Biomedical Research and Therapy* **5**(8), 2572–2580.

Kumar, A., Kumar, M., et al. (2019) Comparison between efficacy of single dose caudal ropivacaine and levobupivacaine for post-operative analgesia following infraumbilical surgeries in paediatric patients. *Journal of Evolution of Medical and Dental Sciences* 8(37), 2841–2845.

Kumar, R. and Joshi, D. (2017) Awareness of dental hygiene amongst the primary school children of low socio-economic strata. *International Journal of Contemporary Pediatrics* 4(1), 28–35.

Lisanti, A.J., Demianczyk, A.C., Costarino, A., et al. (2020) Skin-to-skin is a safe and effective comfort measure for infants before and after neonatal cardiac surgery. *Pediatric Critical Care Medicine* 21(9), e834–e841.

Malviya, S., Voepel-Lewis, T., Burke, C., Merkel, S. and Tait, A.R. (2006a) The revised FLACC observational pain tool: improved reliability and validity for pain assessment in children with cognitive impairment. *Paediatric Anaesthesia* 16(3), 258–265.

Malviya, S., Voepel-Lewis, T. and Tait, A. (2006b) A comparison of observational and objective measures to differentiate depth of sedation in children from birth to 18 years of age. *Anaesthesia and Analgesia* 102, 389–394.

Marcelino, R., Sawardekar, A. and Suresh, S. (2019) Neuraxial anaesthesia in paediatrics. *Anaesthesia and Intensive Care Medicine* 20(6), 338–343.

Michelet, D., Andreu-Gallien, J., Bensalah, T., et al. (2012) A meta-analysis of the use of nonsteroidal antiinflammatory drugs for pediatric postoperative pain. *Anesthesia and Analgesia* 114(2), 393–406.

Miller-Hoover, S.R. (2019) Using valid and reliable tools for pain and sedation assessment in pediatric patients. *Critical Care Nurse* 39(3), 59–66.

Mucalo, L., Brandow, A.M., Dasgupta, M., et al. (2021) Comorbidities are risk factors for hospitalization and serious Covid 19 illnesses in children and adults with sickle cell disease. *Blood Advances* 5(13), 2717–2724.

Noah, M. and Walters, B. (2019) The efficacy of ketamine for improvement of postoperative pain control in adolescent patients undergoing spinal fusion surgery for idiopathic scoliosis. *Spine Journal* 19(9), 147–148.

Ocay, D.D., Otis, A., Teles, A.R. and Ferland, C.E. (2018) Safety of patient-controlled analgesia after surgery in children and adolescents: concerns and potential solutions. *Frontiers in Pediatrics* 6, 336.

Palmer, G.M., Alcock, M.A., Schug, S.A., Scott, D.A., Mott, J.F. and Halliwell, R. (2020) *Acute Pain Management: Scientific Evidence*, 5th edn. Volume 2, Paediatrics. Australian and New Zealand College of Anaesthetists and Faculty of Pain Medicine, Melbourne. Available at https://www.anzca. edu.au/resources/college-publications/ acute-pain-management/apmse5.pdf

Pancekauskaite, G. and Jankauskaite, L. (2018) Paediatric pain medicine: pain differences, recognition and coping acute procedural pain in paediatric emergency room. *Medicina (Kaunas)* 54(6), 94.

Persino, P.R., Saleh, L. and Walner, D.L. (2017) Pain control following tonsillectomy in children: a survey of patients. *International Journal of Pediatric Otorhinolaryngology* 103, 76–79.

Pope, N., Tallon, M., McConigley, R., Leslie, G. and Wilson, S. (2017) Experiences of acute pain in children who present to a healthcare facility for treatment: a systematic review of qualitative evidence. *JBI Database of Systematic Reviews and Implementation Reports* 15(6), 1612–1644.

Rabbitts, J.M., Palermo, T.M. and Lang, E.A. (2020) A conceptual model of biopsychosocial mechanisms of transition from acute to chronic postsurgical pain in children and adolescents. *Journal of Pain Research* 13, 3071–3081.

Roberts, K., Bridle, M. and McLuckie, D. (2020) Enhanced recovery after surgery in paediatrics: a review of the literature. *Brittish Journal of Anaesthesia* 20(7), 235–241.

Robinson, P.S. and Green, J. (2015) Ambient versus traditional environment in pediatric emergency department. *HERD: Health Environments Research and Design Journal* 8(2), 71–80.

Rosen, D.M., Alcock, M.M. and Palmer, G.M. (2022) Opioids for acute pain management in children. *Anaesthesia and Intensive Care* 50(1–2), 81–94.

Rosenbloom, B.N., Page, M.G., Isaac, L., et al. (2019) Pediatric chronic postsurgical pain and functional disability: a prospective study of risk factors up to one-year after major surgery. *Journal of Pain Research* 12, 3079–3098.

Royal Children's Hospital (RCH), Melbourne (2021a) Assessment of sensory block. https://www.rch. org.au/anaes/pain_management/Assessment_ of_sensory_block/

Royal Children's Hospital (RCH), Melbourne (2021b) Assessment of motor block. https://www.rch. org.au/anaes/pain_management/Assessment_ of_motor_block/

Rudikoff, A.G., Tieu, D., Banzali, F.M., et.al. (2022) Perioperative acetaminophen and dexmedetomidine eliminate post-operative opioid requirement following pediatric tonsillectomy. *Journal of Clinical Medicine* 11(3), 561.

San Diego Patient Safety Council (2014) Tool Kit: Patient Controlled Analgesia (PCA) Guidelines of Care. https://www.bd.com/documents/ continuing-education/BD_Patient-Safety-Council-PCA-Toolkit_CE_EN.pdf

Schlechter, J.A., Gornick, B.R., Harrah, T. and Sherman, B. (2022) Do continuous peripheral nerve blocks decrease home opioid use following anterior cruciate ligament reconstruction in children and adolescents? The envelope please. *Journal of Pediatric Orthopedics* 42(4), e356–e361.

Schoolman-Anderson, K., Lane, R.D., Schunk, J.E., Mercham, N., Thomas, R. and Adelgais, K. (2018) Pediatric emergency department triage-based pain guideline utilizing intranasal fentanyl: effects of implementation. *Emergency Medicine* 36(9), 1603–1607.

Schug, S.A., Palmer, G.M., Scott, D.A., Alcock, M., Halliwell, R. and Mott, J.F. (2020) *Acute Pain*

Management: Scientific Evidence, 5th edn. Australian and New Zealand College of Anaesthetists and Faculty of Pain Medicine, Melbourne. Available at https://www.anzca.edu.au/resources/college-publications/acute-pain-management/apmse5.pdf (accessed 2 June 2023).

Setlur, A. and Friedland, H. (2018) Treatment of pain with intranasal fentanyl in pediatric patients in an acute care setting: a systematic review. *Pain Management* 8(5), 341–352.

Shinnick, J.K., Short, H.L. and Heiss, K.F. (2016) Enhanced recovery in pediatric surgery: a review of the literature. *Journal of Surgical Research* 202(1), 165–176.

Staveski, S.L., Boulanger, K., Erman, L., et al. (2018) The impact of massage and reading on children's pain and anxiety after cardiovascular surgery: a pilot study. *Pediatric Critical Care Medicine* 19(8), 725–732.

Taddio, A., McMurtry, C.M., Bucci, L.M., et al. (2019) Overview of a knowledge translation (KT) project to improve the vaccination experience at school: the CARD™ system. *Paediatrics and Child Health* 24(Suppl. 1), S3–S18.

Temby, S.E, Palmer, G.M., Penrose, S., Peachey, D.M. and Johnson, M.B. (2021) Implementation of an enhanced recovery pathway in Australia after posterior spinal fusion for adolescent idiopathic scoliosis delivers improved outcomes. *Spine Deformity* 9, 1371–1377.

Varga, A.G., Maletz, S.N., Dossat, A.M., Reid, B.T. and Levitt, E.S. (2022) A neuromodulatory system that links opioid-induced sedation and respiratory depression. *FASEB Journal* 36(S1), R4105.

Verhoeven, K., Goubert, L., Jaaniste, T., Van Ryckeghem, D.M. and Crombez, G. (2012) Pain catastrophizing influences the use and the effectiveness of distraction in schoolchildren. *European Journal of Pain* 16(2), 256–267.

Vittinghoff, M., Lonnqvist, P., Mossetti, V., et al. (2018) Postoperative pain management in children: guidance from the Pain Committee of the European Society for Paediatric Anaesthesiology (ESPA Pain Management Ladder Initiative). *Pediatric Anesthesia* 28(6), 493–506.

World Health Organization (2020) *Guidelines on the Management of Chronic Pain in Children*. WHO, Geneva. Available at https://www.who.int/publications/i/item/9789240017870

Wright, J., Louttit, E., Pasternak, E., Madison, M.S. and Spruit, J. (2021) Pain management in pediatrics. *Advances in Family Practice Nursing* 3, 195–214.

8 The Prevention and Treatment of Neuropathic and Visceral Pain

Krista Baerg and Giulia Mesaroli

This chapter defines and describes the main types of neuropathic and visceral pain experienced by children and young people (CYP). The approaches to assessment and the current evidence-based methods for treating and preventing these types of pain are also discussed.

Neuropathic Pain

Neuropathic pain is pain caused by a lesion or disease of the central or peripheral somatosensory nervous system (International Association for the Study of Pain (IASP) 2017). Neuropathic pain is one of three pain mechanisms (neuropathic pain, nociplastic pain, nociceptive pain) recognised by the IASP (2017).

- Neuropathic pain can be acute or chronic (persistent or recurrent for longer than three months) (Scholz et al. 2019).
- It may radiate or travel along a neuroanatomical pathway.
- It is secondary to an underlying neurological lesion (e.g. abnormal diagnostic imaging or obvious trauma) or disease (e.g. stroke, metabolic and genetic disorders) (IASP 2017).

- The onset and location of pain and sensory signs are consistent with the neurological lesion or disease (Scholz et al. 2019).
- Neuropathic pain is classified as central (originating from damage to the brain or spinal cord) or peripheral (originating from damage to the peripheral nerve, plexus, dorsal root ganglion or nerve root) (Scholz et al. 2019).

CYP with neuropathic pain:

- often describe the quality of pain as burning, tingling, pins and needles, shooting, sharp or more sensitive to touch (Askew et al. 2016; McCarthy and Rastogi 2017; Yeung et al. 2017)
- report that pain may be spontaneous or evoked by movement or touch (Scholz et al. 2019)
- often have other changes in sensation in the painful area (e.g. allodynia, paraesthesia, dysaesthesia, hyperalgesia or hyperpathia)
- depending on the underlying cause, other neurological changes may be present (e.g. numbness or weakness).

Managing Pain in Children and Young People: A Clinical Guide, Third Edition. Edited by Alison Twycross, Jennifer Stinson, William T. Zempsky, and Abbie Jordan.

An overview of common terms used to describe sensory changes associated with neuropathic pain is provided in Table 8.1.

Causes of Neuropathic Pain

Neuropathic pain accounts for 10–30% of CYP attending paediatric pain clinics (Walker 2020). However, the prevalence of neuropathic pain in children is unknown (McCarthy and Rastogi 2017; Morgan and Anghelescu 2017).

Causes of neuropathic pain are generally categorised by the level of the lesion or disease within the somatosensory nervous system (Table 8.2). This classification system is intended to be comprehensive, but some neurological lesions or diseases are relatively uncommon in CYP (e.g. trigeminal neuralgia, post-herpetic neuralgia) (Headache Classification Committee 2018; Weinmann et al. 2019). Another method of classification is by the type of disease (e.g. cancer, genetic, infectious) or type of trauma (e.g. postsurgical).

Conditions of the Central Nervous System

Central neuropathic pain arises from damage or disease to the CNS including the brain and spinal cord. Pain and sensory signs are present in the body

Table 8.1 Terms used to describe sensory changes that may be associated with pain.

Term	Definition
Allodynia	Pain due to a stimulus that does not generally provoke pain
Hyperalgesia	Increased pain from a stimulus that generally provokes pain
Hypoalgesia	Diminished pain in response to a generally painful stimulus
Hyperaesthesia	Increased sensitivity to stimulation, excluding the special senses
Hypoaesthesia	Decreased sensitivity to stimulation, excluding the special senses
Hyperpathia	A painful syndrome characterised by an abnormally painful reaction to a stimulus, particularly a repetitive stimulus, as well as an increased threshold
Paraesthesia	An abnormal sensation that is not unpleasant (e.g. pins and needles), which may be spontaneous or evoked
Dysaesthesia	An unpleasant abnormal sensation (e.g. shooting, tingling sensations), which may be spontaneous or evoked

Source: IASP (2017).

Table 8.2 Classification of neuropathic pain by level of lesion or disease in the somatosensory nervous system.

Origin	Classification
Central nervous system	Brain injury
	Spinal cord injury
	Central post-stroke pain
	Multiple sclerosis
Peripheral nervous system	Painful polyneuropathy
	Post amputation
	Peripheral nerve injury
	Painful radiculopathy
	Trigeminal neuralgia
	Post-herpetic neuralgia

Source: Scholz et al. (2019).

corresponding to the CNS lesion or disease (Scholz et al. 2019). An overview of the clinical presentation of some CNS conditions that can cause neuropathic pain in CYP can be found in Table 8.3.

Conditions of the Peripheral Nervous System

Peripheral neuropathic pain may involve one or more peripheral or cranial nerves, nerve plexus or roots, dorsal root ganglia or cranial nerve ganglia (World Health Organization (WHO) 2020a). Pain and sensory signs are experienced in the anatomical region corresponding to the peripheral nervous system injury or disease (Scholz et al. 2019).

An overview of peripheral neuropathic pain conditions, their presentation and common causes is provided in Table 8.4. Additional details regarding common causes of peripheral neuropathic pain conditions in CYP are presented in Table 8.5.

Table 8.3 Examples of central neuropathic pain.

Central nervous system condition	Example
Traumatic brain injury (TBI)	Approximately 24% of CYP with TBI develop chronic pain. This may result from a combination of pain mechanisms (neuropathic, nociplastic and nociceptive); the prevalence of neuropathic pain is not defined (Tham et al. 2013)
Spinal cord injury (SCI)	Examples include syringomyelia, spinal cord tumour, spina bifida or traumatic spinal cord injury (Sandoval-Garcia and Iskandar 2020). Syringomyelia is caused by a syrinx or fluid-filled cavity within the spinal cord that progressively expands and may lead to neurological deficits. Syringomyelia has been identified in almost 25% of CYP with Chiari I malformation (Sandoval-Garcia and Iskandar 2020)
Stroke	Central post-stroke pain can develop when stroke involves the thalamus or spino-thalamic tract (Hauer and Houtrow 2017; Scholz et al. 2019)

Table 8.4 Peripheral neuropathic pain conditions in children and young people.

Classification	Clinical presentation	Common causes
Painful polyneuropathy: pain associated with damage or disease of multiple peripheral nerves	Pain and burning sensation in the hands or feet as well as tingling or numbness. Often associated with impaired temperature sensation and autonomic function due to small-fibre involvement (Misra et al. 2008)	Neurotoxic drugs, metabolic disorders, genetic disorders (e.g. Fabry disease, Charcot–Marie–Tooth), autoimmune disorders (e.g. Guillain–Barré syndrome), infectious diseases (e.g. HIV), toxins (e.g. arsenic) (Kliegman et al. 2011; Scholz et al. 2019; Walker 2020)
Post-amputation pain: pain associated with damage of the peripheral nerves at the site of amputation	Pain may be in the residual limb or be phantom limb pain. Pain onset is often within the first week after amputation and persists beyond 1 year in 10–38% (DeMoss et al. 2018)	Prevalence of neuropathic pain after amputation is 3.7–20% for congenital amputations, 12–83% for trauma and 48–90% in paediatric oncology (DeMoss et al. 2018)
Painful peripheral neuropathy: pain associated with damage or disease to a peripheral nerve	Painful area follows the pattern of a peripheral nerve distribution and is typically associated with negative sensory signs (e.g. hypoaesthesia, hypoalgesia) (Scholz et al. 2019)	Peripheral nerve injuries in CYP are most commonly due to glass and knife lacerations or complicated fractures (Costales et al. 2019)

Table 8.4 (Continued)

Classification	Clinical presentation	Common causes
Painful radiculopathy: pain caused by a lesion or disease involving the cervical, thoracic, lumbar or sacral nerve roots	Pain is often triggered by a particular movement and follows a dermatomal distribution (Scholz et al. 2019)	Some common causes include degenerative diseases of the spine, trauma (e.g. disc herniation, after injection therapy or surgery), tumour and infection (e.g. discitis, meningitis) (Scholz et al. 2019)

Table 8.5 Examples of peripheral neuropathic pain.

Example	Description
Chemotherapy-induced polyneuropathy	Chemotherapy-induced polyneuropathy is the most common cause of painful polyneuropathy in CYP, affecting 2–40% of CYP receiving chemotherapy (Smith et al. 2020)
Fabry disease	Fabry disease is an X-linked disease with median age of onset of 6 years in boys. Girls may have classic features but onset is slightly later (Germain et al. 2019)
Erythromelalgia	Pain and heat in the hands or feet are most commonly triggered by heat or exercise and refractory to multiple treatments. Nearly half of young people with inherited erythromelalgia report symptom onset before age 6 years (McDonnell et al. 2016). Small-fibre dysfunction has been demonstrated in CYP with inherited erythromelalgia (Leroux 2018; Arthur et al. 2019).

Visceral Pain

Visceral pain is pain that originates from internal organs of the head or neck region and the thoracic, abdominal or pelvic cavities (Aziz et al. 2019). Visceral pain occurs because the viscera are innervated by sensory afferent nerves extending to the spinal cord.

Visceral pain:

- can be acute or chronic (Aziz et al. 2019);
- is perceived as a deep, vague or poorly localised midline pain
- may be classified as primary or secondary pain
- is typically related to nociplastic or nociceptive mechanisms, or both (Aziz et al. 2019).

CYP with visceral pain may also experience referred pain (described below) and may experience associated symptoms such as cramping, nausea, vomiting, pallor, sweating, dizziness or emotional reactions (e.g. distress and anxiety) (Aziz et al. 2019).

Referred pain describes pain originating in the visceral organ but experienced in another area, such as the abdominal wall, shoulder or jaw (Aziz et al. 2019). Referred pain may occur when somatic nerves are supplied by the same neurosegment as the sensory nerves from the affected organ. Physical examination of the somatic tissues in the referred area may demonstrate pain or sensory signs such as hyperaesthesia, hyperalgesia or allodynia (Aziz et al. 2019).

The classification of visceral pain is outlined in Table 8.6.

Causes of Visceral Pain in CYP

Abdominal pain is the most common type of visceral pain in childhood (Aziz et al. 2019;

Table 8.6 Classification of visceral pain.

Classification	Description
Acute visceral pain	Sharp or intense visceral pain with sudden onset. Related to activation of nociceptors due to tissue injury caused by disease, trauma, surgery, interventions or disease treatments (IASP 2021)
Chronic secondary visceral pain	Persistent or recurrent pain that lasts 3 months or more in a distinct anatomical location compatible with typical referral patterns from specific internal organs, and history compatible with dysfunction or disease. Primarily related to activation of nociceptive pain mechanisms: persistent inflammation, mechanical (e.g. traction, obstruction) or vascular (ischaemia and thrombosis) (Aziz et al. 2019)
Chronic primary visceral pain	Persistent or recurrent pain that lasts 3 months or more that is believed to originate from the internal organs but is not better accounted for by a diagnosis of secondary visceral pain after appropriate medical investigation. Associated with emotional distress or interference with physical or social function. Primarily related to nociplastic pain mechanisms (Aziz et al. 2019)

Table 8.7 Causes of acute and chronic visceral pain in children and young people by body region.

Body region	Examples
Head and neck	Tonsillitis
Thorax	Oesophagitis
Abdomen	Appendicitis
	Bowel obstruction
	Meckel diverticulitis
	Gastroenteritis
	Henoch–Schönlein purpura
	Mesenteric adenitis
	Coeliac disease
	Peptic ulcer disease
	Inflammatory bowel disease (IBD)
	Pancreatitis
	Gallstones
	Renal stones
	Constipation
	Abdominal pain syndromes (e.g. irritable bowel syndrome (IBS) and abdominal migraine)[a]
Pelvis	Primary dysmenorrhoea[a]
	Endometriosis
	Urinary tract infection
	Ovarian cyst
	Pelvic inflammatory disease
	Pelvic pain syndrome[a]
Any region	Sickle cell vaso-occlusive crisis
	Surgery
	Trauma
	Systemic lupus erythematosus
	Cancer (tumours)

[a], chronic primary visceral pain disorders.
Sources: Tsao and Tinsley Anderson (2017); Aziz et al. (2019).

Treede et al. 2019). Information about the common causes of acute and chronic visceral pain in CYP is provided in Table 8.7.

Acute visceral pain (e.g. acute abdominal pain) may be due to surgical and non-surgical conditions. Examples include (Kim 2013; Raymond et al. 2022):

- acute appendicitis
- abdominal trauma
- intussusception
- gastroenteritis
- constipation
- mesenteric adenitis.

PRACTICE POINT

- Acute appendicitis is the most common surgical cause of acute abdominal pain in CYP.
- Acute appendicitis often presents with vague visceral pain in the periumbilical area. As inflammation progresses, the pain becomes parietal and localises to the right lower quadrant over 6–48 hours.
- Because CYP may have an atypical presentation, consider acute appendicitis in children who present with abdominal pain and vomiting, with or without fever or focal abdominal tenderness.

Sources: Kim (2013); Raymond et al. (2022)

Chronic secondary visceral pain due to persistent inflammation includes conditions such as (Aziz et al. 2019):

- endometriosis
- inflammatory bowel disease (IBD)
- chronic pancreatitis

- systemic lupus erythematosus
- chronic tonsillitis
- post-infective enteropathies
- oesophagitis.

There are consensus guidelines for the treatment of some common conditions associated with chronic secondary visceral pain due to inflammation. However, evidence to support best practice is limited. Additional information for some types of chronic secondary visceral pain conditions due to inflammation can be found in Table 8.8.

Chronic secondary visceral pain due to mechanical obstruction may occur when a hollow viscera is obstructed or with external compression of internal organs. Some examples include obstruction by renal stones or gallstones, and bowel obstruction (Aziz et al. 2019).

Chronic secondary visceral pain due to vascular mechanisms may occur when there is reduced blood flow to the viscera (e.g. vascular disease, hypercoagulability, thrombosis formation). Recurrent crises due to sickle cell disease (SCD) is an example (Aziz et al. 2019). Information about visceral pain in SCD is shown in Box 8.1.

Table 8.8 Chronic secondary visceral pain conditions due to inflammation.

Visceral pain condition	Description
Endometriosis	- Endometriosis affects 15% of menstruating women and is the most common cause of secondary dysmenorrhoea. Secondary dysmenorrhoea refers to painful menses due to pelvic pathology or a recognised medical condition - Endometriosis is considered when clinically significant dysmenorrhoea persists despite treatment with hormonal agents and NSAIDs, and history, physical examination and pelvic ultrasonography do not reveal another cause (ACOG Committee 2018)
Inflammatory bowel disease (IBD)	- In North America, the incidence of IBD in children, including Crohn's disease and ulcerative colitis, is approximately 10 per 100 000 (Mack et al. 2019) - Classic symptoms include weight loss, abdominal pain and bloody diarrhoea, but CYP may also present with poor growth, anaemia or extraintestinal manifestation (Ruemmele et al. 2014; Mack et al. 2019)
Pancreatitis	- Incidence of pancreatitis in children is 12 per 100 000. Most patients have risk factors (e.g. anatomical risk factors, medication triggers, genetic factors) (Uc and Husain 2019) - Acute recurrent pancreatitis is defined as at least two attacks within a year, with at least 1-month pain-free interval between and interval normalisation of lipase/amylase (Párniczky et al. 2018) - Chronic pancreatitis is an irreversible chronic disease, often involving treatment-refractory abdominal pain (Párniczky et al. 2018)

BOX 8.1 PAIN ASSOCIATED WITH SICKLE CELL DISEASE

- SCD is a multisystem disorder associated with acute, chronic and procedural pain due to a wide array of complications.
- Vaso-occlusive crisis is the most common and debilitating manifestation of SCD.

CYP hospitalised with sickle cell vaso-occlusive crisis have been shown to have moderate to severe pain scores throughout hospitalisation despite medication dosing within accepted guidelines.

Sources: Ender et al. (2014); Tanabe et al. (2019)

Assessing Neuropathic and Visceral Pain

As with other forms of pain, a complete assessment should be undertaken to ensure serious conditions (e.g. malignancy, inflammatory conditions, surgical conditions and degenerative disorders) are not missed. Assessment should include the following:

- complete medical history, including history of presenting illness, review of symptoms, past medical and surgical history, family history and medication use.
- complete physical examination, including assessment of general appearance, growth parameters and vital signs.
- review of the results of any past investigations (e.g. blood tests, diagnostic imaging) (Aziz et al. 2019; Scholz et al. 2019).
- multidimensional pain assessment, including:
  - a thorough pain history
  - assessment of the impact of pain on the family and CYP's sleep, mood, school attendance and social function (McCarthy and Rastogi 2017).

PRACTICE POINT

- All children with pain require a comprehensive medical assessment to ensure that a serious underlying condition is not missed.
- Signs and symptoms that could indicate an underlying pathology, or *red flags*, should prompt further investigation to diagnose any underlying disease (Rajindrajith et al. 2018; Frosch et al. 2022).
- Any further investigations or referrals that are indicated to address the CYP's medical condition should be initiated promptly.

More information about the assessment of pain can be found in Chapter 6.

Additional Considerations When Assessing Neuropathic Pain

For some CYP, neuropathic pain may be the first presenting symptom of a neurological disease or

PRACTICE POINT

Some examples of 'red flags' for CYP with back pain

- Young age (under 10 years)
- History of other medical condition (e.g. trauma, glucocorticoid use, exercise-related onset of pain)
- Neurological symptoms (e.g. radicular pain, altered bowel or bladder function, sensory changes)
- Other clinical signs (e.g. fever, hypertension, hypermobility)
- Clinical findings suggestive of malignancy or inflammatory disease
- Abnormal physical examination
- Pain at multiple sites

Source: Adapted from Frosch et al. (2022)

lesion. If a pain history and physical examination suggest possible neuropathic pain (e.g. abnormal neurological examination) but there is no known history of disease or injury, further examination and testing is required.

For CYP with neuropathic pain the following are required for diagnosis (Finnerup et al. 2016):

- *history* of a lesion or disease of the somatosensory nervous system
- *onset* of pain coincides with the onset of the nervous system injury or disease
- *location* of pain and sensory symptoms consistent with the lesion or disease
- *quality* of pain may be described as burning, tingling, pins and needles, shooting or lancinating
- *associated symptoms* may include other sensory symptoms (e.g. numbness)
- pain may *radiate*, or travel, along the neuroanatomical pathway
- *temporally*, the pain may be spontaneous or evoked by movement or touch.

Two self-report pain assessment tools can be used with CYP with cancer-related neuropathic pain:

- Pediatric-Modified Total Neuropathy Score (Schouten et al. 2020; Smith et al. 2020)
- Pediatric Neuropathic Pain Scale©-Five (PNPS©-5) (Lavoie Smith et al. 2015).

There are no validated screening tools to differentiate neuropathic pain symptoms from non-neuropathic pain symptoms in CYP (Morgan and Anghelescu 2017). There are several screening tools developed for use in adults, including:

- PROMIS PQ-Neuro Neuropathic Pain Quality Scale (Askew et al. 2016)

- Self-report Leeds Assessment of Neuropathic Symptoms and Signs (S-LANSS) (Bennett et al. 2005)
- PainDETECT (Freynhagen et al. 2006).

PRACTICE POINT

- Caution should be observed if using these tools with CYP as the patterns of pain experiences and aetiology of neuropathic pain in CYP differs from those in adults.
- A children's specific neuropathic pain screening tool has been developed (Pediatric PainSCAN©), but has not yet been validated (Mesaroli et al. 2021).

CYP with severe neurological impairment may exhibit persistent pain behaviours such as irritability and agitation. The term 'neuro-irritability' may be used if no source of pain is identified and treatment of potential nociceptive sources is unhelpful (Hauer and Houtrow 2017). Differentiating neuropathic pain from neuro-irritability pain presents a clinical challenge when caring for non-verbal CYP (Friedrichsdorf 2015).

During the neurological examination special attention should be paid to:

- cognitive and emotional function
- fundoscopic examination and assessment of cranial nerves
- sensation
- coordination
- tendon and plantar reflexes
- muscle power, tone and bulk
- any abnormal movements (e.g. dystonia)
- dysmorphic features or neurocutaneous changes (e.g. café au lait spots, ash leaf spots).

When conducting a sensory examination in the area of pain, always explain to the CYP what to expect and start in an area where sensation is normal to determine the baseline (McCarthy and Rastogi 2017). The aim of bedside sensory testing is to determine whether there are differences in sensation in the painful area (pain, increased or decreased sensation, or other abnormal sensations). Some practical tips for carrying out a bedside sensory examination are described below.

PRACTICE POINT

- Bedside sensory examinations commonly include touch using a cotton ball or tissue, and pin prick using a pin or toothpick.
- Additional, but less common, examination tools include vibration (tuning fork) and warm or cold temperature (metal, tube of water or wet cloth).
- Bedside sensory testing should look for qualitative differences between affected and non-affected body regions.

It is helpful to refer to the appropriate neuro-anatomical pattern of associated sensory signs (e.g. for lesions of a peripheral nerve, reference a peripheral nerve map; for lesions of the spinal cord, reference a dermatome map). The sensory examination should map the location of pain and sensory signs and compare this to known neuro-anatomical patterns (see Table 8.9 for examples), including:

- dermatomes
- peripheral nerve map
- stocking–glove pattern

PRACTICE POINT

If a CYP has pain, a relevant neurological lesion or disease, and the location of pain is consistent with the neuroanatomical pattern of the nerve lesion or disease, they are likely to have neuropathic pain.

- cranial nerve pattern.

As part of the diagnostic process, tests will need to be carried out. These may include:

- diagnostic tests to confirm the lesion or disease
- nerve conduction studies and electromyography (EMG)
- disease-specific tests (e.g. MRI, genetic testing)
- enables the measurement of changes in sensitivity to different types of sensations such as temperature, touch or pressure (https://www.gosh.nhs.uk/conditions-and-treatments/procedures-and-treatments/quantitative-sensory-testing/).
- can be performed on CYP as young as five years but requires specific expertise and is not available in all clinical settings (McCarthy and Rastogi 2017; Morgan and Anghelescu 2017)
- Other tests should be carried out as needed to support diagnosis and prognostication.

Additional Considerations When Assessing Visceral Pain

For some CYP, visceral pain may be the first presenting symptom of visceral dysfunction or disease. If a pain history and physical examination suggest possible visceral pain but there is no known diagnosis, further examination and testing is required to ensure that a serious underlying condition which requires medical or surgical treatment is not missed.

Signs and symptoms that could indicate an underlying pathology or 'red flags' for CYP with visceral pain should prompt further investigation (Devanarayana and Rajindrajith 2018; Rajindrajith et al. 2018).

Table 8.9 Common patterns of neuropathic pain and sensory signs.

Neuropathic pain condition	Neuroanatomically plausible distribution of pain and sensory signs	Illustration of typical distribution
Trigeminal neuralgia	Within the facial or intraoral trigeminal territory	
Post-herpetic neuralgia	Unilaterally distributed in one or more spinal dermatomes or the trigeminal ophthalmic division	
Peripheral nerve injury pain	In the innervation territory of the lesioned nerve, typically distal to a trauma, surgery or compression	
Post-amputation pain	In the missing body part and/or in the residual limb	
Painful polyneuropathy	In feet, may extend to involve lower legs, thighs and hands	
Painful radiculopathy	Distribution consistent with the innervation territory of the nerve root	
Neuropathic pain associated with spinal cord injury	At and/or below the level of the spinal cord lesion	
Central post-stroke pain	Contralateral to the stroke. In lateral medullary infarction, the distribution can also involve the ipsilateral side of the face	
Central neuropathic pain associated with multiple sclerosis	Can be a combination of distributions seen in spinal cord injury and stroke	

Source: Reproduced with permission from Finnerup et al. (2016).

PRACTICE POINT

Examples of 'red flags' for CYP with abdominal pain

- Unexplained fever
- Growth failure (e.g. involuntary weight loss, slowed linear growth, delayed puberty)
- Significant vomiting or diarrhoea
- Gastrointestinal bleeding
- Persistent localised tenderness in right upper or lower quadrant
- Perirectal disease
- Difficult or painful swallowing
- Arthritis
- Family history of bowel disease (e.g. IBD, coeliac disease, peptic ulcer disease)

Sources: Adapted from Rajindrajith et al. (2018); Devanarayana and Rajindrajith (2018)

PRACTICE POINT

The HEEADSSS assessment is one screening approach that can be helpful in assessing for psychosocial risk factors.

- Home
- Education/employment
- Eating
- Activities
- Drugs
- Sexuality
- Suicide/depression
- Safety

Source: McCarthy and Rastogi (2017)

Exposure to traumatic life events (e.g. physical, sexual or emotional abuse) affects pain severity and perpetuation (Rajindrajith *et al.* 2018). Approximately 20% of women with chronic abdominal or pelvic pain report past history of abuse during childhood (McCarthy and Rastogi 2017). When assessing visceral pain, older CYP should also be interviewed on their own to assess for psychosocial risk factors and safety (e.g. HEEADSSS Assessment Guide) (McCarthy and Rastogi 2017). For CYP, special attention should be made to reviewing their psychosocial risk factors (including sexual history) in a safe space with active listening technique (McCarthy and Rastogi 2017). To ensure patient safety, follow professional and jurisdictional requirements for reporting of child maltreatment.

When taking a pain history with a CYP with visceral pain, you may find:

- *onset* of pain may be associated with menarche, onset of systemic disease, or an inciting event such as trauma, infection or medication use (Aziz et al. 2019)
- *location* of pain is consistent with the anatomical location of an organ or expected location for referred pain from an organ (Aziz et al. 2019)
- *quality* of pain is consistent with the cause (mechanical, inflammatory, vascular) (Aziz et al. 2019)
- *associated symptoms* such as diarrhoea, constipation, nausea, fatigue, loss of appetite, cramping, bowel or voiding symptoms, dyspareunia or low back pain (Devanarayana and Rajindrajith 2018; Rajindrajith *et al.* 2018)
- *temporally* pain may be related to eating, bowel movements or menstrual cycles (Devanarayana and Rajindrajith 2018; Rajindrajith *et al.* 2018)

pain progression may follow a classic pattern, e.g. the pain of appendicitis is initially felt in the periumbilical area but later, with illness progression, it may be felt in the right lower quadrant (Raymond et al. 2022).

Physical examination of the head, neck, thorax, abdomen and, if applicable, the pelvis or perianal area is required to assess visceral pain (Raymond et al. 2022). The examination should determine if tenderness is present at the anatomical location of visceral origin. In the area of referred pain, hyperaesthesia (superficial or deep), hyperalgesia or allodynia may be present (Aziz et al. 2019).

CASE STUDY: PART 1

Sarah is a 12-year-old female with osteosarcoma in her left proximal tibia. She is scheduled for surgical resection in six months. She is complaining of pain and burning on the outer area of her leg, around the area of the tumour and down the side of her leg to her foot. Having reviewed an approach to assessing neuropathic pain, reflect on the following.

1. What questions do you want to ask Sarah about her pain and sensation?
2. How would you approach a sensory examination?
3. What neuroanatomical pattern might her pain and sensory symptoms follow?

Treatments for Neuropathic and Visceral Pain

When treating neuropathic or visceral pain, a multimodal approach combining pharmacological approaches and physical and psychological interventions is needed (Harrison et al. 2019) (see Chapter 1). Multimodal approaches to the treatment of nociceptive and chronic pain are outlined in Chapters 7 and 9–11, respectively.

Since neuropathic and visceral pain may have multiple aetiologies and the pathophysiology differs based on the underlying cause, no single treatment is effective in all cases. Once there is an explanation for the pain, joint goal setting with the CYP and family should be undertaken. When co-producing a clinical plan, remember:

- treatment is aimed at managing pain and associated symptoms as well as reducing pain-related disability
- when possible, disease-modifying treatments should be provided with pathophysiology guiding treatment
- neuropathic pain may be from more than one source alongside nociceptive pain
- the need for close follow-up to monitor for response and adverse events (Scottish Government 2018)
- at follow-up, decisions about whether to continue treatment should be based on outcome measures, such as pain intensity and functional outcomes (Baumbauer et al. 2016)
- new symptoms or changes in pattern of illness require assessment as further investigations may be warranted
- CYP with pain conditions should continue to have regular care for comorbid medical conditions.

The current evidence available to inform treatment is very limited, with many studies being of low quality (Birnie et al. 2020; WHO 2020b). Very few studies focus specifically on neuropathic or visceral pain. Guidelines and systematic reviews of the literature have identified the need for more research. See

Chapter 1 for more details about the physical and psychological strategies used to manage CYP's pain.

Physical Interventions

The main aim of physical interventions is to optimise CYP's participation in functional activities (e.g. attending school and participating in sport and leisure activities) and focus on developing self-management strategies (Scottish Government 2018).

To achieve these aims, it is often useful to involve (Kempert et al. 2017; Harrison et al. 2019):

- occupational therapists to focus on participation in activities of daily living (e.g. school and leisure activities)
- physiotherapists (physical therapists) to focus on the CYP's mobility and participation in physical activity.

Despite the lack of evidence to guide treatment, physical interventions are seen as essential components of treatment of CYP with neuropathic or visceral pain. The interventions with some, albeit limited, evidence to support their use in practice are highlighted in Box 8.2.

Psychological Interventions

Psychological therapies remain a cornerstone of multimodal pain management, although more research is needed in this area. Psychological interventions can be delivered face to face or online (Scottish Government 2018; Birnie et al. 2020; WHO 2020b). These interventions help CYP with neuropathic or visceral pain to manage and cope with their pain. Examples of psychological pain-relieving interventions which have evidence to support their use are listed in Box 8.3.

BOX 8.2   PHYSICAL STRATEGIES FOR MANAGING NEUROPATHIC AND VISCERAL PAIN

- Individualised exercise programmes targeting physical impairments (Scottish Government 2018; Harrison et al. 2019; WHO 2020b)
- Daily physical activity (Scottish Government 2018)
- Relaxation (Scottish Government 2018)
- Transcutaneous electrical nerve stimulation (TENS) (Scottish Government 2018)
- Activity pacing (Kempert 2021)
- Mirror therapy has limited evidence supporting its use for phantom limb pain (Moseley 2006; Anghelescu et al 2016).
- Graded motor imagery (Moseley 2006)
- Passive modalities, including massage therapy and acupuncture (Tsao 2007; Golianu et al. 2014)

BOX 8.3   COMMON PSYCHOLOGICAL INTERVENTIONS FOR CHRONIC PAIN SELF-MANAGEMENT[a]

- Acceptance and commitment therapy
- Biofeedback
- Cognitive behavioural therapy (CBT): small case studies suggest there may be benefit from CBT and hypnotherapy for young people with IBD, but results are mixed for mindfulness-based therapies (Person and Keefer 2019)
- Distraction
- Exposure-based therapies
- Hypnotherapy: gut-directed hypnotherapy relies on induction of the hypnotic state and post-hypnotic suggestions aimed to reduce frequency and intensity of gastrointestinal pain, normalise bowel activity and increase the CYP's overall sense of physical well-being (Palsson and Ballou 2020)

- Mindfulness
- Psychotherapy: has been used in paediatric phantom limb pain with success but prospective controlled trials are necessary (DeMoss et al. 2018)
- Sleep hygiene strategies

a As recommended by Scottish Government (2018), Birnie et al. (2020) and WHO (2020b)

CASE STUDY: PART 2

Sarah is having trouble coping with her cancer diagnosis and her pain. She doesn't want to see her friends and avoids them at school. When she walks, she is limping and avoids putting weight on her left leg. Her leg is sensitive to touch, so she won't let the bed sheets touch her leg, and it takes her a long time to fall asleep at night. Having reviewed evidence-based approaches to multimodal treatment, reflect on the following.

1. What physical interventions may help her cope with her pain?
2. What strategies might help her fall asleep at night?
3. What psychological strategies might help her cope with her pain and engage socially?

Pharmacological Interventions

The use of pharmacological interventions for chronic pain are only recommended as part of a wider supported self-management approach (Scottish Government 2018; WHO 2020b). Current recommendations include:

- short courses of paracetamol and/or NSAIDs are recommended (Scottish Government 2018)

- adjuvant analgesics may act as primary analgesics in the treatment of neuropathic and chronic visceral pain (Friedrichsdorf and Goubert 2020)
- 5% lidocaine patches may be used in the management of CYP with localised neuropathic pain (Scottish Government 2018)
- a few case reports suggest potential benefit from neuromodulation for neuropathic pain in young people, but there are confounding factors and mixed results and a need for quality evidence (Tyagi et al. 2016; Kim and Cucchiaro 2017; Kim et al. 2018)
- for chronic non-cancer pain, opioids should only be used for appropriate indications and prescribed and monitored by trained providers, after weighing benefits and risks; a clear plan for continuation, tapering or discontinuation of opioids is recommended (Scottish Government 2018; WHO 2020b).

Suggested pharmacological interventions for specific diseases are outlined in Table 8.10. An overview of the pharmacology of commonly used analgesics and adjuvant medications is provided in Chapter 5. Details of drug dosages are given in the Appendix.

CASE STUDY: PART 3

Sarah has been using a multimodal approach to pain management, and her mood and physical function are improving. Her pain and sensory signs are persistent, and she rates her pain intensity on average 6/10 on the numerical pain rating scale. She sometimes uses paracetamol and ibuprofen, but they don't seem to help much.

1. What analgesic drugs would you prescribe/administer for Sarah?
2. Are there any side effects you need to consider?

Table 8.10 Disease-specific guidelines for pharmacological treatment.

Type of pain	Recommended pharmacological treatment
Primary dysmenorrhea	■ NSAIDs are most effective if started 1–2 days before onset of menses and continued for the first 2–3 days afterwards ■ The efficacy and safety means ibuprofen is recommended as the optimal over-the-counter analgesic for primary dysmenorrhea (Nie et al. 2020) ■ Opioids are not recommended (ACOG Committee 2018; Sauvan et al. 2018)
Acute pancreatitis	■ For mild pain, scheduled paracetamol and ibuprofen are recommended and the oral route is preferred, if tolerated ■ For moderate or severe pain, a strong opioid is necessary and intramuscular routes should be avoided (Abu-El-Haija et al. 2018)
Chronic pancreatitis	■ Non-opioid analgesics are recommended as the first line of therapy ■ Centrally acting agents (e.g. gabapentin) are also commonly prescribed (Párniczky et al. 2018) ■ Intercostal and coeliac plexus blocks have been used for chest pain and pancreatitis (Drewes et al. 2017)
Sickle cell disease (SCD)	■ Health professionals caring for CYP with SCD should become familiar with local guidelines and follow established protocols to ensure timely assessment (and reassessment) and initiation of acute pain management and supportive care (National Institute for Health and Care Excellence 2017; Brandow et al. 2020)

Spiritual Considerations

A correlation between spiritual coping and quality of life in CYP with chronic illness has been established (Friedrichsdorf and Goubert 2020). Recognising and respecting diverse spiritual, religious and cultural differences, the healthcare practitioner is advised to explore lifestyle strategies and consider with the CYP and family an approach that supports their overall well-being.

Summary

- Neuropathic pain occurs in a subset of CYP with lesions or diseases of the peripheral or central nervous system.
- Sensory assessments are an important component of a comprehensive pain assessment for neuropathic pain.
- Visceral pain arises from the internal organs of the head or neck region and the thoracic, abdominal or pelvic cavities.
- Abdominal pain is the most common visceral pain in CYP.
- Treatment of visceral and neuropathic pain in CYP uses a multimodal approach, including pharmacological, physical and psychological interventions.

Key to Case Study

Part 1

1. You may want to ask Sarah when the pain started, where the pain is, what it feels like, how it changes over the course of the day, and if she has any other symptoms in the painful area (e.g. numbness). To help her explain the pain location, you can use a body diagram, and Sarah can draw the distribution of her pain. She may use different colours to show different types of pain.
2. First, provide instructions to Sarah so she knows what to expect. You may use a soft item (e.g. cotton ball) and a sharp item (e.g. toothpick). Apply the textures to the affected side and the unaffected side and assess for qualitative differences. Classify any sensory changes noted in the affected area (see Table 8.1).
3. Based on the description of the pain location, the peroneal nerve may be affected.

Part 2

1. An individualised exercise programme with regular activity tailored to her ability and interests is recommended (e.g. swimming, yoga). The programme should be paced to avoid exacerbating her pain and allow for gradual progression. If she finds warmth soothing, she might use a warm bath in the evening or after activity to soothe her pain while relaxing. Consultation with a local physiotherapist may be helpful in determining if she might benefit from TENS for pain management or a mobility aid to support social engagement.

2. First-line approach would include sleep hygiene strategies (e.g. keeping a regular bedtime schedule and routine). If sleep does not improve, she may benefit from CBT.
3. A first-line approach to pain management will include pain education (psychoeducation). Referral to a health psychologist for CBT may also be helpful for supporting pain management and coping. A school meeting may be helpful for encouraging school attendance and for devising a modified plan that will support both academic and social goals at school. Sarah may need a quiet place to rest at school.

Part 3

1. A pain modulator for neuropathic pain may be more helpful for Sarah's tumour-related pain than paracetamol and ibuprofen, such as amitriptyline at bedtime to help with pain and sleep. Gabapentin may be added during the day. Medication counselling will include off-label use and potential risks and benefits.
2. Gabapentin may increase appetite so it will be important to counsel her on healthy eating and portion sizes. Gabapentin may cause daytime sleepiness, which may impact focus at school and safety when operating equipment. Both medications may cause a dry mouth so it may be helpful for her to carry a water bottle. Consultation with a local pain physician or clinical pharmacist may be helpful as medication will require titration and monitoring for side effects.

Multiple Choice Questions

1. Which one of the following statements describing neuropathic pain is true?
   a. Neuropathic pain may be due secondary to an underlying neurological lesion or disease
   b. Neuropathic pain is always chronic, lasting longer than three months
   c. Neuropathic pain is classified according to the level of the neurological lesion or disease (central or peripheral)
   d. All children and young people with neurological injury or disease will experience neuropathic pain
   e. (a) and (c)

2. When assessing neuropathic pain in children and young people, which one of the following statements is false?
   a. Pain often described as a dull ache
   b. Pain can be evoked or spontaneous
   c. Pain is in a region corresponding with a nerve lesion or disease
   d. Changes in sensation may be present in the painful area (such as allodynia or hyperalgesia)

3. What is the correct definition of visceral pain?
   a. Pain that spreads from one visceral organ to another visceral organ
   b. Pain that originates in a visceral organ but is experienced in a different area of the body

   c. Pain that originates from a visceral organ but spreads to a larger area
   d. Pain in the viscera that is evoked by activity

4. What might you find when taking a history of a child or young person with visceral pain?
   a. Pain described in the area of the visceral organ may radiate distally
   b. Onset of pain coincides with onset of tissue trauma or disease in the viscera (e.g. infection)
   c. Pain often described as numbness and tingling
   d. Pain is often triggered by activity and relieved with rest
   e. (a) and (b)

5. Which of the following statements regarding management of visceral pain in children and young people is true?
   a. Psychological interventions are only indicated when there is no underlying pathology
   b. Physical and psychological interventions should be initiated when disease-modifying medications fail
   c. Multimodal treatment, including disease-modifying medications, aim to manage pain and symptoms
   d. Physical interventions include activity pacing, ice/heat, acceptance and commitment therapy

Acknowledgements

Dr Megan Crone, Division of Pediatric Neurology, University of Saskatchewan reviewed an earlier version of neuropathic pain content in this chapter. Dr David Burnett, Assistant Professor, Division of Pediatric Gastroenterology, Hepatology and Nutrition, University of Saskatchewan reviewed an earlier version of visceral pain content this chapter.

ADDITIONAL RESOURCES

- American Academy of Pediatrics, Section on Integrative Medicine (2016) Mind–body therapies in children and youth. *Pediatrics* 138(3), e20161896. doi: 10.1542/peds.2016-1896
- Facial Pain Association: `https://fpa-support.org/`
- Genetic and Rare Diseases Information Center: `https://rarediseases.info.nih.gov`
- Hereditary Neuropathy Foundation: `https://www.hnf-cure.org/`

References

Abu-El-Haija, M., Kumar, S., Quiros, J.M., et al. (2018) Management of acute pancreatitis in the pediatric population: a clinical report from the North American Society for Pediatric Gastroenterology, Hepatology and Nutrition Pancreas Committee. *Journal of Pediatric Gastroenterology and Nutrition* 66(1), 159–176.

ACOG Committee (2018) Opinion No. 760. Summary: dysmenorrhea and endometriosis in the adolescent. *Obstetrics and Gynecology* 132(6), e249–258.

Anghelescu, D.L., Kelly, C.N., Steen, B.D., et al. (2016) Mirror therapy for phantom limb pain at a pediatric oncology institution. *Rehabilitation Oncology* 34(3), 104–110.

Arthur, L., Keen, K., Verriotis, M., et al. (2019) Pediatric erythromelalgia and SCN9A mutations: systematic review and single-center case series. *Journal of Pediatrics* 206, 217–224.e9.

Askew, R.L., Cook, K.F., Keefe, F.J., et al. (2016) A PROMIS measure of neuropathic pain quality. *Value in Health* 19(5), 623–630.

Aziz, Q., Giamberardino, M.A., Barke, A., et al. (2019) The IASP classification of chronic pain for ICD-11: chronic secondary visceral pain. *Pain*, 160(1), 69–76.

Baumbauer, K.M., Young, E.E., Starkweather, A.R., Guite, J.W., Russell, B.S. and Manworren, R.C.B. (2016) Managing chronic pain in special populations with emphasis on pediatric, geriatric, and drug abuser populations. *Medical Clinics of North America* 100(1), 183–197.

Bennett, M.I., Smith, B.H., Torrance, N. and Potter, J. (2005) The S-LANSS score for identifying pain of predominantly neuropathic origin: validation for use in clinical and postal research. *Journal of Pain* 6(3), 149–158.

Birnie, K.A., Ouellette, C., Do Amaral, T. and Stinson, J.N. (2020) Mapping the evidence and gaps of interventions for pediatric chronic pain to inform policy, research, and practice: a systematic review and quality assessment of systematic reviews. *Canadian Journal of Pain* 4(1), 129–148.

Brandow, A.M., Carroll, C.P., Creary, S., et al. (2020) American Society of Hematology 2020 guidelines for sickle cell disease: management of acute and chronic pain. *Blood Advances* 4(12), 2656–2701.

Costales, J.R., Socolovsky, M., Lázaro, J.A.S. and García, R.A. (2019) Peripheral nerve injuries in the pediatric population: a review of the literature. Part I: traumatic nerve injuries. *Child's Nervous System* 35(1), 29–35.

DeMoss, P., Ramsey, L.H. and Karlson, C.W. (2018) Phantom limb pain in pediatric oncology. *Frontiers in Neurology* 9, 219.

Devanarayana, N.M. and Rajindrajith, S. (2018) Irritable bowel syndrome in children: current knowledge, challenges and opportunities. *World Journal of Gastroenterology* 24(21), 2211–2235.

Drewes, A.M., Bouwense, S.A.W., Campbell, C.M., et al. (2017) Guidelines for the understanding and management of pain in chronic pancreatitis. *Pancreatology* 17(5), 720–731.

Ender, K., Krajewski, J.A., Babineau, J., et al. (2014) Use of a clinical pathway to improve the acute management of vaso-occlusive crisis pain in pediatric sickle cell disease. *Pediatric Blood and Cancer* 61, 693–696.

Finnerup, N.B., Haroutounian, S., Kamerman, P., et al. (2016) Neuropathic pain: an updated grading system for research and clinical practice. *Pain* 157(8), 1599–1606.

Freynhagen, R., Baron, R., Gockel, U. and Tölle, T.R. (2006) painDETECT: a new screening questionnaire to identify neuropathic components in patients with back pain. *Current Medical Research and Opinion* 22(10), 1911–1920.

Friedrichsdorf, S. (2015) Advanced management of neuropathic pain in pediatric palliative care: the concept of multimodal analgesia (SA544). *Journal of Pain and Symptom Management* 49(2), 403.

Friedrichsdorf, S.J. and Goubert, L. (2020) Pediatric pain treatment and prevention for hospitalized children. *Pain Reports* 5(1), e804.

Frosch, M., Mauritz, M.D., Bielack, S., et al. (2022) Etiology, risk factors, and diagnosis of back pain in children and adolescents: evidence- and consensus-based interdisciplinary recommendations. *Children (Basel, Switzerland)* 9(2), 192.

Germain, D.P., Fouilhoux, A., Decramer, S., et al. (2019) Consensus recommendations for diagnosis, management and treatment of Fabry disease in paediatric patients. *Clinical Genetics* 96(2), 107–117.

Golianu, B., Yeh, A.M. and Brooks, M. (2014) Acupuncture for pediatric pain. *Children (Basel, Switzerland)* 1(2), 134–148.

Harrison, L.E., Pate, J.W., Richardson, P.A., Ickmans, K., Wicksell, R.K. and Simons, L.E. (2019) Best-evidence for the rehabilitation of chronic pain. Part 1: pediatric pain. *Journal of Clinical Medicine* 8(9), 1267.

Hauer, J. and Houtrow, A.J. (2017) Pain assessment and treatment in children with significant impairment of the central nervous system. *Pediatrics* 139(6), e20171002.

Headache Classification Committee (2018) *The International Classification of Headache Disorders*, 3rd edn. Available at https://ichd-3.org/ (accessed 25 September 2020).

International Association for the Study of Pain (2017) Terminology. Available at https://www.iasp-pain.org/resources/terminology/ (accessed 30 November 2021).

International Association for the Study of Pain (2021) What is acute pain? Available at https://www.iasp-pain.org/resources/topics/acute-pain/ (accessed 26 May 2023).

Kempert, H. (2021) Teaching and applying activity pacing in pediatric chronic pain rehabilitation using practitioner feedback and pace breaks. *Pediatric Pain Letter* 23(2), 31–42.

Kim, E. and Cucchiaro, G. (2017) Unique considerations in spinal cord stimulator placement in pediatrics: a case report. *A&A Case Reports* 9(4), 112–115.

Kim, E., Gamble, S., Schwartz, A. and Cucchiaro, G. (2018) Neuromodulation in pediatrics: case series. *Clinical Journal of Pain* 34(11), 983–990.

Kim, J.S. (2013) Acute abdominal pain in children. *Pediatric Gastroenterology, Hepatology and Nutrition* 16(4), 219–224.

Kliegman, R.M., Stanton, B.M.D., St. Geme, J., Schor, N.F. and Behrman, R.E. (2011) *Nelson Textbook of Pediatrics*, 19th edn. Elsevier Health Sciences Division, Philadelphia, PA.

Lavoie Smith, E.M., Li, L., Chiang, C., et al. (2015) Patterns and severity of vincristine-induced peripheral neuropathy in children with acute lymphoblastic leukemia. *Journal of the Peripheral Nervous System* 20(1), 37–46.

Leroux, M.B. (2018) Erythromelalgia: a cutaneous manifestation of neuropathy? *Anais Brasileiros de Dermatologia* 93(1), 86–94.

McCarthy, K.F. and Rastogi, S. (2017) Complex pain in children and young people. Part I: assessment. *BJA Education* 17(10), 317–322.

McDonnell, A., Schulman, B., Ali, Z., *et al.* (2016) Inherited erythromelalgia due to mutations in SCN9A: natural history, clinical phenotype and somatosensory profile. *Brain* 139(4), 1052–1065.

Mack, D.R., Benchimol, E.I., Critch, J., et al. (2019) Canadian Association of Gastroenterology Clinical Practice Guideline for the medical management of pediatric luminal Crohn's disease. *Journal of the Canadian Association of Gastroenterology* 2(3), e35–e63.

Mesaroli, G., Campbell, F., Hundert, A., et al. (2021) Development of a screening tool for pediatric neuropathic pain and complex regional pain syndrome: Pediatric PainSCAN. *Clinical Journal of Pain* 38(1), 15–22.

Misra, U.K., Kalita, J. and Nair, P.P. (2008) Diagnostic approach to peripheral neuropathy. *Annals of the Indian Academy of Neurology* 11(2), 89–97.

Morgan, K.J. and Anghelescu, D.L. (2017) A review of adult and pediatric neuropathic pain assessment tools. *Clinical Journal of Pain* 33(9), 844–852.

Moseley, G.L. (2006) Graded motor imagery for pathologic pain: a randomized controlled trial. *Neurology* 67(12), 2129–2134.

National Institute for Health and Care Excellence (2017) Sickle cell disease: acute painful episode overview. Available at https://pathways.nice.org.uk/pathways/sickle-cell-disease-acute-painful-episode

Nie, W., Xu, P., Hao, C., Chen, Y., Yin, Y. and Wang, L. (2020) Efficacy and safety of over-the-counter analgesics for primary dysmenorrhea: a network meta-analysis. *Medicine (Baltimore)* 99(19), e19881.

Palsson, O.S. and Ballou, S. (2020) Hypnosis and cognitive behavioral therapies for the management of gastrointestinal disorders. *Current Gastroenterology Reports* 22(7), 31.

Párniczky, A., Abu-El-Haija, M., Husain, S., et al. (2018) EPC/HPSG evidence-based guidelines for the management of pediatric pancreatitis. *Pancreatology* 18(2), 146–160.

Person, H. and Keefer, L. (2019) Brain–gut therapies for pediatric functional gastrointestinal disorders and inflammatory bowel disease. *Current Gastroenterology Reports* 21(4), 12.

Rajindrajith, S., Zeevenhooven, J., Devanarayana, N.M., Perera, B.J.C. and Benninga, M.A. (2018) Functional abdominal pain disorders in children. *Expert Review of Gastroenterology and Hepatology* 12(4), 369–390.

Raymond, M., Marsicovetere, P. and DeShaney, K. (2022) Diagnosing and managing acute abdominal pain in children. *Journal of the American Academy of Physician Assistants* 35(1), 16–20.

Ruemmele, F.M., Veres, G., Kolho, K.L., et al. (2014) Consensus guidelines of ECCO/ESPGHAN on the medical management of pediatric Crohn's disease. *Journal of Crohn's and Colitis* 8(10), 1179–1207.

Sandoval-Garcia, C. and Iskandar, B. (2020) Syringomyelia in children. International Society for Pediatric Neurosurgery. Available at https://www.ispn.guide/congenital-disorders-of-the-nervous-system-in-children/syringomyelia-in-children-homepage/ (accessed 11 November 2020).

Sauvan, M., Chabbert-Buffet, N., Geoffron, S., Legendre, G., Wattier, J.M. and Fernandez, H. (2018) Management of painful endometriosis in adolescents: CNGOF-HAS Endometriosis Guidelines. *Gynecologie, Obstetrique, Fertilite et Senologie* 46(3), 264–266.

Scholz, J., Finnerup, N.B., Attal, N., et al. (2019) The IASP classification of chronic pain for ICD-11: chronic neuropathic pain. *Pain* 160(1), 53–59.

Schouten, S.M., van de Velde, M.E., Kaspers, G.J.L., et al. (2020) Measuring vincristine-induced peripheral neuropathy in children with cancer: validation of the Dutch pediatric-modified Total Neuropathy Score. *Supportive Care in Cancer* 28(6), 2867–2873.

Scottish Government (2018) *Management of Chronic Pain in Children and Young People: A National Clinical Guideline.* Scottish Government, Edinburgh. Available at http://www.gov.scot/Resource/0053/00533194.pdf.

Smith, E.M.L., Kuisell, C., Kanzawa-Lee, G.A., et al. (2020) Approaches to measure paediatric chemotherapy-induced peripheral neurotoxicity: a systematic review. *Lancet Haematology* 7(5), e408–e417.

Tanabe, P., Spratling, R., Smith, D., Grissom, P. and Hulihan, M. (2019) CE: understanding the complications of sickle cell disease. *American Journal of Nursing* 119(6), 26–35.

Tham, S.W., Palermo, T.M., Wang, J., et al. (2013) Persistent pain in adolescents following traumatic brain injury. *Journal of Pain* 14(10), 1242–1249.

Treede, R.D., Rief, W., Barke, A., et al. (2019) Chronic pain as a symptom or a disease: the IASP Classification of Chronic Pain for the International Classification of Diseases (ICD-11). *Pain* 160(1), 19–27.

Tsao, J.C.I. (2007) Effectiveness of massage therapy for chronic, non-malignant pain: a review. *Evidence-based Complementary and Alternative Medicine* 4(2), 165–179.

Tsao, K. and Tinsley Anderson, K. (2017) Evaluation of abdominal pain in children. *BMJ Best Practice.* Available at https://bestpractice.bmj.com/topics/en-us/787/

Tyagi, R., Kloepping, C. and Shah, S. (2016) Spinal cord stimulation for recurrent tethered cord syndrome in a pediatric patient: case report. *Journal of Neurosurgery Pediatrics* 18(1), 105–110.

Uc, A. and Husain, S.Z. (2019) Pancreatitis in children. *Gastroenterology* 156(7), 1969–1978.

Walker, S.M. (2020) Neuropathic pain in children: steps towards improved recognition and management. *EBioMedicine* 62, 103124.

Weinmann, S., Naleway, A.L., Koppolu, P., et al. (2019) Incidence of herpes zoster among children: 2003–2014. *Pediatrics* 144(1), e20182917.

World Health Organization (2020a) *International Classification of Diseases*, 11th revision. WHO, Geneva. Available at `https://icd.who.int/en` (accessed 28 February 2021).

World Health Organization (2020b) *Guidelines on the Management of Chronic Pain in Children*. WHO, Geneva. Available at `https://www.who.int/publications/i/item/9789240017870`

Yeung, K.-K., Engle, L., Rabel, A., Keith Adamson, K., Schwellnus, H. and Evans, C. (2017) It just feels weird!: a qualitative study of how children aged 10–18 years describe neuropathic pain. *Disability and Rehabilitation* 39(17), 1695–1702.

9 Musculoskeletal Pain in Children and Young People

Sara Klein, Karen Chiu, Jacqui Clinch, and Christina Liossi

Musculoskeletal (MSK) pain is common in children and young people (CYP). The World Health Organization (WHO) Global Burden of Disease project indicated that MSK conditions, particularly back and neck pain, are responsible for around 10% of years lived with disability among 15–19 year olds, and 5% in 10–14 year olds (WHO 2015). When MSK pain persists and/or becomes widespread, it can have a detrimental impact on physical and psychological well-being, along with how CYP function and participate in social, academic and family settings (Baweja and Walco 2020).

Patients can experience a lengthy search for diagnosis and effective treatment, often seeing multiple health professionals and specialists, undergoing many investigations and receiving several diagnoses (Kaufman and Sherry 2017). This challenging and difficult cycle can increase vulnerability for the CYP to overuse medication and result in numerous trips to the emergency department, thereby creating a drain on family and healthcare resources (Fleegler and Schecter 2015; Kaufman and Sherry 2017).

This chapter reviews the epidemiology of specific types of MSK pain common to CYP, exploring contributing factors and the impact on various aspects of their lives. We describe the general characteristics of MSK pain and discuss chronic widespread pain (CWP) and complex regional pain syndrome (CRPS). Recommendations for assessment and treatment with a focus on a biopsychosocial approach to care, including multidisciplinary rehabilitation and self-management, are also discussed.

What is Musculoskeletal Pain?

MSK pain is defined as pain coming from MSK structures, such as muscles, ligaments, bones, tendons or joints. It can be localised to the limbs or spine, or it can be widespread and in multiple locations. Chronic MSK pain is persistent pain that has lasted longer than three months or longer than what would be expected for a particular condition. The International Association for the Study of Pain (IASP) differentiates between chronic primary and secondary MSK pain (Figures 9.1 and 9.2). IASP acknowledges that chronic MSK pain can be a primary disorder and a condition in its own right where there is not an identifiable underlying disease process or injury that is causing the pain. This type of pain is often associated with impact on physical and psychological function (Nicholas et al. 2019). Examples of chronic primary MSK

Managing Pain in Children and Young People: A Clinical Guide, Third Edition. Edited by Alison Twycross, Jennifer Stinson, William T. Zempsky, and Abbie Jordan.

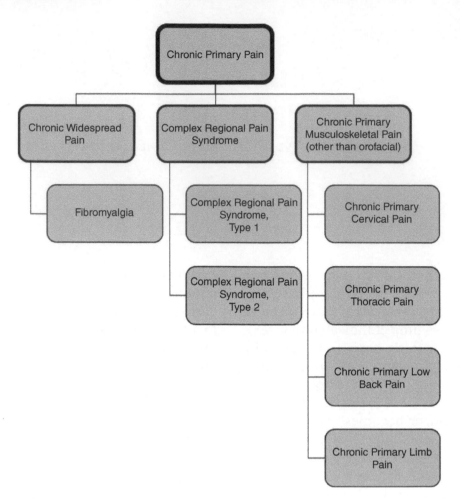

Figure 9.1 Classification of chronic primary pain.

Source: Adapted with permission from the IASP (Nicholas et al. 2019).

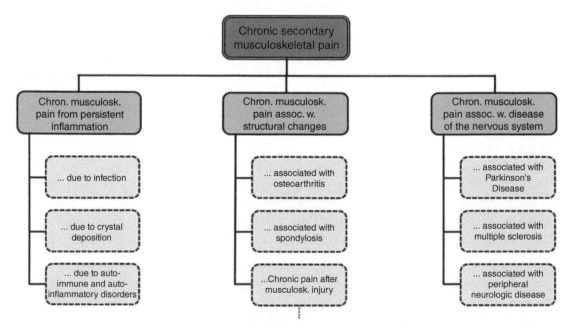

Figure 9.2 Classification of chronic secondary MSK pain.

Source: Adapted with permission from the IASP (Perrot et al. 2019).

pain are chronic low back pain and primary limb pain.

Chronic secondary MSK pain is chronic pain in the MSK structures that arises from an underlying disease (Perrot et al. 2019). Chronic secondary MSK pain can arise in soft tissue, joints, bones, tendons or spine, and may be related to either localised or systemic conditions or deep somatic lesions. There are three main causes for chronic secondary MSK pain:

- persistent inflammation related to an underlying inflammatory condition, such as juvenile idiopathic arthritis (JIA)
- local MSK structural changes related to osteoarthritis or fracture where there may be bony deformities
- diseases of the nervous system (e.g. cerebral palsy), where there may be altered motor and sensory function.

Epidemiology and Presentation of MSK Pain for CYP

Estimates of the prevalence of MSK pain in CYP vary.

- The European Agency for Safety at Work (EU-OSHA 2021) found the prevalence of MSK pain to be around 30% among CYP aged 7–26.5 years, with a slightly higher rate of 34% for those aged 15–32 years. However, the report notes that estimates vary greatly between individual studies (0.5–91.0%).
- A study exploring MSK pain in six-year-old children found a three-month prevalence of 10%, of which one-third was chronic pain, with 45% also experiencing pain at other sites (van den Heuvel et al. 2020).
- Another study found that there were 28.6 million visits over a nine-year period

for chronic MSK pain for people under the age of 25 years, equating to an average of 3.2 million visits per year across the USA (Feldman and Nahin 2021).

Table 9.1 shows common types of chronic MSK pain that are found in CYP, which may be either chronic primary or secondary conditions.

Impact of MSK Pain

Pain has a widespread impact on the lives of CYP, affecting physical, psychological, social, developmental and familial functioning. Pain frequently impairs CYP's concentration, mood, anxiety and sleep, in addition to engagement with school and sports (Andreucci et al. 2021; Pourbordbari et al. 2022). CYP who experience persistent MSK pain have an increased likelihood of developing CWP and pain-associated disability in adult life (Walker et al. 2010; Kamper et al. 2016a).

Clinical Features of Chronic MSK Pain

Chronic MSK pain:

- often starts in a localised area of the body and may intensify and radiate to other areas;
- is often associated with hypervigilance to the affected area and reluctance to mobilise due to fear of discomfort and pain.

CYP may guard or protect, or avoid use or contact with affected areas, leading to stiffness, muscular spasms, abnormal posture and gait, and ultimately greatly reduced fitness. This cycle of avoidance can lead to fear of pain and movement, and subsequently amplification of the pain experience (Asmundson et al. 2012).

Table 9.1 Common types of chronic MSK pain in CYP.

Type of MSK pain	Description
Generalised joint hypermobility (GJH)	▪ School-aged children with complaints of joint pain ▪ Normal examination plus findings of joint laxity ▪ Not all patients with joint laxity complain of pain ▪ Typically present after increased activity or end of day ▪ Typically present in bilateral limbs and often found in lower extremity, mainly knees ▪ Common in children under 8 years old affecting 13–20% in some populations (Sperotto et al. 2015) ▪ Hypermobility in joints is scored using the Beighton scale (see Figure 9.3). Tobias et al. (2013) found that young people with a Beighton score greater than 6 at 13.8 years had increased pain at 17.8 years
Benign limb pain of childhood	▪ Lower extremity pain of unknown cause that is typically present in school-aged children with intermittent bilateral hip, calf, thigh or posterior knee pain ▪ Examination is typically normal ▪ May be described as deep, achy, severe ▪ Resolves with rest ▪ Affects up to 49% of children aged 4–14 years (Weiss and Stinson 2018)
Overuse syndromes	▪ Skeletal immaturity combined with high-intensity physical training can cause strain on tendons and MSK structures (Weiss and Stinson 2018) ▪ Common conditions: Osgood–Schlatter disease, Sever's disease, patellofemoral pain syndrome
Juvenile idiopathic arthritis (JIA)	▪ JIA is characterised by recurrent flares or chronic joint inflammation and stiffness ▪ Many CYP experience pain despite adequate medication to manage disease activity; predictors of pain include genetics, negative emotions, family dynamics and parental distress (Brandelli et al. 2023)
Back pain	▪ Less common in younger children but prevalence increases with age and by age 20, 70–80% would have experienced at least one episode of back pain ▪ Most cases are unspecific low back pain related to sprain, strain or muscle spasm (8.9%), scoliosis (4.6%), spondylolysis or spondylolisthesis (< 1%) (Weiss and Stinson 2018)

In some cases, e.g. when there is an inciting event or an underlying disease, pain may start as a result of activation of nociceptive pathways – a protective response to a noxious stimulus. With repeated exposure to the painful stimulus over time, or with activation of the pain pathways for an extended period of time, a phenomenon known as central sensitisation may occur. If central sensitisation occurs there is a heightened state of sensitivity of the central nervous system, resulting in a decreased threshold for activation of the pain pathways. This can result in allodynia, hyperalgesia and secondary hyperalgesia (i.e. increased pain sensitivity outside the area of injury or inflammation; Latremoliere and Woolf 2009). See Chapter 3 for definitions of these terms.

Although a highly heterogeneous population, associated symptoms and signs of chronic MSK pain in CYP include the following:

▪ Greater hypervigilance and pain sensitivity than expected from a given physical trigger (O'Sullivan et al. 2011; Ocay et al. 2022).

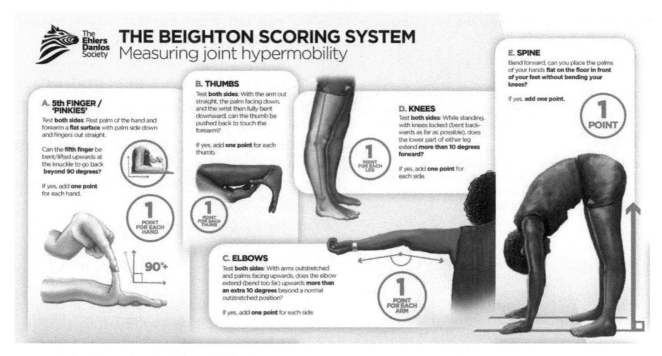

Figure 9.3 How to use the Beighton scoring system to measure joint hypermobility.

Source: Infographics from the Ehlers–Danlos Society, `https://www.ehlers-danlos.com/assessing-joint-hypermobility/`

- Perceived thermodysregulation where limbs may be cool and mottled (Geisser et al. 2003).
- Autonomic dysfunction where pain can heighten sympathetic nervous system activity, with tachycardia, hyperventilation (compounded with panic attacks), cold sweats, blurred vision, abdominal pain and extreme pallor (Evans et al. 2013).
- MSK disequilibrium where MSK pain can permanently affect positioning. With reduced proprioceptive signals from the joints, limbs are held in a fixed position, affecting gait. Resultant asymmetry can lead to other vulnerable bodily sites taking an altered load, causing further discomfort. Over time, affected limbs may adopt flexed positions and tightened soft tissue structures, further exaggerating imbalance and pain (Caes et al. 2018).

Risk Factors for Chronic MSK Pain

Research has examined factors that influence the development and persistence of chronic MSK pain. These include:

- female gender (Kamper et al. 2016b; Kløven et al. 2017)
- having a physical disability (Grøholt et al. 2003)
- living in a low-educated and/or low-income family (Huguet et al. 2016; Andias and Silva 2022)
- being an adolescent, particularly an older adolescent (Kamper et al. 2016a)
- living with common symptoms, such as joint pain, headaches and abdominal pain, which are linked with a moderately increased risk of CWP in adulthood (Jones et al. 2007)
- family history of MSK pain conditions (Dario et al. 2019).

Table 9.2 Common emotional and cognitive aspects of MSK pain.

Factor	Detail
Depressive or anxiety disorder	A bidirectional relationship has been found between MSK pain, depression and anxiety (Cunningham et al. 2015)
Pain catastrophising	Pain catastrophising of the CYP and their parent/carer is associated with maladaptive pain-related outcomes (Miller et al. 2018; Dougherty et al. 2021)
Behavioural avoidance	Common pain avoidant behaviours include lack of engagement in an activity and avoiding specific behaviours due to fear of pain or injury. Avoidance is a crucial factor in the onset and maintenance of pain-related disability, contributing to the cycle of pain, catastrophising and fear (Volders et al. 2015)

Psychological Aspects of Chronic MSK Pain

Negative cognitions and psychological distress frequently coexist with chronic MSK pain in CYP. Common emotional and cognitive aspects of MSK pain in CYP are presented in Table 9.2.

Complex Regional Pain Syndrome and Chronic Widespread Pain

In 2019, IASP revised its definitions to include a more comprehensive definition of pain. In this revision, CRPS and CWP were removed from under the umbrella of chronic MSK pain (Nicholas et al. 2019). They are now each defined as a primary pain condition. We define CRPS and CWP here but emphasise that they are not currently considered MSK pain diagnoses.

Complex Regional Pain Syndrome

CRPS is a pain condition characterised by a collection of pain symptoms, often in a limb, that increases with movement. The Budapest Criteria is a tool to help facilitate an accurate diagnosis (Harden et al. 2010; see Table 9.3),

Table 9.3 Budapest criteria for clinical diagnosis of CRPS.

1. Continuing pain, which is disproportionate to any inciting event

2. Must report at least one symptom in three of the four following categories:
   - *Sensory*: hyperalgesia and/or allodynia
   - *Vasomotor*: temperature asymmetry and/or skin colour changes and/or skin colour asymmetry
   - *Sudomotor/oedema*: oedema and/or sweating changes and/or sweating asymmetry
   - *Motor/trophic*: decreased range of motion and/or motor dysfunction (weakness, tremor, dystonia) and/or trophic changes (hair, nail, skin)

3. Must display at least one sign at time of evaluation in two or more of the following categories:
   - *Sensory*: evidence of hyperalgesia (to pin-prick) and/or allodynia (to light touch and/or deep somatic pressure and/or joint movement)
   - *Vasomotor*: evidence of temperature asymmetry and/or skin colour changes and/or asymmetry
   - *Sudomotor/oedema*: evidence of oedema and/or sweating changes and/or sweating asymmetry
   - *Motor/trophic*: evidence of decreased range of motion and/or motor dysfunction (weakness, tremor, dystonia) and/or trophic changes (hair, nail, skin)

4. There is no other diagnosis that better explains the signs and symptoms

Source: Adapted from Harden et al. (2010).

although it has yet to be validated for use with CYP. In this condition, there may be fear of pain with movement of the painful body part. This can cause sequelae, such as loss of range of motion, abnormal posturing and functional impairment.

There are two types of CRPS.

- CRPS type 1 occurs after an injury or trauma to the body but without any findings of nerve lesions; sometimes there can be no injury present at all. It is most commonly observed in young girls and in the lower limb (Weissmann and Uziel 2016).
- CRPS type 2 occurs after damage to a nerve (Weiss and Stinson 2018).

Type 1 is more common in CYP, with the prevalence being 1.2 per 100 000 in children 5–15 years old (Weiss and Stinson 2018). The clinical presentations of CRPS type 1 and type 2 are similar, with the primary distinguishing factor being the mechanism of the pain. Differentiating the subtypes does not change the therapeutic approach (Harden et al. 2022). In CRPS, CYP may report burning, shooting or electrical pain, most often in a limb. They may display muscle atrophy or weakness as well as autonomic and trophic changes to the limb, for example swelling, shiny skin, hair or nail changes, and mottled skin colour. Motor symptoms include decreased range of motion but could also involve dystonia, tremors or jerks (Weiss and Stinson 2018).

PRACTICE POINT

To make a diagnosis of CRPS, the signs and symptoms cannot be better explained by any other disease or condition.

Chronic Widespread Pain

The mechanism of pain is nociplastic – the pain messages are not a sign of underlying damage or tissue injury but rather due to an altered pain messaging system (Kashikar-Zuck and Ting 2014). Pain is typically present in four out of five body regions (upper and lower left and right, and axial skeleton) and in at least three body quadrants (Kashikar-Zuck and Ting 2014). It is associated with fatigue, cognitive dysfunction and mood issues (e.g. anxiety and depression). The prevalence of CWP in CYP is 7–15% and is seen mostly in young females (Arnold et al 2019). Central sensitisation is hypothesised to be the underlying mechanism for this condition.

Diagnosing, Assessing and Treating Chronic Musculoskeletal Pain

History-taking

One objective of taking a thorough pain history is to determine if there are comorbid conditions or organic causes of the pain, which is essential to making the diagnosis. Recognising the biopsychosocial model and the multiple dimensions that create the pain experience, the clinician should ask a series of questions related to school, sleep, mood and participation in physical and social activities to better understand the impact of pain on function and quality of life. It is also important to identify red flags, including symptoms of malignancy, trauma or infection, and advise immediate medical attention. Table 9.4 provides a list of suggested questions in reference to the biopsychosocial framework when taking a history from a CYP presenting with MSK pain.

Table 9.4 Considerations for taking history in the context of MSK pain.

Consideration	Questions to ask
How is the pain characterised?	Use 'PQRST' ■ *Provoking and relieving*: What makes the pain better or worse? ■ *Quality*: How would you describe the pain? ■ *Region and radiation*: What body part or areas are painful? ■ *Severity*: How would you rate the pain: now, lowest, worst? How much does the pain bother you? How does your pain impact your daily activities? ■ *Time*: Are there times in the day when the pain is better or worse?
Associated symptoms	■ Does the painful area look swollen, discoloured or have nail or hair changes? ■ Is the painful area sensitive to touch? ■ Nausea, vomiting, light-headedness, vision changes, weakness, fatigue? ■ Rashes, fever, weight loss, night sweats? ■ Gastrointestinal symptoms? ■ Upper or lower respiratory tract symptoms? ■ Changes in bowel or bladder function?

Biological factors	■ What medications are you taking?
	■ Have you had previous injuries or illness?
	■ Is there a family history of related conditions:
	  ■ Ankylosing spondylitis/axial spondyloarthropathy, reactive arthritis, rheumatoid arthritis
	  ■ Inflammatory bowel disease
	  ■ Psoriasis
	  ■ Chronic pain back, fibromyalgia, CRPS

Psychological factors	■ What are your sleep routines? ■ How would you describe your mood? ■ How would the parents/caregivers describe the CYP's personality? ■ Are there identifiable stressors in school, family or peer group?
Social factors	■ Do you like school? How do you perform in school? ■ What activities do you like to do? ■ Do you spend time with friends or family?
Environmental factors	■ Have there been any recent significant events or life changes? ■ Who do you live with at home? ■ How do you navigate your home, neighbourhood or school environments?

CASE STUDY: PART 1

Samantha is a 15-year-old female who presents with chronic right ankle pain, one year post lateral ankle sprain. Imaging including X-ray, ultrasound and MRI are all normal. She reports sharp and achy pain in the ankle joint as well as pain in the toes and calf. She was previously a high-performing athlete who puts a lot of pressure on herself to do well in school and sports. She has a history of generalised anxiety disorder. Samantha explains that her treatments to date include taking paracetamol when she is in pain, which is daily, and physiotherapy that includes massage, laser and ultrasound treatments. She does not currently have any formal psychological intervention.

1. What questions would you ask about Samantha's pain and symptoms to help determine what type of pain she has?
2. What questions would you ask to help determine how much her pain is impacting her function?

Assessment of Musculoskeletal Pain

MSK pain in CYP has historically been measured using self-reported pain scales (e.g. numerical and visual analogue scales). These provide a subjective measure of pain intensity. However, they do not capture the impact of pain on physical, psychological and social functioning. Consequently, multidimensional tools have been developed and validated in CYP with chronic pain conditions; some examples include the following:

- Bath Adolescent Pain Questionnaire (BAPQ) designed for young people with chronic pain, which has been validated in rheumatology and pain management clinics (Eccleston et al. 2005).
- Patient Reported Outcomes Measurement Information System (PROMIS®) with seven domains studied in CYP aged 8–17 years with chronic MSK pain: Pain Interference, Fatigue, Anxiety, Depression, Mobility, Upper Extremity Function and Peer Relationships (Kashikar-Zuck et al. 2016).
- Pediatric Quality of Life Inventory (PedsQL), which has been validated in paediatric chronic health conditions (Varni et al. 1999).

More detailed information on pain assessment is provided in Chapter 6.

After obtaining a thorough history of the CYP's pain experience, a physical examination should be conducted to complete the comprehensive pain assessment. Findings from the subjective history and physical examination will formulate the diagnosis and guide effective treatment planning. The paediatric Gait Arms Legs Spine (pGALS) is a simple and validated MSK examination to screen for abnormal joints, alignment, gait or motor milestones. pGALS is commonly used in paediatric rheumatology and is crucial for the early diagnosis of rheumatic diseases in CYP (Foster and Jandial 2013).

ADDITIONAL INFORMATION

More information about pGALS can be found in the article by Foster and Jandial (2013), available at `https://ped-rheum.biomedcentral.com/articles/10.1186/1546-0096-11-44`

Other common assessment tools include the Beighton scoring system to measure for generalised joint hypermobility (Figure 9.3) and the Budapest criteria for clinically diagnosing CRPS (Table 9.3). During a MSK focused physical examination, clinicians should observe for signs of deconditioning, muscular imbalances, altered gait mechanics, abnormal postures and compensations that may be organic or related to disuse, overprotection or fear of pain and movement. It is important to note that focusing on functional movements shifts the focus from a test to regular daily tasks (e.g. walking, sit to stand, donning and doffing shoes, or picking up an object from the ground), which may reduce hypervigilance to pain and sensations during movement.

CASE STUDY: PART 2

With further questioning, you determine that Samantha's functional pain-related disability is quite high. She is missing two to three days of school per week, misses six out of ten social opportunities, takes two hours to fall asleep and has stopped all sports. She is tearful when she talks about not being able to be on her basketball team as this was previously a large part of her identity and socialisation. She denies any numbness, tingling or burning and has no sensitivity to light touch.

She denies any changes in hair growth, nail growth or skin.

1. What would your physical assessment entail?
2. What would you rule in/rule out?
   On observation, Samantha stands with 75% of her weight on her left side. Comparison of her bilateral lower extremities displays decreased muscle bulk in her right gastrocnemius muscle compared to left. There is no swelling, redness or skin changes. She has poor active and passive range of motion of her right ankle joint and toes and is grimacing a lot as she moves. She does not have any allodynia or hyperalgesia in the right lower extremity. She does have tenderness to palpation over the right ankle joint and Achilles.
3. What is your pain diagnosis?
4. How would you explain this to the patient and family?

Treatment of Chronic Musculoskeletal Pain

The multidisciplinary approach to chronic pain treatment, which acknowledges the biopsychosocial model and addresses the biological, psychological and social factors contributing to pain and disability, has been shown to be the most effective approach to treating chronic MSK pain. There is a role for pharmacology when prescribed alongside physical and psychological rehabilitation with the view of promoting function, although there are limited high-quality trials to support use of analgesics or interventional treatment for children's chronic MSK pain (Scottish Government 2018).

There is increasing evidence to suggest that the combination of physiotherapy, pain neuroscience education and psychological treatment is more effective in reducing pain and disability than physiotherapy alone (Booth et al. 2017; Scottish Government 2018). The gold standard for chronic pain management is the multidisciplinary '3-P' approach involving pharmacology, physiotherapy and psychology (Fisher et al. 2022). In addition to reducing pain-related disability, treatment should also focus on inclusion of the family to encourage optimal uptake of the treatment plan and address CYP's experiences of medicalisation and preconceived ideas about pain (Scottish Government 2018; Health Standard Organization 2023).

Typically, rehabilitation approaches share features, including:

- pain neuroscience education
- symptom management
- physiotherapy
- psychological therapy
- complementary and alternative therapies.

Early recognition and intervention in an outpatient or inpatient setting is key and typically leads to more positive outcomes. Including parents/carers in treatment is important since optimal CYP functioning has been shown to be associated with changing parent behaviour and responses to their CYP's pain (Gauntlett-Gilbert and Jordan 2020). More information about physical and psychological pain-relieving interventions is provided in Chapter 1.

Pain Neuroscience Education

A first step in rehabilitation is to provide an understanding of how one's body may be working to maintain pain. The goal of education is to teach CYP and families about the basic neuroscience of pain and the differences between acute and chronic pain (Harrison et al. 2019). This can be challenging due to a dominant view that pain in joints and muscles represents a warning sign of disease or abnormality.

Education can reduce fear, providing information to counter CYP's beliefs that symptoms are related to an underlying serious disease. In the case of chronic pain, it is important to reassure that increased pain is not equivalent to greater damage to the body. Use of rhetorical devices (e.g. metaphors, infographics, stories) and explaining the case of phantom limb experiences can challenge the idea that brain signals indicate peripheral damage (Koechlin et al. 2020).

Symptom Management

Physical strategies (e.g. superficial heat applications and cryotherapy) are commonly used for symptom management and pain relief and are recommended in the 2023 Canadian Pain Management Standards (Health Standards Organization 2023). Heat and cold can also be used as an adjunct to exercise therapy. At the physiological level, heat can increase blood flow to the treatment area and increase tissue extensibility, whereas cold can manage oedema and inflammation by reducing blood flow (Malanga et al. 2015). However, no high-quality studies support these treatment modalities.

Physiotherapy

Physical activity and exercise are crucial components in the management of chronic MSK pain (Caes et al. 2018; Scottish Government 2018; Health Standards Organization 2023). Typical physiotherapy treatment, including range of motion exercises, stretching, aerobic and resistance training and motor and postural re-education, can be prescribed to optimise muscular balance and functioning as well as activity participation (Caes et al. 2018). However, most of the recommendations are based on adult populations and there are limited studies that robustly evaluate the effect of physiotherapy in childhood pain conditions. There are no standardised guidelines for exercise or treatment protocols for CYP with chronic MSK pain (Caes et al. 2018).

In one rather dated randomised controlled pilot trial, CYP aged 8–18 years with fibromyalgia experienced significant improvements in physical function, quality of life, symptoms and pain after participating in a 12-week aerobic programme consisting of gentle stretches of the upper and lower body, low-impact aerobic cardio-dance and boxing movements (Stephens et al. 2008).

When initiating treatment, it is helpful to establish a SMART (specific, measurable, attainable, relevant, timely) goal that is functional and meaningful to CYP. With guidance from a physiotherapist, the functional goal can be broken down into achievable short-term goals, and the progression of physical activity should follow a gradual, consistent, graded activity plan (Caes et al. 2018). Research suggests the following.

- In many MSK conditions, increasingly active MSK systems are associated with reductions in muscle spasms and tightening (Cunningham and Kashikar-Zuck 2013).
- Most of the evidence supporting exercise for chronic MSK pain is based on aerobic and resistance exercise studies (Booth et al. 2017).
- Besides potential gains in physical performance, gradual exposure to exercise is beneficial in reducing maladaptive cognitions such as pain catastrophising, kinesiophobia and fear of pain (Booth et al. 2017).
- Where possible, CYP should devise their own fitness plan related to daily enjoyable activities rather than exercising in a hospital gym, and be encouraged to participate in self-management strategies (Scottish Government 2018; Health Standards Organization 2023).

■ Promotion of self-management can have a positive impact on self-efficacy and return to function and hence there is an emphasis on active over passive treatments (Harrison et al. 2019).

Graded Exercise

For CYP with myalgic encephalomyelitis/chronic fatigue syndrome (ME/CFS) or post-acute COVID sequelae (long COVID), graded exercise is no longer recommended as it has been shown to make symptoms worse over time (National Institute for Health and Care Excellence 2021a,b). For other CYP with MSK pain (Kempert 2021):

■ a graded exercise plan should identify a baseline level of activity and gradually increase intensity each week

■ it is imperative for clinicians and parents to reinforce activity pacing and coping skills (see section Psychological treatments) for self-management and continued functioning despite pain

■ graded exercise programmes implemented with pacing are an effective strategy for helping to minimise entrapment in an overactivity–underactivity cycle, also referred to as the boom or bust cycle

■ if the CYP experiences post-exertional malaise or symptom exacerbation, there needs to be a plan to maintain gentle activities at a reduced intensity

■ although the definition of activity pacing varies, many agree that pacing involves balancing activity and rest based on a plan rather than symptoms, breaking down tasks, and bringing awareness to one's posture and body mechanics.

In cases where there are structural changes in bone or joint, contractures or joint hypermobility, physiotherapists or occupational therapists may recommend splints or foot orthoses (Dunbar et al. 2017; Health Standards Organization 2023). However, these strategies should not be used in isolation, but in combination with graded exercise and physical activity, with the goal of eventually weaning off additional supports. While research supports the use of splints for joint protection, pain reduction and improving function for adults with rheumatoid arthritis, there are no known studies that have investigated the use of splints in CYP with chronic pain (Caes et al. 2018). Further, the potential risks of long-term immobilisation and range restriction must be considered and such supports prescribed at the discretion of the multidisciplinary team.

PRACTICE POINT

■ Physiotherapy is a key component of the interdisciplinary treatment of chronic MSK pain. However, there is a lack of research on CYP.

■ Treatment planning is based on the SMART goal that is functional and meaningful and identified by the CYP.

■ Structured graded activity programmes and pacing progress physical activity based on a plan and encourage implementation of coping skills to manage post-exertional malaise or symptom exacerbation.

■ Graded exercise is not recommended for CYP with ME/CFS or long COVID.

Psychological Treatments

Multicomponent psychological interventions, such as cognitive behavioural therapy (CBT) or acceptance and commitment therapy (ACT), combined with coping skills, are widely used by psychologists working in chronic pain services (Coakley and Wihak 2017). These can be delivered face to face, online or in a hybrid format

(Fisher et al. 2019). Psychologists will start by introducing the connection between thoughts, feelings and pain, and the bidirectional relationships. Negative thoughts that pain is a sign of damage, and avoidant behaviours, whether intentional or unintentional, can perpetuate pain and must be addressed (Caes et al. 2018).

Pain flares may occur as the CYP participates in physiotherapy and gradually returns to social activities and therefore the teaching and implementation of coping strategies is valuable. Coping skills can be distraction or active strategies including breathing, relaxation or imagery (Caes et al. 2018).

Another component of psychological treatment is parent and family education and counselling (Palermo et al. 2016; Caes et al. 2018). It is well established that parents play a crucial role in chronic pain management. Parents can be trained in operant conditioning, recognising stress and negative emotions, encouraging use of coping strategies, promoting sleep hygiene, supporting school plans and enhancing communication (Palermo et al. 2016).

Although psychological interventions are generally effective in chronic pain management, there is limited data on their effectiveness specifically for MSK pain and, importantly, which component parts are most effective (Fisher et al. 2018, 2019). According to systematic reviews, pain-focused psychology demonstrates small to moderate effects on reducing pain and disability in CYP for up to 12 months (Caes et al. 2018). Moreover, most CYP with MSK pain have more than one pain condition and many psychological comorbidities (Coakley and Wihak 2017) that require an individualised approach to their psychosocial management (Liossi and Howard 2016).

Complementary Interventions

Complementary and alternative medicine (CAM) involves diverse approaches to healthcare that are not presently considered part of conventional medicine. Within the domain of CAM, use of massage, yoga, acupuncture, art and music therapy and hypnosis are increasingly popular amongst CYP with chronic pain. CYP with higher pain intensity and more significant functional disability tend to use behavioural CAM (e.g. hypnosis, relaxation training, biofeedback), which is correlated with accommodative coping skills (Vinson et al. 2014; Caes et al. 2018). Although evidence is sparse concerning the effectiveness of CAM approaches to MSK pain in CYP, interventions are consistent with a biopsychosocial approach and should be considered.

Pharmacotherapy

While there may be a role for pharmacological intervention in targeted areas, it is of utmost importance that this is for a fixed period of time, with regular reviews by the prescribing physician or nurse practitioner, and used alongside a multidisciplinary treatment programme.

Many analgesic drugs, given in different modalities, have been used for CYP with chronic MSK pain. These are not supported by well-controlled clinical trials. Indeed, recent Cochrane reviews evaluating data on paracetamol, opioids, antidepressants and anticonvulsants concluded that there were insufficient data in all groups for meaningful analysis (Eccleston et al. 2019). Worryingly, CYP are increasingly using over-the-counter medications and recreational substances to alleviate pain (Skarstein et al. 2016).

Similarly, there is no robust evidence supporting the use of spinal cord stimulation or therapeutic blocks in chronic MSK pain conditions, including CRPS, in CYP (Williams and Howard 2016). When considering which analgesic drugs to use with this patient group, it is sensible to follow the WHO (2020) guidelines. Details of drug dosages are provided in the Appendix.

PRACTICE POINT

- If considering a trial of medication, always consider the nature of the pain that is presenting and consider comorbidities.
- Paracetamol and, assuming no contraindications, non-steroidal anti-inflammatory drugs (NSAIDs) are a reasonable first line for most pain conditions.
- If there is a neuropathic element, then gabapentin or pregabalin can be considered, but one needs to caution the lack of robust evidence and potential side effects. These drugs should be started at a low dose and titrated up if tolerated and shown to have an effect.
- Amitriptyline is an antidepressant that is still used, despite lack of robust data, to address both generalised chronic pain and sleep-onset insomnia. Again, if considered, this should be started at a low dose and titrated up if felt to be helpful.
- Opioids are sometimes prescribed for significant breakthrough pain. The types of opioids considered vary between centres and countries.
- It is vital that any young person prescribed an opioid-based medication for chronic pain has frequent medication check-ins. There is growing concern regarding opioid misuse and, in the absence of trial data, it is important to be cautious.

CASE STUDY: PART 3

You have diagnosed Samantha with chronic primary MSK pain in her right lower limb. You explain that this is a diagnosis in its own right and not a sign of ongoing injury or damage in her body. You educate her about the biopsychosocial model and the contributory factors that may keep pain persisting, including her fear of pain, disuse and deconditioning of the limb and body, anxiety and poor function (sleep, school attendance, physical activity and socialisation). You suggest a multimodal approach with a focus on regaining function, and a graded return to school, sleep, socialisation and exercise.

1. What pharmacological, psychological and physiotherapy treatments would you recommend?

Treatment of Chronic Regional Pain Syndrome

Early diagnosis and timely access to treatment is crucial for the complete recovery of CRPS symptoms and for reducing disability. In CYP with CRPS, the first-line treatment uses a multidisciplinary approach with physiotherapy, occupational therapy and CBT, with the overall focus on return to function (Weissmann and Uziel 2016; Lascombes and Mamie 2017; Vescio et al. 2020; Broman et al. 2021). Intense physical and psychological rehabilitation in the form of three- to six-week treatment blocks with weekly sessions and home exercise programmes has been shown to be effective for CRPS in CYP (Weissman and Uziel 2016). (More information about physical and psychological pain-relieving interventions is provided in Chapter 1.)

For CYP who continue to experience persistent pain and functional impairments despite treatment in outpatient settings, there are more intensive programmes emerging in the form of day hospital or inpatient programmes (Brooke and Janselewitz 2012; Logan et al. 2012; Cucchiaro et al. 2017). An example of this is provided by

Logan et al. (2012) who completed a longitudinal case series on CYP in a day hospital programme. Daily physical, occupational and psychological therapies provided for eight hours a day for five days per week, with a three-week length of stay demonstrated:

- reductions in pain intensity
- reduced medication use
- reduced reliance on assistive devices
- improvements in self-reported occupational performance and functional abilities
- maintained improvements at follow-up appointment (median of 10 months post discharge).

The multidisciplinary approach is widely recognised and implemented in clinical settings globally. However, there is no standard treatment protocol and the efficacy in CYP is not yet supported by high-quality evidence (Weissmann and Uziel 2016).

If physical and psychological rehabilitation are not successful, pharmacological interventions can be used as an adjunct (Cucchiaro et al. 2017; Vescio et al. 2020). As prescribed for neuropathic pain in adults, amitriptyline and gabapentin are equally demonstrated to reduce pain intensity and improve sleep outcomes for CYP with CRPS type 1 or neuropathic pain who were part of a multidisciplinary pain programme (Brown et al. 2016). Interventional treatment with continuous regional anaesthetic provided through an epidural or peripheral catheter was studied retrospectively in children who participated in an inpatient multidisciplinary rehabilitation programme (Donado et al. 2017). At four months after discharge, there continued to be improvements in pain, function and disability scores (Donado et al. 2017). These are promising results that highlight the need for further research examining the long-term outcomes in pain, function and quality of life.

Intensive Multidisciplinary Pain Programmes

For CYP with significant pain-related disability, treatment in an outpatient medical setting may not be sufficient to support return to function. For patients and families who continue to struggle with pain and disability, intensive multidisciplinary pain rehabilitation programmes are indicated and may include inpatient admission and/or daily outpatient programming (Liossi et al. 2019; Claus et al. 2022). Daily treatment may include but not be limited to (Bruce et al. 2017; Liossi et al. 2019; Hurtubise et al. 2020; Claus et al. 2022):

- group and individualised exercise and recreational activity
- occupational therapy
- physiotherapy
- psychological therapies
- nursing
- psychiatry
- family therapy
- parental training.

Treatment is integrated, with shared goals focusing on improvements in functional activities (e.g. school attendance, sleep, physical activity and socialisation). The addition of an interdisciplinary graded exposure programme has been found to lead to a significant and clinically relevant decrease in functional disability compared with usual care interdisciplinary outpatient rehabilitation care (Dekker et al. 2020). Overall, at 12 months post intervention, intensive multidisciplinary pain programmes result in clinically significant improvements in pain intensity, disability and school absenteeism, as well as moderate improvements in anxiety and depression (Liossi et al. 2019; Claus et al. 2022). However, there are cost and access barriers as most of the inpatient and day hospital programmes are in the UK and USA, which makes outpatient programmes the more feasible option for timely treatment for those in many other countries.

Long-term Outcomes in CYP with Chronic Musculoskeletal Pain

Although there is a high prevalence of chronic MSK pain in CYP, studies concerning outcomes and predictive factors for persistence and recurrence of pain are scarce.

- Early multidisciplinary input in specific conditions has been associated with improved outcomes. Across MSK pain

conditions, female gender, older age group (11+), coexistence of psychosomatic symptoms, having high disability index, and multisite pain are associated with long-term persistence of pain (Holden et al. 2021).

- CRPS in CYP typically has a favourable prognosis if early physiotherapy is initiated with psychological support, alongside parental involvement in rehabilitation (Liossi et al. 2015; Weissman and Uziel 2016).

However, it is recognised that a minority of young people, even after specialised pain management interventions, do not improve significantly and suffer from persistent or recurrent pain. Further understanding of all aspects of pain behaviours and pain mechanisms in CYP is key to improving treatment outcomes for those with chronic MSK pain conditions.

Summary

- MSK pain is defined as pain originating from muscles, ligaments, bones, tendons or joints.
- When MSK pain persists for over three months or beyond what would be expected for a particular condition, it becomes chronic MSK pain, which is an increasing concern.
- Chronic MSK pain can be distinguished as chronic primary or secondary MSK pain. Chronic MSK pain in CYP has a detrimental impact on function, school participation and psychological well-being, and it is costly for families and the healthcare system.
- CYP who experience chronic MSK pain have a higher likelihood of developing persistent pain as adults.
- Assessment and treatment should follow the biopsychosocial model, which recognises the complexity of chronic pain and

the impact of chronic pain on function and well-being.

- It is common for CYP with chronic MSK pain to present with muscular imbalances, deconditioning, abnormal gait and compensations due to disuse, fear or avoidant/ protective behaviours.
- First line of treatment is the multidisciplinary approach that includes pharmacology, physiotherapy, psychology and pain neuroscience education. Inclusion of the family is crucial.
- The use of complementary and alternative medicine is increasingly popular. However, there is no evidence to demonstrate its impact on CYP's chronic MSK pain.
- If pain and disability persist despite treatment, there are intensive inpatient programmes available, primarily located in the UK and USA.

■ Over the past decade, there has been a greater recognition of chronic MSK pain in CYP, yet a gap in evidence-based treatment remains.

■ Further research is needed to support the multidisciplinary approach and establish standardised treatment protocols for CYP with chronic MSK pain.

Key to Case Study

Part 1

1. What is the location of the pain? Is it localised or does it radiate to other areas? How would you describe the pain? Is it worse or better at certain times of the day? What are the aggravating and easing factors? Do you experience other symptoms such as swelling, colour changes, skin changes, changes in hair or nail growth?

2. Are you attending school and how many days have you missed because of pain or pain-related symptoms? Do you have trouble falling asleep or do you wake up through the night? Does pain interfere with social outings and, if so, what is the percentage of missed opportunities? Are you engaged in any physical activities currently, and are there previous activities that you have stopped or modified because of pain? What is your sitting, standing, walking tolerance?

See also Table 9.4.

Part 2

1. Components of physical assessment:
   a. Observation of gait, posture, weight bearing, protective behaviours
   b. Inspect colour, skin, hair, nail, muscle bulk and quality of tissue of the affected versus unaffected limb
   c. Active and passive range of motion of affected joint and the joints above and below, compare with the unaffected limb
   d. Muscle strength and flexibility tests
   e. Balance tests

   f. Functional movements such as sit to stand, lie to sit, squats, picking up an object from the ground, removing socks and shoes
   g. Sensory assessment for light touch and pin-prick
   h. Palpation of muscles to assess for tension and tenderness.

2. Rule in type of pain: determine the source of pain is the MSK system or nerves, and whether it is primary or secondary MSK pain. Rule out acute injury (e.g. fracture), CRPS, compartment syndrome, infection.

3. Chronic primary MSK pain of the right ankle with significant pain-related disability.

4. We acknowledge that your pain is very real. There is a difference between acute versus chronic pain, where chronic pain is not a sign of ongoing damage and it is produced or amplified by signals sent through your nervous system. Chronic pain is a diagnosis in its own right. Chronic pain is complex and there is a link between pain, emotions, sleep and deconditioning. Chronic pain is not a lifelong condition and the gold standard for treatment is functional rehabilitation using a multidisciplinary approach.

Part 3

1. The 3-P approach to treatment

Pharmacological
The aim of pharmacotherapy in the context of persistent or recurring pain is to potentially give

some relief while the young person is engaging with the meaningful interdisciplinary rehabilitation that improves function. If there is no relief from the medications, then safely stop them. Avoid polypharmacy.

- It is very important that Samantha and her family understand that, at best, medications aimed at reducing pain in a chronic pain setting generally have very limited effect. They are best utilised as part of a dedicated interdisciplinary rehabilitation plan. The Cochrane reviews clearly show a lack of evidence in this area (Eccleston et al. 2019).
- Regular paracetamol and NSAIDs (unless a contraindication) can be given regularly in the first instance (WHO 2020).
- If there is neuropathic pain, then consider gabapentin/pregabalin, but again this must be in the context of an overarching rehabilitation plan. Counsel regarding side effects and potential lack of efficacy (de Leeuw et al. 2020).
- Amitriptyline can be considered if there is a mixed picture of poor sleep, low mood and nociceptive pain. Side effects (including fatigue and headaches) are common (de Leeuw et al. 2020).

- If there is significant breakout pain that is overwhelming, then opioids are an option but only under the guidance of a dedicated pain physician and with regular reviews (WHO 2020).

Physiotherapy
- Focus on active strategies including an individualised exercise programme with stretching, strengthening, proprioception training, walking and aerobic components.
- Create a graded activity plan with the goal of returning to a functional activity that is identified as important and meaningful by the CYP.
- Use of hydrotherapy for movement and progressive loading.

Psychology
- CBT to work on anxiety which can heighten the nervous system and, therefore, increase pain signals.
- Mind body strategies to calm the body to help with sleep and performance of progressive physiotherapy.
- Exposure therapy to address fear avoidance of particular activities or situations.
- Education on sleep hygiene.
- Develop a return to school plan in collaboration with CYP, family and teachers.

Multiple Choice Questions

1. Which of the following is not part of the multidisciplinary approach to treating chronic MSK pain?
   a. Pharmacological strategies
   b. Psychological strategies
   c. Resting until the pain is gone
   d. Physical strategies
2. Which of the following is considered an example of MSK pain?
   a. CRPS
   b. CWP

   c. Fibromyalgia
   d. Low back pain
3. Which of the following outcome measures is *not* considered a comprehensive and sufficient evaluation of the impact of MSK pain in CYP?
   a. Visual analogue scale (VAS)
   b. Bath Adolescent Pain Questionnaire (BAPQ)
   c. Patient Reported Outcomes Measurement Information System (PROMIS®)

d. Pediatric Quality of Life Inventory (PedsQL)

4. Which of the following factors are not associated with increased risk for developing chronic MSK pain?

a. Female gender
b. Having an operation on the upper extremity as a child
c. Being an adolescent
d. Family history of MSK pain conditions

Acknowledgement

Jo-Anne Marcuz, Physiotherapist, Department of Rheumatology, The Hospital for Sick Children, Toronto, Canada reviewed an earlier version of this chapter.

References

Andias, R. and Silva, A.G. (2022) The onset of chronic musculoskeletal pain in high school adolescents: associated factors and the role of symptoms of central sensitization. *Physical Therapy* 102(4), pzab286.

Andreucci, A., Groenewald, C.B., Rathleff, M.S. and Palermo, T.M. (2021) The role of sleep in the transition from acute to chronic musculoskeletal pain in youth: a narrative review. *Children* 8(3), 241.

Arnold, L.M., Bennett, R.M., Crofford, L.J., et al. (2019) AAPT diagnostic criteria for fibromyalgia. *Journal of Pain* 20(6), 611–628.

Asmundson, G.J., Noel, M., Petter, M. and Parkerson, H.A. (2012) Pediatric fear-avoidance model of chronic pain: foundation, application and future directions. *Pain Research and Management* 17(6), 397–405.

Baweja, R. and Walco, G. (2020) Chronic pain and its impact on pediatric mental health. *Journal of the American Academy of Child and Adolescent Psychiatry* 59(10 Suppl.), S41.

Booth, J., Moseley, G.L., Schiltenwolf, M., Cashin, A., Davies, M. and Hübscher, M. (2017) Exercise for chronic musculoskeletal pain: a biopsychosocial approach. *Musculoskeletal Care* 15(4), 413–421.

Brandelli, Y.N., Chambers, C.T., Mackinnon, S.P., et al. (2023) A systematic review of the psychosocial factors associated with pain in children with juvenile idiopathic arthritis. *Pediatric Rheumatology Online Journal* 21(1), 57.

Broman, J., Weigel, C., Hellmundt, L. and Persson, A. (2021) A descriptive study on the treatment of pediatric CRPS in the Nordic countries and Germany. *Paediatric and Neonatal Pain* 3(4), 163–169.

Brooke, V. and Janselewitz, S. (2012) Outcomes of children with complex regional pain syndrome after intensive inpatient rehabilitation. *Pain Research and Management* 4(5), 349–354.

Brown, S., Johnston, B., Amaria, K., et al. (2016) A randomized controlled trial of amitriptyline versus gabapentin for complex regional pain syndrome type I and neuropathic pain in children. *Scandinavian Journal of Pain* 13, 156–163.

Bruce, B.K., Weiss, K.E., Ale, C.M., Harrison, T.E. and Fischer, P.R. (2017) Development of an interdisciplinary pediatric pain rehabilitation program: the first 1000 consecutive patients. *Mayo Clinic Proceedings Innovations, Quality and Outcomes* 1(2), 141–149.

Caes, L., Fisher, E., Clinch, J. and Eccleston, C. (2018) Current evidence-based interdisciplinary treatment options for pediatric musculoskeletal pain. *Current Treatment Options in Rheumatology* 4(3), 223–234.

Claus, B.B., Stahlschmidt, L., Dunford, E., et al. (2022) Intensive interdisciplinary pain treatment for children and adolescents with chronic non-cancer pain: a preregistered systematic review and individual patient data meta-analysis. *Pain* 163(12), 2281–2301.

Coakley, R. and Wihak, T. (2017) Evidence-based psychological interventions for the management of pediatric chronic pain: new directions in research and clinical practice. *Children* 4(2), 9.

Cucchiaro, G., Craig, K., Marks, K., Cooley, K., Cox, T.K.B. and Schwartz, J. (2017) Short- and long-term results of an inpatient programme to manage complex regional pain syndrome in children and adolescents. *British Journal of Pain* 11(2), 87–96.

Cunningham, N.R. and Kashikar-Zuck, S. (2013) Non-pharmacological treatment of pain in rheumatic diseases and other musculoskeletal pain conditions. *Current Rheumatology Reports* 15(2), 306.

Cunningham, N.R., Tran, S.T., Lynch-Jordan, A.M., et al. (2015) Psychiatric disorders in young adults diagnosed with juvenile fibromyalgia in adolescence. *Journal of Rheumatology* 42(12), 2427–2433.

Dario, A.B., Kamper, S.J., O'Keeffe, M., et al. (2019) Family history of pain and risk of musculoskeletal pain in children and adolescents: a systematic review and meta-analysis. *Pain* 160(11), 2430–2439.

Dekker, C., van Haastregt, J.C.M., Verbunt, J.A.M.C.F., et al. (2020) Pain-related fear in adolescents with chronic musculoskeletal pain: process evaluation of an interdisciplinary graded exposure program. *BMC Health Services Research* 20(1), 213.

de Leeuw, T.G., van der Zanden, T., Ravera, S., et al. (2020) Diagnosis and treatment of chronic neuropathic and mixed pain in children and adolescents: results of a survey study amongst practitioners. *Children* 7(11), 208.

Donado, C., Lobo, K., Velarde-Álvarez, M.F., et al. (2017) Continuous regional anesthesia and inpatient rehabilitation for pediatric complex regional pain syndrome. *Regional Anesthesia and Pain Medicine* 42(4), 527–534.

Dougherty, B.L., Zelikovsky, N., Miller, K.S., Rodriguez, D., Armstrong, S.L. and Sherry, D.D. (2021) Longitudinal impact of parental catastrophizing on child functional disability in pediatric amplified pain. *Journal of Pediatric Psychology* 46(4), 474–484.

Dunbar, C., McMahon, A.M., Leach, S. and Hawley, D.P. (2017) Splinting in children with inflammatory joint disease and hypermobility: a survey of current practice in the United Kingdom. *Rheumatology* 56(Suppl. 7), kex390.035.

Eccleston, C., Jordan, A., McCracken, L.M., Sleed, M., Connell, H. and Clinch, J. (2005) The Bath Adolescent Pain Questionnaire (BAPQ): development and preliminary psychometric evaluation of an instrument to assess the impact of chronic pain on adolescents. *Pain* 118(1–2), 263–270.

Eccleston, C., Fisher, E., Cooper, T.E., et al. (2019) Pharmacological interventions for chronic pain in children: an overview of systematic reviews. *Pain* 160(8), 1698–1707.

Ehlers–Danlos Society (2023) Assessing joint hypermobility. Available at `https://www.ehlers-danlos.com/assessing-joint-hypermobility/` (accessed 17 May 2023).

EU-OSHA (2021) Musculoskeletal disorders among children and young people: prevalence, risk factors, preventive measures. Available at `https://osha.europa.eu/en/publications/musculoskeletal-disorders-among-children-and-young-people-prevalence-risk-factors-preventive-measures` (accessed 5 June 2023).

Evans, S., Seidman, L.C., Tsao, J.C., Lung, K.C., Zeltzer, L.K. and Naliboff, B.D. (2013) Heart rate variability as a biomarker for autonomic nervous system response differences between children with chronic pain and healthy control children. *Journal of Pain Research* 6, 449–457.

Feldman, D.E. and Nahin, R.L. (2021) National estimates of chronic musculoskeletal pain and its treatment in children, adolescents, and young adults in the United States: data from the 2007–2015 National Ambulatory Medical Care Survey. *Journal of Pediatrics* 233, 212–219.e1.

Fisher, E., Law, E., Dudeney, J., Palermo, T.M., Stewart, G. and Eccleston, C. (2018) Psychological therapies for the management of chronic and recurrent pain in children and adolescents. *Cochrane Database of Systematic Reviews* (9), CD003968.

Fisher, E., Law, E., Dudeney, J., Eccleston, E and Palermo, T.M. (2019) Psychological therapies (remotely delivered) for the management of chronic and recurrent pain in children and adolescents. *Cochrane Database of Systematic Reviews* (4), CD011118.

Fisher, E., Villanueva, G., Henschke, N., et al. (2022) Efficacy and safety of pharmacological, physical, and psychological interventions for the management of chronic pain in children: a WHO systematic review and meta-analysis. *Pain* 163(1), e1–e19. Erratum in *Pain* 2023, 164(2), e121.

Fleegler, E.W. and Schechter, N.L. (2015) Pain and prejudice. *JAMA Pediatrics* 169(11), 991–993.

Foster, H.E. and Jandial, S. (2013) pGALS: paediatric Gait Arms Legs and Spine: a simple examination of the musculoskeletal system. *Pediatric Rheumatology Online Journal* 11(1), 44.

Gauntlett-Gilbert, J. and Jordan, A. (2020) Fear, boldness, and caution: parent effects on how children manage chronic pain. *Pain* 161(6), 1127–1128.

Geisser, M.E., Casey, K.L., Brucksch, C.B., Ribbens, C.M., Appleton, B.B. and Crofford, L.J. (2003) Perception of noxious and innocuous heat stimulation among healthy women and women with fibromyalgia: association with mood, somatic focus, and catastrophizing. *Pain* 102(3), 243–250.

Grøholt, E.K., Stigum, H., Nordhagen, R. and Köhler, L. (2003) Recurrent pain in children, socioeconomic factors and accumulation in families. *European Journal of Epidemiology* 18(10), 965–975.

Harden, N.R., Bruehl, S., Perez, R.S.G.M., et al. (2010) Validation of proposed diagnostic criteria (the 'Budapest Criteria') for complex regional pain syndrome. *Pain* 150(2), 268–274.

Harden, N.R., McCabe, C.S., Goebel, A., et al. (2022) Complex regional pain syndrome: practical diagnostic and treatment guidelines, 5th edition. *Pain Medicine* 23(Suppl. 1), S1–S53.

Harrison, L.E., Pate, J.W., Richardson, P.A., Ickmans, K., Wicksell, R.K. and Simons, L.E. (2019) Best-evidence for the rehabilitation of chronic pain part 1: pediatric pain. *Journal of Clinical Medicine* 8(9), 1267.

Health Standards Organization (2023) Pediatric pain management. Available at https://store.healthstandards.org/products/pediatric-pain-management-can-hso-13200-2023-e (accessed 26 May 2023).

Holden, S., Roos, E.M., Straszek, C.L., et al. (2021) Prognosis and transition of multi-site pain during the course of 5 years: results of knee pain and function from a prospective cohort study among 756 adolescents. *PLoS One* 16(5), e0250415.

Huguet, A., Tougas, M.E., Hayden, J., McGrath, P.J., Stinson, J.N. and Chambers, C.T. (2016) Systematic review with meta-analysis of childhood and adolescent risk and prognostic factors for musculoskeletal pain. *Pain* 157(12), 2640–2656.

Hurtubise, K., Blais, S., Noel, M., et al. (2020) Is it worth it? A comparison of an intensive interdisciplinary pain treatment and a multimodal treatment for youths with pain-related disability. *Clinical Journal of Pain* 36(11), 833–844.

Jones, G.T., Silman, A.J., Power, C. and Macfarlane, G.J. (2007) Are common symptoms in childhood associated with chronic widespread body pain in adulthood? Results from the 1958 British birth cohort study. *Arthritis and Rheumatism* 56(5), 1669–1675.

Kamper, S.J., Henschke, N., Hestbaek, L., Dunn, K.M. and Williams, C.M. (2016a) Musculoskeletal pain in children and adolescents. *Brazilian Journal of Physical Therapy* 20(3), 275–284.

Kamper, S.J., Yamato, T.P. and Williams, C.M. (2016b) The prevalence, risk factors, prognosis and treatment for back pain in children and adolescents: an overview of systematic reviews. *Best Practice and Research in Clinical Rheumatology* 30(6), 1021–1036.

Kashikar-Zuck, S. and Ting, T.V. (2014) Juvenile fibromyalgia: current status of research and future developments. *Nature Reviews Rheumatology* 10(2), 89–96.

Kashikar-Zuck, S., Carle, A., Barnett, K., et al. (2016) Longitudinal evaluation of patient-reported outcomes measurement information systems measures in pediatric chronic pain. *Pain* 157(2), 339–347.

Kaufman, T.J. and Sherry, D.D. (2017) Trends in medicalization of children with amplified musculoskeletal pain syndrome. *Pain Medicine* 18(5), 825–831.

Kempert, H. (2021) Teaching and applying activity pacing in pediatric chronic pain rehabilitation using practitioner feedback and pace breaks. *Pediatric Pain Letter* 23(2), 31–42.

Kløven, B., Hoftun, G.B., Romundstad, P.R. and Rygg, M. (2017) Relationship between pubertal timing and chronic nonspecific pain in adolescent girls: the Young-HUNT3 study (2006–2008). *Pain* 158(8), 1554–1560.

Koechlin, H., Locher, C. and Prchal, A. (2020) Talking to children and families about chronic pain: the importance of pain education. An introduction for pediatricians and other health care providers. *Children* 7(10), 179.

Lascombes, P. and Mamie, C. (2017) Complex regional pain syndrome type I in children: what is new? *Orthopaedics and Traumatology, Surgery and Research* 103(1S), S135–S142.

Latremoliere, A. and Woolf, C.J. (2009) Central sensitization: a generator of pain hypersensitivity by central neural plasticity. *Journal of Pain* 10(9), 895–926.

Liossi, C. and Howard, K. (2016) Pediatric chronic pain: biopsychosocial assessment and formulation. *Pediatrics* 138(5), e20160331.

Liossi, C., Clinch, J. and Howard, R. (2015) Need for early recognition and multidisciplinary management of paediatric complex regional pain syndrome. *British Medical Journal* 351, h4748.

Liossi, C., Johnstone, L., Lilley, S., Caes, L., Williams, G. and Schoth, D.E. (2019) Effectiveness of interdisciplinary interventions in paediatric chronic pain management: a systematic review and subset meta-analysis. *British Journal of Anaesthesia* 123(2), e359–e371.

Logan, D.E., Carpino, E.A., Chiang, G., et al. (2012) A day-hospital approach to treatment of pediatric complex regional pain syndrome: initial functional outcomes. *Clinical Journal of Pain* 28(9), 766–774.

Malanga, G.A., Yan, N. and Stark, J. (2015) Mechanisms and efficacy of heat and cold therapies for musculoskeletal injury. *Postgraduate Medicine* 127(1), 57–65.

Miller, M.M., Meints, S.M. and Hirsh, A.T. (2018) Catastrophizing, pain, and functional outcomes for children with chronic pain: a meta-analytic review. *Pain* 159(12), 2442–2460.

National Institute for Health and Care Excellence (2021a) *Myalgic Encephalomyelitis (or Encephalopathy)/Chronic Fatigue Syndrome: Diagnosis and Management.* NICE Guideline NG206. Available at https://www.nice.org.uk/guidance/ng206

National Institute for Health and Care Excellence (2021b) *COVID-19 Rapid Guideline: Managing the Long-term Effects of COVID-19.* Available at https://www.nice.org.uk/guidance/ng188/resources/covid19-rapid-guideline-managing-the-longterm-effects-of-covid19-pdf-51035515742

Nicholas, M., Vlaeyen, J.W.S., Rief, W., et al. (2019) The IASP classification of chronic pain for ICD-11: chronic primary pain. *Pain* 160(1), 28–37.

Ocay, D.D., Ye, D.L., Larche, C.L., Potvin, S., Marchand, S. and Ferland, C.E. (2022) Clusters of facilitatory and inhibitory conditioned pain modulation responses in a large sample of children, adolescents, and young adults with chronic pain. *Pain Reports* 7(6), e1032.

O'Sullivan, P., Beales, D., Jensen, L., Murray, K. and Myers, T. (2011) Characteristics of chronic non-specific musculoskeletal pain in children and adolescents attending a rheumatology outpatients clinic: a cross-sectional study. *Pediatric Rheumatology Online Journal* 9(1), 1–9.

Palermo, T.M., Law, E.F., Fales, J., Bromberg, M.H., Jessen-Fiddick, T. and Tai, G. (2016) Internet-delivered cognitive-behavioral treatment for adolescents with chronic pain and their parents: a randomized controlled multicenter trial. *Pain* 157(1), 174–185.

Perrot, S., Cohen, M., Barke, A., Korwisi, B., Rief, W. and Treede, R.D. (2019) The IASP classification of chronic pain for ICD-11: chronic secondary musculoskeletal pain. *Pain* 160(1), 77–82.

Pourbordbari, N., Jensen, M.B., Olesen, J.L., Holden, S. and Rathleff, M.S. (2022) Bio-psycho-social characteristics and impact of musculoskeletal pain in one hundred children and adolescents consulting general practice. *BioMed Central Primary Care* 23(1), 20.

Scottish Government (2018) *Management of Chronic Pain in Children and Young People. A National Clinical Guideline.* Scottish Government, Edinburgh. Available at https://www.gov.scot/publications/management-chronic-pain-children-young-people/ (accessed 16 May 2023).

Skarstein, S., Lagerløv, P., Kvarme, L.G. and Helseth, S. (2016) High use of over-the-counter analgesic: possible warnings of reduced quality of life in adolescents. A qualitative study. *BioMed Central Nursing* 15(1), 1–11.

Sperotto, F., Brachi, S., Vittadello, F. and Zulian, F. (2015) Musculoskeletal pain in schoolchildren across puberty: a 3-year follow-up study. *Pediatric Rheumatology* 15, 13–16.

Stephens, S., Feldman, B.M., Bradley, N., et al. (2008) Feasibility and effectiveness of an aerobic exercise program in children with fibromyalgia: results of a randomized controlled pilot trial. *Arthritis and Rheumatism* 59(10), 1399–1406.

Tobias, J.H., Deere, K., Palmer, S., Clark, E.M. and Clinch, J. (2013) Joint hypermobility is a risk factor for musculoskeletal pain during adolescence: findings of a prospective cohort study. *Arthritis and Rheumatism* 65(4), 1107–1115.

van den Heuvel, M.M., Jansen, P.W., Bindels, P.J.E., Bierma-Zeinstra, S.M.A. and van Middelkoop, M. (2020) Musculoskeletal pain in 6-year-old children: the Generation R Study. *Pain* 161(6), 1278–1285.

Varni, J.W., Seid, M. and Rode, C.A. (1999) The PedsQL™: measurement model for the pediatric quality of life inventory. *Medical Care* 37(2), 126–139.

Vescio, A., Testa, G., Culmone, A., et al. (2020) Treatment of complex regional pain syndrome in children and adolescents: a structured literature scoping review. *Children* 7(11), 245.

Vinson, R., Yeh, G., Davis, R.B. and Logan, D. (2014) Correlates of complementary and alternative medicine use in a pediatric tertiary pain center. *Academic Pediatrics* 14(5), 491–496.

Volders, S., Boddez, Y., De Peuter, S., Meulders, A. and Vlaeyen, J.W. (2015) Avoidance behavior in chronic pain research: a cold case revisited. *Behaviour Research and Therapy* 64, 31–37.

Walker, L.S., Dengler-Crish, C.M., Rippel, S. and Bruehl, S. (2010) Functional abdominal pain in childhood and adolescence increases risk for chronic pain in adulthood. *Pain* 150(3), 568–572.

Weiss, J.E. and Stinson, J.N. (2018) Pediatric pain syndromes and noninflammatory musculoskeletal pain. *Pediatric Clinics of North America* 65(4), 801–826.

Weissmann, R. and Uziel, Y. (2016) Pediatric complex regional pain syndrome: a review. *Pediatric Rheumatology Online Journal* 14(1), 29.

Williams, G. and Howard, R. (2016) The pharmacological management of complex regional pain syndrome in pediatric patients. *Paediatric Drugs* 18(4), 243–250.

World Health Organization (2015) GBD Compare VizHub. Institute for Health Metrics and Evaluation. Available at `https://vizhub.healthdata.org/gbd-compare/` (accessed 5 June 2023)

World Health Organization (2020) *WHO Guideline for the Management of Chronic Pain in Children*, pp. 1–11. WHO, Geneva. Available at `https://apps.who.int/iris/bitstream/handle/10665/337999/9789240017870-eng.pdf` (accessed 16 May 2023).

10 Preventing and Treating Chronic Headache Disorders in Children and Young People

Naiyi Sun, Christina Liossi, and Jacqui Clinch

Chronic headaches are common in children and young people (CYP). The third edition of the International Classification of Headache Disorders (ICHD-3) divides headaches into primary and secondary headaches (Headache Classification Committee of the International Headache Society 2018). Primary headaches are idiopathic with no known secondary causes, while secondary headaches are caused by an underlying condition. Table 10.1 provides details of some commonly encountered headache diagnoses in CYP. A complete list of headache disorders can be found in the ICHD-3 at https://ichd-3.org/.

In this chapter we examine some common chronic headache conditions, describing their epidemiology, comorbidities and treatment options.

Definitions

Chronic Daily Headache

■ Diagnosed when headache is present for a minimum of 15 days in one month over a period of three consecutive months, with no underlying organic pathology.

Table 10.1 Headache aetiologies.

Primary headaches
Migraine headache
Without aura
With aura
Tension-type headache (TTH)
Trigeminal autonomic cephalalgias
Cluster headache
Secondary headaches
Non-vascular intracranial disorder
Tumour
Intracranial hypertension
Chiari 1 malformation
Infection
Vascular disorder
Vascular malformation
Cerebral sinovenous thrombosis
Substance withdrawal
Medication overuse headache
Post-traumatic headache
Painful lesions of the cranial nerves

Managing Pain in Children and Young People: A Clinical Guide, Third Edition. Edited by Alison Twycross, Jennifer Stinson, William T. Zempsky, and Abbie Jordan.
© 2024 John Wiley & Sons Ltd. Published 2024 by John Wiley & Sons Ltd.

- Typically, the headaches last for more than four hours per day.

It is common for CYP with chronic daily headache to have a combination of chronic migraine and chronic tension-type headache (TTH). The prevalence of chronic daily headache ranges from 0.9 to 7.8% in studies of CYP, in which girls are disproportionally more affected than boys (Seshia 2012; Wöber-Bingöl 2013; Connelly and Sekhon 2019).

Chronic Migraine

- Chronic migraine is diagnosed when individuals report migraine features on at least eight days per month.
- Of CYP experiencing chronic daily headache, 67% also describe chronic migraine (Blume 2017; Youssef and Mack 2020).

Tension-type Headache

- TTH is considered chronic when it occurs on at least 15 days per month for more than three months (Headache Classification Committee of the International Headache Society 2018).
- TTH affects about 31% (range 10–72%) of CYP based on several prevalence studies (Monteith and Sprenger 2010, Genizi et al. 2021).

Symptoms of Chronic Migraine

Chronic migraine is complex, with typical symptoms including both severe intermittent pain and continuous background pain.

Severe Intermittent Headaches

- Overwhelming pulsating and throbbing pain
- With or without aura (as with acute migraines)
- Nausea and/or vomiting

- Photophobia, phonophobia, osmophobia
- Extreme tiredness
- Persistent headache after rest.

Continuous Background Headache

- Worse at beginning or end of day
- Crushing and band-like (akin to tension headache)
- Less severe but always present.

Symptoms of Chronic Tension-type Headache

- Last hours to days, or are unremitting
- Bilateral location
- Pressing or tightening, non-pulsating quality
- Mild or moderate in intensity
- Not aggravated by routine physical activity (e.g. walking or climbing stairs)
- No more than one of photophobia, phonophobia or mild nausea.

Comorbidities Associated with Chronic Headache Disorders

As with many chronic pain states, it is very common that CYP with persistent headaches and migraines also report co-occurring physical and emotional symptoms (Blume 2017; Youssef and Mack 2020). These include:

- dizziness, often secondary to deconditioning, occasionally orthostatic
- blurred vision
- sleep disturbance
- musculoskeletal and abdominal pain
- fatigue
- anxiety
- low mood
- concentration difficulty.

Impact of Headaches

Chronic headaches significantly impact CYP's quality of life, affecting their education, socialisation and family life (Philipp et al. 2019; Youssef and Mack 2020). Further, CYP who suffer from headaches often experience significant sleep disturbance, which may be a risk factor for poor physical, academic and emotional functioning, such as increased anxiety (Clementi et al. 2020). Importantly, all aspects of symptomatology should be addressed as often the headaches do not improve unless other key symptoms are addressed (e.g. sleep, anxiety, low mood) (Youssef and Mack 2020).

Assessment of Pain in CYP with Headaches

A thorough history and focused neurological examination are critical for distinguishing between primary and secondary headache disorders. Further investigations (e.g. neuroimaging, lumbar puncture) as well as consultation with a paediatric neurologist may be needed.

In terms of headache characteristics, it would be helpful to ask about:

- pain intensity
- duration of headaches
- time of day of headache occurrences
- experience of nausea and/or vomiting
- whether the headaches occur with the presence of aura
- experience of pins and needles
- experience of visual disturbance
- slurred speech
- somnolence (feeling drowsy) post headache
- family history of migraine and/or other type of headaches.

Red flag questions to ask include:

- Do you vomit with the headache, particularly in the morning?
- Do you have visual disturbance that continues?
- Have you noticed personality change after headache?
- Does your headache ever stop?
- Does the headache wake you from sleep or is it present first thing on awakening?

Differential possible diagnoses include:

- idiopathic intracranial hypertension
- white matter abnormalities, arachnoid cysts, pineal cysts
- space-occupying lesions (e.g. tumours)
- infections of the central nervous system (e.g. meningitis, encephalitis).

When assessing CYP with chronic headaches, it is important to note:

- the nature of the headache
- sleep
- postural changes
- the impact of pain on daily activities
- general physical and emotional well-being.

A headache diary completed for a minimum of eight weeks can be helpful in (National Institute for Health and Care Excellence 2021):

- diagnosis
- identifying triggers (e.g. stress, diet, dehydration, menstrual cycle, sleep, bruxism, poor posture, weather changes)
- recording frequency and severity of episodes
- evaluating treatment efficacy.

Various headache diaries are available, including paper-based and electronic. There is some limited evidence supporting the reliability and validity of both, but also criticisms relating to effort and time required from both patients and professionals, and limited patient adherence (Stinson et al. 2013; Kellier et al. 2022). Other measures, such as the Pediatric Migraine Disability Assessment (PedMIDAS), a six-item questionnaire tested and validated for ages 4 to 18 and intended to be self-administered by the patient and their parent/carer (Hershey et al. 2001), have been developed for assessing migraine-related disability and quality of life in CYP.

Psychological Assessment

Primary headache is often associated with comorbid psychopathology, and therefore the CYP should be screened for anxiety and mood disorders at a minimum, while clinicians must remain alert to the presence of other psychiatric disorders. Other important constructs that are useful assessments include (Liossi and Howard 2016):

- locus of control (i.e. individual's perception of the level of control they have over the occurrence of headache)
- self-efficacy (i.e. individual's belief that they can successfully manage their headache and improve their quality of life)
- attitudes towards headaches, social stigma, catastrophising, coping and acceptance.

After the initial assessment, there should be a multidisciplinary reassessment within three months. Many CYP and their families also benefit from dedicated pain management programmes to reduce the impact of pain and pain-associated disability (Liossi et al. 2019; Claus et al. 2022).

CASE STUDY: PART 1

Daniel, age 13, attends your clinic with a two-year history of increasingly frequent headaches. He describes them as starting as a dull ache around his head and then spreading backwards, particularly over the right side of his head. Daniel feels sick with them and occasionally vomits. Currently, he is managing these headaches with rest and occasional use of paracetamol. He is missing one to two days of school each week due to these headaches.

1. What other characteristics of Daniel's headaches are you interested in?
2. Are there any 'red flag' questions you would like to ask Daniel?

Management of Chronic Headache Disorders

Unlike acute headaches and migraines, the chronic forms can be more challenging to understand and treat (Rastogi et al. 2018). Chronic migraines are extremely disabling (Gazerani 2021), and many families become increasingly frustrated and anxious that nothing is found on scans or other investigations, often seeking multiple clinical opinions.

The cornerstones of treatment include (Eigenbrodt et al. 2021):

- education
- lifestyle modifications
- preventive medications
- abortive medications
- psychological strategies
- physiotherapy (physical therapy)
- addressing pain-associated disability including sleep.

Examples of current best practice guidelines for the treatment of migraine in CYP are provided in Box 10.1.

Education

Time spent with families explaining the nature of chronic migraine/daily headaches, the aetiopathology and demonstrating lack of pathology in the results is invaluable, since chronic migraine/daily headache are primary pain conditions rather than diagnoses of exclusion. Relevant educational resources, including some specific to chronic headaches, are available (e.g. `https://www.deutsches-kinderschmerzzentrum.de/en/about-us/videos/#c2975`).

Lifestyle Modifications

Like other pain conditions, families need to understand the comorbidities, including sleep deprivation, anxiety and low mood, that can complicate the impact of headaches on a CYP's well-being; therefore, although these comorbidities are not causative, they also need to be addressed. The improvement of lifestyle is a central element in the management of CYP's headaches and is consequently central to education. Lifestyle modifications aim to improve the CYP's quality of life, reduce the severity of headache episodes and improve their well-being into adulthood. Such lifestyle modifications include:

- sleep hygiene
- eating regularly (avoiding skipping meals)
- adequate hydration, particularly in CYP who are also suffering with dizziness
- reducing caffeine intake (e.g. iced tea, soda, chocolate)
- reducing alcohol, tobacco and vaping consumption
- reducing screen time
- engaging in low-impact aerobic exercise.

Preventive Medications

Conventional pain medicines are often not as effective as hoped for the treatment of headache and migraine. Medications need to be used in a structured insightful way, alongside other physical and psychological pain management interventions (Quresh et al. 2019; Powers et al. 2021).

Most randomised controlled trials (RCTs) studying the efficacy of preventive medications fail to demonstrate superiority to placebo for migraine in CYP (Oskoui et al. 2019). In chronic daily headache and chronic migraines, a reasonable short-term therapeutic goal would be to reduce the frequency of severe intermittent headaches and reduce the intensity of the continuous background headache. An overview of medications to consider can be found in Table 10.2. Regular medication check-ins should be done to review efficacy and potential side effects.

Nutraceutical treatments including vitamin B_2 (riboflavin), vitamin D, magnesium and melatonin, can be useful preventive headache treatments in CYP. Although evidence supporting the use of these substances is weak, they are well tolerated with a low side-effect profile (Orr and Venkateswaran 2014; Szperka 2021).

Neuromodulation is another emerging treatment option for migraine. It aims to reduce pain by targeting structures in the nervous system that are commonly involved in headache pathophysiology. There are several non-invasive neuromodulating devices approved

Table 10.2 Brief overview of preventive medications for treating chronic headache disorders in CYP.

Type of medication	Example of medication	Potential impacts of medication use for CYP
Tricyclic antidepressants	Amitriptyline	■ May improve sleep and stabilise mood at higher doses ■ Recent RCT did not show superiority of amitriptyline over placebo in migraine in CYP (Powers et al. 2017)
Anticonvulsants	Topiramate	■ In the USA, topiramate is the only FDA-approved treatment option for preventive therapy for chronic migraine in young people over the age of 12 ■ Licensed for young people 16 years and older for migraines in the UK ■ Has been shown to reduce the severity of the constant headache ■ However, an RCT has questioned the efficacy of topiramate in migraine in CYP (Powers et al. 2017)
Botulinum neurotoxin	Onabotulinum toxin A (Botox)	■ May reduce the severity of daily headaches ■ Should only be considered as a treatment option in a dedicated centre (Marcelo and Freund 2020)
Anti-CGRP monoclonal antibodies (mAbs)	Erenumab Fremanezumab Epinezumab Galcanezumab	■ Treatment trials of anti-CGRP mAbs in adults have demonstrated efficacy for migraine prevention (Hershey 2017). ■ Clinical trials investigating this class of medication in CYP are currently underway ■ An expert consensus guideline from the American Headache Society suggests that CGRP ligand/receptor antibodies can be considered in postpubertal young people experiencing relatively frequent migraines, i.e. eight or more headache days per month with moderate or severe migraine-related disability (Szperka et al. 2018)

CGRP, calcitonin gene-related peptide.
Note: Please consult the NICE British National Formulary for Children (BNFc) at https://bnfc.nice.org.uk/ for dosing recommendations for children and adolescents.

for the treatment of migraine in young people, including:

■ remote electrical neuromodulation (REN)
■ non-invasive vagal nerve stimulation (nVNS)
■ single pulse transcranial magnetic stimulation (sTMS).

Evidence to support their use in CYP is currently limited (Irwin et al. 2018; Hershey et al. 2022). However, they provide a promising non-pharmacological acute treatment option for young people with migraine.

Abortive Medications

For more severe intermittent headache episodes with migrainous qualities, abortive analgesics can be considered. They should be given as early as possible during an attack and include the following.

■ Over-the-counter (OTC) medications, such as non-steroidal anti-inflammatory drugs (NSAIDs, e.g. ibuprofen, naproxen, diclofenac) and/or paracetamol.
■ Triptans (sumatriptan, zolmitriptan, rizatriptan, almotriptan, eletriptan,

naratriptan), available as injections, nasal sprays, tablets and dissolving tablets, are frequently used for patients with moderate to severe migraine headaches unresponsive to OTC therapy.

- Caffeine is used as an adjuvant in combination with OTC analgesics (e.g. paracetamol and ibuprofen) for acute treatment of TTH and migraine. However, when used in excess, caffeine can place patients at risk of medication overuse headache (MOH) and development of chronic headaches (Lipton et al. 2017).

Frequent use of acute pain-relievers such as NSAIDs and paracetamol can complicate the management of primary headache disorders (Powers et al. 2017).

- It is important to determine whether medication overuse is contributing to headache burden leading to MOH.
- It is reasonable to discourage patients from using analgesic drugs to treat the continuous background headache since this may result in analgesic overuse and a potential analgesic rebound headache.
- These pain relievers should be used no more than three days per week to avoid the development of MOH. CYP should also avoid excessive caffeine, barbiturate and opioids, as these may cause rebound headaches.

CASE STUDY: PART 2

Daniel explains in clinic that he is keen to start treatment for his increasingly frequent headaches.

1. What is your advice and suggested treatment at this stage for Daniel?

Psychological Interventions

Psychological therapies aim to modify the cognitive-emotional and cognitive-behavioural processes that influence pain. Three main forms of therapy that have been evaluated in RCTs and reviewed in meta-analyses include:

- relaxation training
- biofeedback
- multimodal cognitive behavioural therapy (CBT).

Evidence demonstrates that these psychological therapies can be efficacious in reducing headache and migraine frequency post treatment (Trautmann et al. 2006; Fisher et al. 2018). So far there is only scarce evidence on hypnosis, mindfulness-based stress reduction (MBSR) and acceptance and commitment therapy (ACT), although these therapeutic approaches are frequently used in clinical practice (Knestrick et al. 2022).

Similarly, digital health interventions including mobile phone headache diary apps and behavioural/therapeutic treatments are increasingly utilised by patients and health professionals. However, there is currently limited data on their effectiveness (Hundert et al. 2014; van de Graaf et al. 2021).

Physiotherapy and Other Physical Interventions

Physiotherapy (physical therapy) for chronic migraine focuses on musculoskeletal dysfunction and vestibular symptoms/postural control impairment. Through a combination of education, manual and exercise therapy, balance exercises and vestibular rehabilitation, the aim is to reduce pain, sensitisation and vestibular symptoms, and optimise function. For TTH, physiotherapy generally takes the form of education and aerobic exercise (Carvalho et al. 2020).

Various other physical interventions have been evaluated in the management of chronic headaches with varying success. Amongst them a multimodal treatment comprising daily practice of mindfulness and qi gong, along with osteopathic manual treatments, was efficacious in decreasing headache frequency, pain intensity and pain restriction in young people with chronic TTH (Przekop et al. 2016).

CASE STUDY: PART 3

On review six months later, Daniel has the headaches less frequently (every four weeks), but he is missing a couple of days of school when the headaches occur.

1. What is your advice and suggested treatment at this stage for Daniel?

Outcomes for CYP who Experience Chronic Headaches and Chronic Migraines

Many studies have explored the long-term outcomes of childhood-onset headaches and migraine in CYP. In community populations of CYP with chronic daily headaches, approximately 75% show improvement after two years, with a minority (12%) reporting ongoing headaches eight years after diagnosis, despite intervention. Findings overall suggest the following are associated with a poorer short- and long-term prognosis of frequent headaches in early adolescents (Wang et al. 2009; Larsson et al. 2018; Sillanpää and Saarinen 2018):

- female gender
- presence of migraine at baseline
- reduced social functioning
- higher levels of depressive symptoms.

Retrospective and prospective follow-up studies of clinical samples of CYP experiencing primary migraine have reported that most patients continue to have headache in adulthood, although the headache classification often changes over time. Most patients report moderate or severe headache and increasingly choose to care for their headaches with medication (Brna et al. 2005; Antonaci et al. 2014). However, such samples typically include young people with complex neurological presentations, severe attacks in terms of frequency and intensity, and significantly impaired quality of life compared with those treated in primary care.

Summary

- Chronic headaches are common in CYP and can be divided into primary and secondary headaches.
- A thorough history and focused neurological examination are critical for distinguishing between primary and secondary headache disorders.
- Chronic headaches significantly impact CYP's quality of life and all aspects of symptomatology should be addressed.
- Cornerstones of headache treatment include education, lifestyle modifications, preventive and abortive medications, psychological strategies, physical strategies, and addressing all areas of pain-associated disability.

- CYP should be reassessed at regular intervals to evaluate effectiveness of treatment and impact of pain.
- Risk factors associated with poorer short- and long-term prognosis of frequent headaches in CYP include female gender, presence of migraine at baseline, reduced social functioning and higher levels of depressive symptoms.
- Consider referral to a specialist paediatric psychologist to teach additional pain-coping strategies and help reduce the impact of headaches on daily life including school attendance.

Key to Case Study

Part 1

1. In terms of headache characteristics, it would be helpful to ask about:
   a. Pain intensity
   b. Duration of headaches
   c. Time of day of headache occurrences
   d. Experience of nausea and/or vomiting
   e. Whether the headaches occur with the presence of aura
   f. Experience of pins and needles
   g. Experience of visual disturbance
   h. Slurred speech
   i. Somnolence (feeling drowsy) post headache
   j. Family history of migraine and/or other type of headaches.

2. Red flag questions to ask include:
   a. Do you vomit with the headache, particularly in the morning?
   b. Do you have visual disturbance that continues?
   c. Have you noticed personality change post headache?
   d. Does your headache ever stop?
   e. Does the headache wake you from sleep or is present first thing on awakening?

It would be important to ask these questions alongside a full examination including neurological and eye examination.

Part 2

1. First, look at lifestyle factors (e.g. sleep and diet) to evaluate any triggering factors for Daniel's headaches. It is important to educate Daniel about making any identified lifestyle changes. Ask Daniel to keep a headache diary and also suggest simple analgesia first and potentially a triptan if you feel appropriate at this stage. Recommend simple breathing techniques and relaxation exercises (e.g. progressive muscle relaxation).

Part 3

1. Review the headache diary to identify any possible triggers and lifestyle changes that Daniel can make to reduce the frequency of headaches. Triptans can be useful if there is a definite pattern.

Multiple Choice Questions

1. Which of the following is not a possible differential diagnosis for a young person with chronic daily headache and/or chronic migraine?
   a. Idiopathic intracranial hypertension
   b. White matter abnormalities, arachnoid cysts, pineal cysts
   c. Space-occupying lesions (tumours, etc.)
   d. Prosopagnosia

2. Chronic daily headache means headache for how many days per month?
   a. 3 days per month
   b. 7 days per month
   c. 10 days per month
   d. 15 days per month

3. Which of the following is not a drug used for prophylactic treatment of migraine?
    a. Tricyclic antidepressants
    b. Anticonvulsants
    c. Diazepam
    d. Botulinum neurotoxin

4. What lifestyle modifications can improve the patient's quality of life and reduce the severity of headache episodes?
    a. Sleep hygiene, eating regularly, remaining hydrated, reducing caffeine intake
    b. Reducing alcohol, tobacco and vaping consumption and engaging in low-impact aerobic exercise
    c. Reducing screen time
    d. All of the above

5. What psychological interventions can be efficacious in the management of chronic daily headaches?
    a. Gestalt therapy, family therapy and multimodal cognitive behavioural therapy
    b. Relaxation training, biofeedback and multimodal cognitive behavioural therapy
    c. Meditation, solution-focused therapy and multimodal cognitive behavioural therapy
    d. Yoga, behaviour therapy, psychoanalytic psychotherapy

Acknowledgement

C.L. is supported by funds from Great Ormond Street Hospital Children's Charity Research Awards (V5118, V4421).

References

Antonaci, F., Voiticovschi-Iosob, C., Di Stefano, A.L., Galli, F., Ozge, A. and Balottin, U. (2014) The evolution of headache from childhood to adulthood: a review of the literature. *Journal of Headache and Pain* 15(1), 15.

Blume, K. (2017) Childhood headache: a brief review. *Pediatric Annals* 46(4), e155–e165.

Brna, P., Dooley, J., Gordon, K. and Dewan, T. (2005) The prognosis of childhood headache: a 20-year follow-up. *Archives of Pediatrics and Adolescent Medicine* 159(12), 1157–1160.

Carvalho, G.F., Schwarz, A., Szikszay, T.M., Adamczyk, W.M., Bevilaqua-Grossi, D. and Luedtke, K. (2020) Physical therapy and migraine: musculoskeletal and balance dysfunctions and their relevance for clinical practice. *Brazilian Journal of Physical Therapy* 24(4), 306–317.

Claus, B.B., Stahlschmidt, L., Dunford, E., et al. (2022) Intensive interdisciplinary pain treatment for children and adolescents with chronic non-cancer pain: a preregistered systematic review and individual patient data meta-analysis. *Pain* 163(12), 2281–2301.

Clementi, M.A., Chang, Y.H., Gambhir, R., Lebel, A. and Logan, D.E. (2020) The impact of sleep on disability and school functioning: results from a tertiary pediatric headache center. *Journal of Child Neurology* 35(3), 221–227.

Connelly, M. and Sekhon, S. (2019) Current perspectives on the development and treatment of chronic daily headache in children and adolescents. *Pain Management* 9(2), 175–189.

Eigenbrodt, A.K., Ashina, H., Khan, S., et al. (2021) Diagnosis and management of migraine in ten steps. *Nature Reviews Neurology* 17(8), 501–514.

Fisher, E., Law, E., Dudeney, J., Palermo, T.M., Stewart, G. and Eccleston, C. (2018) Psychological therapies for the management of chronic and recurrent pain in children and adolescents. *Cochrane Database of Systematic Reviews* (9), CD003968.

Gazerani, P. (2021) Migraine and mood in children. *Behavioral Science* 11(4), 52.

Genizi, J., Bugdnoskya, V., Aboud, A., et al. (2021) Migraine and tension-type headache among children and adolescents: application of International Headache Society criteria in a clinical setting. *Journal of Child Neurology* 36(8), 618–624.

Headache Classification Committee of the International Headache Society (2018) The International Classification of Headache Disorders, 3rd edition. *Cephalalgia* 38(1), 1–211.

Hershey, A.D. (2017) CGRP: the next frontier for migraine. *New England Journal of Medicine* 377(22), 2190–2191.

Hershey, A.D., Powers, S.W., Vockell, A.L., LeCates, S., Kabbouche, M.A. and Maynard, M.K. (2001) PedMIDAS: development of a questionnaire to assess disability of migraines in children. *Neurology* 57(11), 2034–2039.

Hershey, A.D., Irwin, S., Rabany, L., et al. (2022) Comparison of remote electrical neuromodulation and standard-care medications for acute treatment of migraine in adolescents: a post-hoc analysis. *Pain Medicine* 23(4), 815–820.

Hundert, A.S., Huguet, A., McGrath, P.J., Stinson, J.N. and Wheaton, M. (2014) Commercially available mobile phone headache diary apps: a systematic review. *JMIR Mhealth Uhealth* 2(3), e36.

Irwin, S.L., Qubty, W., Allen, I.E., Patniyot, I., Goadsby, P.J. and Gelfand, A.A. (2018) Transcranial magnetic stimulation for migraine prevention in adolescents: a pilot open-label study. *Headache* 58(5), 724–731.

Kellier, D.J., Marquez de Prado, B., Haagen, D., et al. (2022) Development of a text message-based headache diary in adolescents and children. *Cephalalgia* 42(10), 1013–1021.

Knestrick, K.E., Gibler, R.C., Reidy, B.L. and Powers, S.W. (2022) Psychological interventions for pediatric headache disorders: a 2021 update on research progress and needs. *Current Pain and Headache Reports*, 26(1), 85–91.

Larsson, B., Sigurdson, J.F. and Sund, A.M. (2018) Long-term follow-up of a community sample of adolescents with frequent headaches. *Journal of Headache and Pain* 19(1), 79.

Liossi, C. and Howard, R.F. (2016) Pediatric chronic pain: biopsychosocial assessment and formulation. *Pediatrics* 138(5), e20160331.

Liossi, C., Johnstone, L., Lilley, S., Caes, L., Williams, G. and Schoth, D.E. (2019) Effectiveness of interdisciplinary interventions in paediatric chronic pain management: a systematic review and subset meta-analysis. *British Journal of Anaesthesia* 123(2), e359–e371.

Lipton, R.B., Diener, H.-C., Robbins, M.S., Garas, S.Y. and Patel, K. (2017) Caffeine in the management of patients with headache. *Journal of Headache and Pain* 18(1), 107.

Marcelo, R. and Freund, B. (2020) The efficacy of botulinum toxin in pediatric chronic migraine: a literature review. *Journal of Child Neurology* 35(12), 844–851.

Monteith, T.S. and Sprenger, T. (2010) Tension type headache in adolescence and childhood: where are we now? *Current Pain and Headache Reports* 14(6), 424–430.

National Institute for Health and Care Excellence (2021) Scenario: Migraine in young people aged 12–17 years. Available at https://cks.nice.org.uk/topics/migraine/management/young-people-aged-12-17-years/ (accessed 10 July 2022).

Orr, S.L. and Venkateswaran, S. (2014) Nutraceuticals in the prophylaxis of pediatric migraine: evidence-based review and recommendations. *Cephalalgia* 34(8), 568–583.

Oskoui, M., Pringsheim, T., Holler-Managan, Y., et al. (2019) Practice guideline update summary: Acute treatment of migraine in children and adolescents. Report of the Guideline Development, Dissemination, and Implementation Subcommittee of the American Academy of Neurology and the American Headache Society. *Neurology* 93(11), 487–499.

Philipp, J., Zeiler, M., Wöber, C., et al. (2019) Prevalence and burden of headache in children and adolescents in Austria: a nationwide study in a representative sample of pupils aged 10–18 years. *Journal of Headache and Pain* 20(1), 101.

Powers, S.W., Coffey, C.S., Chamberlin, L.A., et al. (2017) Trial of amitriptyline, topiramate, and placebo for pediatric migraine. *New England Journal of Medicine* 376(2), 115–124.

Powers, S.W., Coffey, C.S., Chamberlin, L.A., et al. (2021) Prevalence of headache days and disability 3 years after participation in the childhood and adolescent migraine prevention medication trial. *JAMA Network Open* 4(7), e2114712.

Przekop, P., Przekop, A. and Haviland, M.G. (2016) Multimodal compared to pharmacologic treatments for chronic tension-type headache in adolescents. *Journal of Bodywork and Movement Therapies* 20(4), 715–721.

Qureshi, M.H., Esper, G.J. and Bashir, F.F. (2019) When to consider prophylactic antimigraine therapy in children with migraine. *Current Treatment Options in Neurology* 21(4), 15.

Rastogi, R.G., Borrero-Mejias, C., Hickman, C., Lewis, K.S. and Little, R. (2018) Management of episodic migraine in children and adolescents: a practical approach. *Current Neurology and Neuroscience Reports* 18(12), 103.

Seshia, S.S. (2012) Chronic daily headache in children and adolescents. *Current Pain and Headache Reports* 16(1), 60–72.

Sillanpää, M. and Saarinen, M.M. (2018) Long term outcome of childhood onset headache: a prospective community study. *Cephalalgia* 38(6), 1159–1166.

Stinson, J.N., Huguet, A., McGrath, P., et al. (2013) A qualitative review of the psychometric properties and feasibility of electronic headache diaries for children and adults: where we are and where we need to go. *Pain Research and Management* 18(3), 142–152.

Szperka, C. (2021) Headache in children and adolescents. *Continuum (Minneap Minn)* 27(3), 703–731.

Szperka, C.L., VanderPluym, J., Orr, S.L., et al. (2018) Recommendations on the use of anti-CGRP monoclonal antibodies in children and adolescents. *Headache* 58(10), 1658–1669.

Trautmann, E., Lackschewitz, H. and Kröner-Herwig, B. (2006) Psychological treatment of recurrent headache in children and adolescents: a meta-analysis. *Cephalalgia* 26(12), 1411–1426.

van de Graaf, D.L., Schoonman, G.G., Habibović, M. and Pauws, S.C. (2021) Towards eHealth to support the health journey of headache patients: a scoping review. *Journal of Neurology* 268(10), 3646–3665.

Wang, S.J., Fuh, J.L. and Lu, S.R. (2009) Chronic daily headache in adolescents: an 8-year follow-up study. *Neurology* 73(6), 416–422.

Wöber-Bingöl, C. (2013) Epidemiology of migraine and headache in children and adolescents. *Current Pain and Headache Reports* 17(6), 341.

Youssef, P.E. and Mack, K.J. (2020) Episodic and chronic migraine in children. *Developmental Medicine and Child Neurology* 62(1), 34–41.

11 Chronic Postsurgical Pain in Children and Young People

Christina Liossi, Jacqui Clinch, and Brittany N. Rosenbloom

Chronic postsurgical pain (CPSP) is a frequent and often highly disabling complication of children's surgery. The definition originally proposed by Macrae (2008) and subsequently refined by Werner and Kongsgaard (2014) informed the International Classification of Diseases (ICD-11) definition (Schug et al. 2019) and is currently used in paediatric clinical practice and research. This definition maintains that CPSP exists when the criteria in Box 11.1 are met.

A meta-analysis of 628 patients revealed that approximately 20% of children and young people (CYP) who undergo surgery go on to develop CPSP pain 12 months after surgery (Rabbitts et al 2017). However, the prevalence rate for CPSP ranges between 11 and 54% (Rabbitts et al. 2017; Rosenbloom and Katz 2022). Such wide-ranging prevalence rates may be explained by studies being underpowered, combining a variety of surgical procedures, using various definitions of CPSP, having high attrition rates and long durations between time of surgery and report.

Key factors underlying the transition from acute to chronic postsurgical pain are complex, reflecting the interplay of biological, psychological and socioenvironmental factors (Chapman and Vierck 2017; Rabbitts et al. 2020;

> **BOX 11.1 DEFINITION OF CHRONIC POSTSURGICAL PAIN**
>
> - Pain develops or increases in intensity after a surgical procedure and persists at least three months after surgery.
> - Pain was not present preoperatively or is substantially different in character and intensity to any preoperative pain.
> - Pain interferes significantly with health-related quality of life.
> - Pain experienced is a continuation of acute postsurgical pain or develops after an asymptomatic period.
> - Pain is localised to the surgical site and/or projected to dermatome innervated by a nerve in the surgical field or Head's zone (after surgery to deep somatic and visceral tissues).
> - The cause of pain cannot be attributed to other causes (e.g. cancer recurrence, infection).
>
> Sources: Werner and Kongsgaard (2014); Schug et al. (2019).

Dourson et al. 2022; Newton-John 2022; Rosenbloom and Katz 2022; Walker 2022). To date, numerous risk factors that could be associated with the development of CPSP in CYP have been proposed and investigated with mixed results. These include:

- older age (Sieberg et al. 2013)
- female sex (Connelly et al. 2014)
- higher levels of preoperative pain (Batoz et al. 2016; Rosenbloom et al. 2019)
- higher levels of postoperative pain (Pagé et al. 2013; Rabbitts et al. 2015)
- higher levels of CYP catastrophic thinking about pain (Birnie et al. 2017)
- higher levels of parent/carer catastrophic thinking about pain (Rabbitts et al. 2015)
- higher levels of preoperative functional disability (Rosenbloom et al. 2019).

A systematic review identified presurgical increased pain intensity, high child anxiety, low child pain coping efficacy and high parental pain catastrophising as the only presurgical factors predictive of CPSP. Unexpectedly, the biological and medical factors assessed were not associated with CPSP in any of the reviewed studies (Rabbitts et al. 2017). Through preclinical research, it is hypothesised that biological factors (e.g. genetic, epigenetic, immune) play a role in the development of CPSP (Walker 2022; Dourson et al. 2022). However, more clinical research is needed in this area.

Postsurgical Pain Trajectories and Impact

There are significant differences in pain trajectories both between different surgical procedures and between subgroups of CYP undergoing the same procedure (Sieberg et al. 2013; Rabbitts et al. 2015; Chidambaran et al. 2017; Rosenbloom et al. 2019; Bailey et al. 2021). The number of trajectories range from two (e.g. low-pain group and high-pain group) to five pathways after surgery. A better understanding of pain trajectories after surgery and

how they are shaped by presurgical patient characteristics, and in turn affect functional outcomes, may facilitate the development of strategies to educate families, prevent CPSP and improve outcomes for CYP.

Bailey et al. (2021) identified three distinct postsurgical pain trajectories after scoliosis correction, characterised by:

- moderate to severe pain in the immediate postoperative period that sharply declined over the first few weeks and stabilised to mild or no pain by 12 months
- mild to moderate pain in the immediate postoperative period that gradually declined over the first few weeks and stabilised to mild or no pain by 12 months
- moderate to severe pain in the immediate postoperative period that gradually declined over the first few weeks and stabilised to moderate pain that remained at 12 months.

It is evident that frequency, intensity and functional disability associated with CPSP can vary widely across subgroups of CYP. After surgery some CYP can continue with their lives relatively unaffected while others become increasingly disabled and require referral to specialist pain services (Kachko et al. 2014; Birnie et al. 2022).

Management of Chronic Postsurgical Pain

There is no specific management plan for CPSP and little data to guide individual treatment decisions. The pain management plan tends to be generic across chronic pain diagnoses and informed by the patient's

CASE STUDY: PART 1

Jane is a 14-year-old girl with idiopathic scoliosis who underwent surgery three months
ago. She complains of excruciating pain across
the surgical scar. She is on a combination of
ibuprofen plus paracetamol and opioids that
make her feel drowsy and constipated but do
not 'touch the pain'.

1. What questions would you ask Jane
   about her pain to help with diagnosis
   and treatment?
2. What additional specialist assessments
   would you request to help with diagnosis and treatment of Jane's pain at
   this point?

biopsychosocial assessment and formulation
(Liossi and Howard 2016).

Biopsychosocial Assessment and Formulation

The initial assessment of CPSP includes pain-
specific characteristics, symptoms and behaviours, in addition to a psychosocial assessment
of the CYP and their family.

After a comprehensive assessment, a biopsychosocial formulation of the CPSP is
constructed jointly with the family and provides the framework for the individualised
treatment plan (Rajapakse et al. 2014; Liossi
and Howard 2016).

Treatment of Chronic Postsurgical Pain

CPSP management plans are multidisciplinary
and generally include a combination of pain
education, relevant therapeutic interventions
(pharmacological, psychological and physical)
and setting developmentally appropriate,

meaningful, functional outcome goals. Once
in place, the treatment plan requires reassessment at predetermined intervals and CYP
may require further assessment, formulation
or referral if symptoms are not resolved (Rajapakse et al. 2014).

Systematic reviews of interdisciplinary
interventions combining at least two or three
disciplines (Hechler et al. 2015; Liossi et al.
2019) in outpatient and intensive inpatient settings have shown them to reduce pain intensity and disability in children with chronic
pain, with the effects maintained at one year
follow-up. However, these findings are not
specific to CPSP.

Transitional pain services (TPS) have
emerged in adult tertiary care as an innovative and effective health service model to identify and address risk factors for CPSP (Azam
et al. 2017; Clarke et al. 2018; Katz et al. 2018;
Mikhaeil et al. 2020). TPS consist of comprehensive care provided by pain physicians,
advanced practice nurses, psychologists and
physiotherapists. There is a system readiness
for such a service to be adopted into children's care (Birnie et al 2022). However, more
research is needed on how to implement an
integrated pain service for CYP.

Pain Education

Pain education is a widely used first-line
treatment approach for chronic pain that aims
to challenge pre-existing beliefs of CYP and
their families around pain as a biomedical
phenomenon, instead introducing pain as a
biopsychosocial phenomenon. Tailored individualised education works best and, even if
brief, should always accompany the diagnosis
of chronic pain. In adults with low back pain,
education has been found to improve disability
and pain in the short term (Wood and Hendrick 2019). Adults in receipt of pain education
described the following educational concepts as

important for improvement from persistent pain (Leake et al. 2021):

- pain does not equal body damage
- thoughts, emotions and experiences affect, and are affected by, pain
- an overprotective pain system can be retrained.

When providing pain education within the context of surgery, it is important to incorporate any physical limitations required for healing. These physical limitations are often provided by the surgeon. A conversation about postsurgical activity/movement limitations should take place prior to surgery so that it reduces stress and anxiety after surgery as limitations are predictable.

Pharmacological Interventions

Despite the lack of evidence for the efficacy of pharmacological interventions for managing CPSP in CYP (Eccleston et al. 2019; Wang et al. 2020), over-the-counter and prescription medications are used to manage CPSP. Analgesics should be introduced on a trial basis and stopped if not effective or in the presence of unacceptable side effects. The choice of analgesic for CPSP in CYP is typically determined by:

- presumed underlying mechanism of pain (nociceptive, neuropathic, mixed)
- previous medication use
- adult data
- clinician experience.

In some cases, multimodal analgesia may be appropriate (Williams et al. 2017). Details of drugs that can be used to manage CPSP are provided in Table 11.1.

Basic analgesics such as paracetamol or non-steroidal anti-inflammatory drugs (NSAIDs) are not generally effective for CPSP.

- NSAIDs, such as ibuprofen or naproxen, can be effective in certain chronic pain conditions in adults but no similar evidence is available for children (Eccleston et al. 2017).
- If effective, for a child, basic analgesics can be used singly or in combination on an as-needed (PRN) or regular basis.
- However, the use of these drugs must be monitored over time and, particularly for NSAIDs, gastric protection should be prescribed.

Interventional Strategies

Interventional strategies have a limited role to play in the treatment of CPSP in CYP. Williams et al. (2017) reported that if the nature and location of the pain is favourable, local anaesthetic blockade (with or without steroid) can have an analgesic effect significantly beyond the duration of action of the analgesic agents for some patients. Often repeated blocks are required and appropriate patient selection alongside a robust risk–benefit analysis is needed (Williams et al. 2017).

Psychological Interventions

Multicomponent cognitive behavioural therapy (CBT) augmented by strategies such as relaxation, hypnosis, biofeedback, sleep management and operant strategies aimed at parents, is evidence-based and recommended as first-line treatment of CPSP (Coakley and Wihak 2017; Fisher et al. 2018).

PRACTICE POINT

- The core premise of CBT is that maladaptive cognitions (i.e. thoughts or visual images) contribute to the maintenance of emotional distress and behavioural problems (Hofmann et al. 2012).
- A randomised controlled trial showed that a novel strategy designed to reframe pain memories was effective at reducing CPSP interference among young people undergoing spinal fusion and pectus repair (Pavlova et al. 2022).

Table 11.1 Pharmacological management of chronic postsurgical pain in CYP.

Type of medication	Use and evidence of effectiveness
Anti-neuropathic agents (if pain is assumed to be neuropathic)	■ Tricyclic antidepressants and gabapentinoids are often used in CYP ■ Low-dose amitriptyline is often chosen where there is accompanying sleep disturbance ■ There is no good evidence from randomised controlled trials concerning the efficacy of antidepressants and antiepileptics in the treatment of chronic non-cancer pain in CYP (Cooper et al. 2017a,b)
Topical lidocaine and capsaicin	■ Lidocaine and capsaicin applications are commonly used for neuropathic pain in adults (Derry et al. 2017; Maloney et al. 2021) ■ There is anecdotal evidence for their efficacy in CYP, but the pain associated with application of high-concentration preparations of capsaicin requires the administration of additional oral analgesia and cooling during and after the application, to make the capsaicin more tolerable
Melatonin	■ Melatonin is safe and effective in treating primary sleep disorders and sleep disorders associated with CPSP (Esposito et al. 2019) ■ It has analgesic, anti-inflammatory and anxiolytic effects (Marseglia et al. 2015)
Opioids	■ Opioids are typically ineffective for treating CPSP in CYP due to side effects associated with their long-term use (Friedrichsdorf et al. 2016) ■ Due to the lack of evidence concerning the efficacy of opioids in treating chronic non-cancer pain in CYP (Cooper et al. 2017c), most clinicians will wean off patients from opioids if they have not been discontinued after surgery

Other popular psychologically informed therapeutic approaches include acceptance and commitment therapy (ACT), a third-wave behaviour therapy approach that aims to increase engagement in activities valued by the individuals experiencing chronic pain and associated distress. Additional information about CBT and ACT can be found in Chapter 1.

Limited evidence exists about the use of psychological interventions for CPSP in CYP. Evidence from other types of chronic pain that can be applied to CPSP is summarised below.

PRACTICE POINT

- Unlike classic CBT, ACT does not strive to directly alter maladaptive cognitions, but to increase the repertoire of responses to these cognitions and pain sensations (Pielech et al. 2017).
- Further, ACT targets six psychological processes, including acceptance, cognitive defusion, being present, self as context, values and committed action. Therefore, the initial assessment should involve a discussion of values and hobbies as they are important in motivating young people to move towards functioning and creating psychological flexibility.

- A systematic review of psychological interventions delivered face to face found them to be efficacious at reducing pain frequency in CYP with headache, and pain intensity and anxiety in CYP with other chronic pain conditions post treatment (Fisher et al. 2018). However, these effects were not maintained at follow-up.
- Psychological therapies were beneficial for reducing disability in CYP with mixed chronic pain conditions at post-treatment and follow-up, and for CYP with headache at follow-up (Fisher et al. 2018).

■ Among adults undergoing surgery, psychological interventions delivered by psychologists and provided after surgery were effective at reducing CPSP (Nadinda et al. 2022).

Despite the benefits of face-to-face interventions, there are barriers to attending multidisciplinary pain services, where these exist, for CYP and parents. These include:

■ physical limitations recommended after surgery (e.g. avoidance of long car rides)
■ school and work absence
■ financial costs of travel
■ logistics of organising family life around appointments.

Even though CYP and parents view online interventions positively (Hurley-Wallace et al. 2021), there are only a small number of trials where the remote delivery of psychological therapies via the internet was investigated. Notably, a meta-analysis by Fisher et al. (2019) of 10 studies that delivered remote treatment found that:

■ headache severity was reduced post treatment, but the effect was not maintained at follow-up
■ there were no effects of psychological therapies delivered remotely for disability, anxiety and depression post treatment or at follow-up
■ for mixed pain conditions, there were no beneficial effects of psychological therapies for reducing pain intensity, disability, anxiety or depression post treatment or at follow-up.

Murray et al (2022) published a pilot feasibility trial of an internet-delivered CBT intervention designed for young people undergoing spinal fusion surgery, which showed that this type of intervention is acceptable to young people for managing their perioperative pain. However, more research is needed to examine the efficacy of internet-based CBT interventions for CPSP.

Physical Interventions

Physiotherapy and other physical interventions are an integral part of the multidisciplinary management of CPSP in CYP (Ayling Campos et al. 2011). The combination of aerobic exercises, strengthening and stretching is individualised after a comprehensive history-taking and physical examination. Incorporating Pilates exercises into physiotherapy has been shown to be more effective in decreasing pain intensity, and improving cardiorespiratory fitness, functional ability and quality of life in children with polyarticular juvenile idiopathic arthritis than physiotherapy alone (Azab et al. 2022).

Local heat or cold applications, transcutaneous electrical nerve stimulation (TENS), massage therapy and desensitisation techniques are often used along with complementary medicine interventions such as acupuncture, though evidence for any of these interventions alone is weak (Rajapakse et al. 2014).

CASE STUDY: PART 2

Jane reports her pain to be 12/10; the pain is both superficial and deep. Jane cannot tolerate water on her back when showering and does not allow her mum to touch the skin on or around the scar. She finds it difficult to fall asleep at night and wakes up multiple times during the night in pain.

Specialist psychological assessment reveals low mood, body image dissatisfaction, reduced school attendance and impaired social functioning. Jane's parents are increasingly frustrated and feel helpless, not knowing how best to support Jane.

Specialist physiotherapy assessment shows global deconditioning, and loss of flexibility and decreased range of motion of the spine consistent with scoliosis surgery.

1. What analgesic drugs would you wean Jane off at this point? What analgesic drugs would you prescribe for Jane? What additional medications might you add to Jane's treatment plan at this point?
2. What physical and psychological interventions might specialised health professionals want to include in Jane's pain management plan?
3. In educating Jane and her parents about these strategies, what would you take into consideration?

Prevention of Chronic Postsurgical Pain

Although factors that increase the risk of CPSP have been identified, little is known regarding how to prevent the transition from acute to chronic postsurgical pain. Until further research is conducted, and the exact pathophysiological transition pathway is understood, we need a multidisciplinary preventive approach that involves intensive perioperative psychological and physical therapy, and pharmacological management interventions.

A developmentally appropriate screening measure is needed for early identification of CYP at high risk for CPSP to guide treatment and referral for specialised care. One measure designed to predict children's chronic (non-surgical) pain has been tested within a surgical population (Narayanasamy et al. 2022). However, this measure does not capture all known risk factors for CPSP in CYP and was not designed for CYP as it was modified from an adult back pain screening tool.

It is important we intervene in the pre- and post-surgery phases by:

- effectively treating acute pain (Williams et al. 2017)
- targeting the mechanisms that promote CPSP, for example repeated doses of gabapentin after spinal fusion reduce postoperative opioid requirements but its effects on CPSP are unknown (Rusy et al. 2010)
- assessing patient and parental characteristics associated with increased risk of development of CPSP and addressing them through targeted psychological interventions (Rabbitts et al. 2021).

Summary

- CPSP is a frequent and often highly disabling complication of surgery in CYP.
- Presurgical factors predictive of CPSP include increased pain intensity, high CYP anxiety, low CYP pain coping efficacy, and high parental pain catastrophising.
- Pain management for CPSP in CYP is informed by the patient's biopsychosocial assessment and formulation and includes a combination of education, medications, psychological strategies, physical strategies, and addressing all areas of pain-associated disability.
- To prevent CPSP it is important we intervene in the pre- and post-surgery phases by effectively treating acute pain, targeting

the mechanisms that promote CPSP, assessing patient and parental characteristics associated with increased risk of development of CPSP, and addressing them through targeted psychological interventions.

Key to Case Study

Part 1

1. It would be helpful to ask Jane about the pain location, onset, duration, quality, variability, and exacerbating and alleviating factors. It is important to ask specific questions about any pain before surgery and how pain affects sleep.
2. It is important at this point that you ask for specialist assessments by a psychologist and physiotherapist to ascertain Jane's functioning in key aspects of her life: school, social, hobbies, emotional functioning, activities of daily living, and how the family as a unit manages Jane's condition and pain.

Part 2

1. Jane may benefit from weaning off opioids, discontinuing ibuprofen plus paracetamol if they offer no therapeutic benefit, and introducing amitriptyline at bedtime, starting at a low dose to prevent oversedation. Medication may then be titrated up if required. Lidocaine patches may also be helpful.

2. Early referral to a physiotherapist experienced in managing pain after scoliosis surgery for assessment and intervention would be helpful. Exercises should aim to improve mobility, strength and stamina, as well as desensitise the back to reduce allodynia and hyperalgesia. This can be achieved by having Jane's mum start to gently touch Jane's back with different textures as tolerated until Jane is able to shower without difficulty.

   An early referral to a child psychologist for pain assessment and CBT would be useful. CBT could help by providing pain coping strategies as well as help Jane to improve her mood, body image, sleep hygiene and social and school functioning. Parenting advice and intervention might also be helpful.
3. Explaining the clinical diagnosis, the biopsychosocial model of chronic pain and the reasons for the treatment plan is important for Jane to participate in treatment.

Multiple Choice Questions

1. What is the minimum duration for pain to continue after surgery to enable it to be classified as chronic postsurgical pain?
   a. At least one month
   b. At least two months
   c. At least three months
   d. At least four months

2. Which *two* of the following options are risk factors for the development of CPSP in CYP?
   a. Increasing age and female sex
   b. Laparoscopic surgery
   c. Short operations
   d. Increased presurgical and/or postsurgical pain intensity, high child anxiety, low child pain coping efficacy, and high parental pain catastrophising

3. Which one of the following may help to reduce the incidence of CPSP in CYP?
   a. Steroids
   b. Antibiotics
   c. Pre-emptive analgesia
   d. Amitriptyline
4. Which one of the following statements is *incorrect*?
   a. CPSP management plans are multidisciplinary
   b. Opioids are highly effective in CPSP management and have few side effects
   c. Simple analgesics such as paracetamol and NSAIDs are not generally effective for CPSP
   d. Anti-neuropathic agents such gabapentin and amitriptyline can be prescribed if CPSP is assumed to be neuropathic in nature or mixed

Acknowledgements

C.L. is supported by funds from Great Ormond Street Hospital Children's Charity Research Awards (V5118, V4421). B.N.R. is supported by the Pain in Child Health (PICH) Postdoctoral Fellowship Award supported by the Louise and Alan Edwards Foundation and the Restracomp Fellowship from The Hospital for Sick Children.

References

Ayling Campos, A., Amaria, K., Campbell, F. and McGrath, P.A. (2011) Clinical impact and evidence base for physiotherapy in treating childhood chronic pain. *Physiotherapy Canada* 63(1), 21–33.

Azab, A.R., Kamel, F.H., Basha, M.A., et al. (2022) Impact of clinical Pilates exercise on pain, cardiorespiratory fitness, functional ability, and quality of life in children with polyarticular juvenile idiopathic arthritis. *International Journal of Environmental Research and Public Health* 19(13), 7793.

Azam, M.A., Weinrib, A.Z., Montbriand, J., et al. (2017) Acceptance and commitment therapy to manage pain and opioid use after major surgery: preliminary outcomes from the Toronto General Hospital Transitional Pain Service. *Canadian Journal of Pain* 1(1), 37–49.

Bailey, K.M., Howard, J.J., El-Hawary, R. and Chorney, J. (2021) Pain trajectories following adolescent idiopathic scoliosis correction: analysis of predictors and functional outcomes. *JBJS Open Access* 6(2), e20.00122.

Batoz, H., Semjen, F., Bordes-Demolis, M., Bénard, A. and Nouette-Gaulain, K. (2016) Chronic postsurgical pain in children: prevalence and risk factors. A prospective observational study. *British Journal of Anaesthesia* 117(4), 489–496.

Birnie, K.A., Chorney, J., El-Hawary, R. and PORSCHE Study Group (2017) Child and parent pain catastrophizing and pain from pre-surgery to six weeks post-surgery: examination of cross-sectional and longitudinal actor-partner effects. *Pain* 158(10), 1886–1892.

Birnie, K.A., Stinson, J., Isaac, L., et al. (2022) Mapping the current state of pediatric surgical pain care across Canada and assessing readiness for change. *Canadian Journal of Pain* 6(2), 108–120.

Chapman, C.R. and Vierck, C.J. (2017) The transition of acute postoperative pain to chronic pain: an integrative overview of research on mechanisms. *Journal of Pain* 18(4), 359.e1–359.e38.

Chidambaran, V., Ding, L., Moore, D.L., et al. (2017) Predicting the pain continuum after adolescent idiopathic scoliosis surgery: a prospective cohort study. *European Journal of Pain* 21(7), 1252–1265.

Clarke, H., Azargive, S., Montbriand, J., et al. (2018) Opioid weaning and pain management in post-surgical patients at the Toronto General Hospital Transitional Pain Service. *Canadian Journal of Pain* 2(1), 236–247.

Coakley, R. and Wihak, T. (2017) Evidence-based psychological interventions for the management of pediatric chronic pain: new directions in research and clinical practice. *Children* 4(2), 9.

Connelly, M., Fulmer, R.D., Prohaska, J., et al. (2014) Predictors of postoperative pain trajectories in adolescent idiopathic scoliosis. *Spine* 39(3), E174–E181.

Cooper, T.E., Heathcote, L.C., Clinch, J., et al. (2017a) Antidepressants for chronic non-cancer pain in children and adolescents. *Cochrane Database of Systematic Reviews* (8), CD012535.

Cooper, T.E., Wiffen, P.J., Heathcote, L.C., et al. (2017b) Antiepileptic drugs for chronic non-cancer pain in children and adolescents. *Cochrane Database of Systematic Reviews* (8), CD012536.

Cooper, T.E., Fisher, E., Gray, A.L., et al. (2017c) Opioids for chronic non-cancer pain in children and adolescents. *Cochrane Database of Systematic Reviews* (7), CD012538.

Derry, S., Wiffen, P.J., Kalso, E.A.,et al. (2017) Topical analgesics for acute and chronic pain in adults: an overview of Cochrane Reviews. *Cochrane Database of Systematic Reviews* (5), CD008609.

Dourson, A.J., Willits, A., Raut, N.G.R., et al. (2022) Genetic and epigenetic mechanisms influencing acute to chronic postsurgical pain transitions in pediatrics: preclinical to clinical evidence. *Canadian Journal of Pain* 6(2), 85–107.

Eccleston, C., Cooper, T.E., Fisher, E.,. Anderson, B. and Wilkinson, N.M (2017) Non-steroidal anti-inflammatory drugs (NSAIDs) for chronic non-cancer pain in children and adolescents. *Cochrane Database of Systematic Reviews* (8), CD012537.

Eccleston, C., Fisher, E., Cooper, T.E., et al. (2019) Pharmacological interventions for chronic pain in children: an overview of systematic reviews. *Pain* 160(8), 1698–1707.

Esposito, S., Laino, D., D'Alonzo, R., et al. (2019) Pediatric sleep disturbances and treatment with melatonin. *Journal of Translational Medicine* 17(1), 77.

Fisher, E., Law, E., Dudeney, J., Palermo, T.M., Stewart, G. and Eccleston, C. (2018) Psychological therapies for the management of chronic and recurrent pain in children and adolescents. *Cochrane Database of Systematic Reviews* (9), CD003968.

Fisher, E., Law, E., Dudeney, J., Eccleston, C and Palermo, T.M. (2019) Psychological therapies (remotely delivered) for the management of chronic and recurrent pain in children and adolescents. *Cochrane Database of Systematic Reviews* (4), CD011118.

Friedrichsdorf, S.J., Giordano, J., Desai Dakoji, K., Warmuth, A., Daughtry, C. and Schulz, C.A. (2016) Chronic pain in children and adolescents: diagnosis and treatment of primary pain disorders in head, abdomen, muscles and joints. *Children* 3(4), 42.

Hechler, T., Kanstrup, M., Holley, A.L., et al. (2015) Systematic review on intensive interdisciplinary pain treatment of children with chronic pain. *Pediatrics* 136(1), 115–127.

Hofmann, S.G., Asnaani, A., Vonk, I.J., Sawyer, A.T. and Fang, A. (2012) The efficacy of cognitive behavioral therapy: a review of meta-analyses. *Cognitive Therapy and Research* 36(5), 427–440.

Hurley-Wallace, A., Schoth, D.E., Lilley, S., Williams, G. and Liossi, C. (2021) Online paediatric chronic pain management: assessing the needs of UK adolescents and parents, using a cross-sectional survey. *British Journal of Pain* 15(3), 312–325.

Kachko, L., Ben Ami, S., Lieberman, A., Shor, R., Tzeitlin, E. and Efrat, R. (2014) Neuropathic pain other than CRPS in children and adolescents: incidence, referral, clinical characteristics, management, and clinical outcomes. *Pediatric Anesthesia* 24(6), 608–613.

Katz, J., Weinrib, A.Z. and Clarke, H. (2018) Chronic postsurgical pain: from risk factor identification to multidisciplinary management at the Toronto General Hospital Transitional Pain Service. *Canadian Journal of Pain* 3(2), 49–58.

Leake, H.B., Moseley, G.L., Stanton, T.R., O'Hagan, E.T. and Heathcote, L.C. (2021) What do patients value learning about pain? A mixed-methods survey on the relevance of target concepts after pain science education. *Pain* 162(10), 2558–2568.

Liossi, C. and Howard, R.F. (2016) Pediatric chronic pain: biopsychosocial assessment and formulation. *Pediatrics* 138(5), e20160331.

Liossi, C., Johnstone, L., Lilley, S., Caes, L., Williams, G. and Schoth, D.E. (2019) Effectiveness of interdisciplinary interventions in paediatric chronic pain management: a systematic review and subset meta-analysis. *British Journal of Anaesthesia* 123(2), e359–e371.

Macrae, W.A. (2008) Chronic post-surgical pain: 10 years on. *British Journal of Anaesthesia* 101(1), 77–86.

Maloney, J., Pew, S., Wie, C., Gupta, R., Freeman, J. and Strand, N. (2021) Comprehensive review of topical analgesics for chronic pain. *Current Pain and Headache Reports* 25(2), 7.

Marseglia, L., D'Angelo, G., Manti, S., et al. (2015) Analgesic, anxiolytic and anaesthetic effects of melatonin: new potential uses in pediatrics. *International Journal of Molecular Sciences* 16(1), 1209–1220.

Mikhaeil, J., Ayoo, K., Clarke, H., Wąsowicz, M. and Huang, A. (2020) Review of the Transitional Pain Service as a method of postoperative opioid weaning and a service aimed at minimizing the risk of chronic post-surgical pain. *Anaesthesiology Intensive Therapy* 52(2), 148–153.

Murray, C.B., Bartlett, A., Meyyappan, A., Palermo, T.M., Aaron, R. and Rabbitts, J. (2022) A pilot feasibility and acceptability study of an Internet-delivered psychosocial intervention to reduce postoperative pain in adolescents undergoing spinal fusion. *Canadian Journal of Pain* 6(2), 61–72.

Nadinda, P.G., van Ryckeghem, D.M.L. and Peters, M.L. (2022) Can perioperative psychological interventions decrease the risk of postsurgical pain and disability? A systematic review and meta-analysis of randomized controlled trials. *Pain* 163(7), 1254–1273.

Narayanasamy, S., Yang, F., Ding, L., et al. (2022) Pediatric pain screening tool: a simple 9-item questionnaire predicts functional and chronic postsurgical pain outcomes after major musculoskeletal surgeries. *Journal of Pain* 32(1), 98–111.

Newton-John, T. (2022) Extending the biopsychosocial conceptualization of chronic postsurgical pain in children and adolescents: the family systems perspective. *Canadian Journal of Pain* 6(2), 142–151.

Pagé, M.G., Stinson, J., Campbell, F., Isaac, L. and Katz, J. (2013) Identification of pain-related psychological risk factors for the development and maintenance of pediatric chronic postsurgical pain. *Journal of Pain Research* 6, 167–180.

Pavlova, M., Lund, T., Sun, J., Katz, J., Brindle, M. and Noel, M. (2022) A memory-reframing intervention to reduce pain in youth undergoing major surgery: pilot randomized controlled trial of feasibility and acceptability. *Canadian Journal of Pain* 6(2), 152–165.

Pielech, M., Vowles, K.E. and Wicksell, R. (2017) Acceptance and commitment therapy for pediatric chronic pain: theory and application. *Children* 4(2), 10.

Rabbitts, J.A., Zhou, C., Groenewald, C.B., Durkin, L. and Palermo, T.M. (2015) Trajectories of postsurgical pain in children: risk factors and impact of late pain recovery on long-term health outcomes after major surgery. *Pain* 156(11), 2383–2389.

Rabbitts, J.A., Fisher, E., Rosenbloom, B.N. and Palermo, T.M. (2017) Prevalence and predictors of chronic postsurgical pain in children: a systematic review and meta-analysis. *Journal of Pain* 18(6), 605–614.

Rabbitts, J.A., Palermo, T.M. and Lang, E.A. (2020) A conceptual model of biopsychosocial mechanisms of transition from acute to chronic postsurgical pain in children and adolescents. *Journal of Pain Research* 13, 3071–3080.

Rabbitts, J.A., Zhou, C., de la Vega, R., Aalfs, H., Murray, C.B. and Palermo, T.M. (2021) A digital health peri-operative cognitive-behavioral intervention to prevent transition from acute to chronic postsurgical pain in adolescents undergoing spinal fusion (SurgeryPal™): study protocol for a multisite randomized controlled trial. *Trials* 22(1), 506.

Rajapakse, D., Liossi, C. and Howard, R.F. (2014) Presentation and management of chronic pain. *Archives of Disease in Childhood* 99(5), 474–480.

Rosenbloom, B.N. and Katz, J. (2022) Modeling the transition from acute to chronic postsurgical pain in youth: a narrative review of epidemiologic, perioperative, and psychosocial factors. *Canadian Journal of Pain* 6(2), 166–174.

Rosenbloom, B.N., Pagé, M.G., Isaac, L., et al. (2019) Pediatric chronic postsurgical pain and functional disability: a prospective study of risk factors up to one year after major surgery. *Journal of Pain Research* 12, 3079–3098.

Rusy, L.M., Hainsworth, K.R., Nelson, T.J., et al. (2010) Gabapentin use in pediatric spinal fusion patients: a randomized, double-blind, controlled trial. *Survey of Anesthesiology* 55(1), 45–46.

Schug, S.A., Lavand'homme, P., Barke, A., et al. (2019) The IASP classification of chronic pain for ICD-11: chronic postsurgical or posttraumatic pain. *Pain* 160(1), 45–52.

Sieberg, C.B., Simons, L.E., Edelstein, M.R., et al. (2013) Pain prevalence and trajectories following pediatric spinal fusion surgery. *Journal of Pain* 14(12), 1694–1702.

Walker, S. (2022) Developmental mechanisms of CPSP: clinical observations and translational laboratory evaluations. *Canadian Journal of Pain* 6(2), 49–60.

Wang, G.S., Olsen, H., Severtson, G., Green, J.L. and Dart, R.C. (2020) The impact of the prescription opioid epidemic on young children: trends and mortality. *Drug and Alcohol Dependence* 211, 107924.

Werner, M.U. and Kongsgaard, U.E. (2014) Defining persistent post-surgical pain: is an update required? *British Journal of Anaesthesia* 113(1), 1–4.

Williams, G., Howard, R.F. and Liossi, C. (2017) Persistent postsurgical pain in children and young people: prediction, prevention, and management. *Pain Reports* 2(5), e616.

Wood, L. and Hendrick, P.A. (2019) A systematic review and meta-analysis of pain neuroscience education for chronic low back pain: short- and long-term outcomes of pain and disability. *European Journal of Pain* 23(2), 234–249.

12 Prevention and Management of Procedural Pain

Kaytlin Constantin, Anna Taddio, Deepa Kattail, and C. Meghan McMurtry

Medical procedures are a common source of pain and fear in childhood. Substantial research has focused on the pain and fear related to medical procedures in children and young people (CYP). The goal of this chapter is to provide practical, current and evidence-based guidance for the assessment and management of painful medical procedures in childhood. Using a multimodal approach, we include a review of psychological, physical, procedural and pharmacological interventions. See Chapters 6 and 13 for pain assessment and management in individuals with developmental or learning (intellectual) disabilities and infants.

Procedural Pain

Needles are ubiquitous in healthcare (Box 12.1 lists common procedures). Vaccines are the most common source of needle-related pain, with approximately two dozen injections typically given during childhood (Public Health Agency of Canada 2023). CYP with chronic illness (e.g. arthritis, diabetes, cancer) may undergo many more painful procedures as part of the treatment of their condition, including intravenous injections, finger pokes/pricks and lumbar punctures. CYP who are hospitalised frequently undergo needle procedures: in a Canadian study including almost 4000 hospitalised children, over 78% had experienced a painful procedure in the previous 24 hours (mean number of procedures = 6; Stevens et al. 2011). While 78% of children had a pain management strategy documented within the preceding 24 hours, less than 30% were paired with/documented for a given procedure (Stevens et al. 2011). This is one example of a substantive body of literature which demonstrates that procedural pain is under-recognised and undertreated

> **BOX 12.1 PAINFUL MEDICAL PROCEDURES**
>
> - Immunisations via injection
> - Other injections (e.g. of medicines)
> - Venepuncture, venous cannulation
> - Laceration repair
> - Fracture reduction
> - Heel lance, fingerprick (poke)
> - Dressing changes or wound care
> - Insertion or removal of tubes (e.g. arterial, venous, urinary catheters)
> - Subcutaneous reservoir access (e.g. Port-a-Cath)
> - Lumbar puncture
> - Bone marrow aspiration
>
> Source: Adapted from Reid et al. (2013)

Managing Pain in Children and Young People: A Clinical Guide, Third Edition. Edited by Alison Twycross, Jennifer Stinson, William T. Zempsky, and Abbie Jordan.
© 2024 John Wiley & Sons Ltd. Published 2024 by John Wiley & Sons Ltd.

(Twycross and Collis 2013; Birnie et al. 2014; Friedrichsdorf et al. 2015).

Undertreated procedural pain is associated with negative short-term effects (e.g. unnecessary pain and suffering, longer procedure times, increased use of restraint) and longer-term consequences (e.g. negative memories of the procedure, increased distress and pain at future procedures, need for more analgesic, high levels of needle/procedure-related fear, potential for healthcare avoidance; McMurtry et al. 2015; Friedrichsdorf and Goubert 2020).

> **PRACTICE POINT**
>
> Procedural pain in CYP is under-recognised and undermanaged. Inadequate management of procedural pain and distress is associated with adverse short- and long-term consequences.

Assessing Procedural Pain and Fear

Medical procedures commonly induce pain, fear and anxiety in CYP. Fear is an alarm reaction to a perceived threat and is associated with attempts to escape (e.g. a child flailing, trying to leave). Anxiety is more anticipatory and associated with hypervigilance and avoidance (e.g. child worries, asks their caregiver whether a needle will occur at each doctor's appointment). See McMurtry et al. (2015) for details.

Bidirectional relationships exist between pain and fear and anxiety (Taddio et al. 2012; McMurtry et al. 2011, 2015).

- Higher levels of fear and anxiety relate to increased pain. A negative cycle of increased pain, fear and anxiety can develop and perpetuate future distress related to medical procedures.
- Fear of the pain or other procedure-related factors (e.g. being restrained) escalates pain and fear over time.

- Anxiety about the procedure can lead to focus on threatening aspects of the procedure and heightened pain and fear.

Here, we focus most of this chapter on the assessment and management of fear because:

- pain assessment is described in Chapter 6
- anxiety will be most relevant for only a subset of individuals with high apprehension
- the current readership are likely to be engaging with individuals in close temporal proximity to procedures when fear (not anxiety) is the dominant feature.

Assessment Methods

The process of assessing pain and fear accurately and reliably is a logical precursor to selecting appropriate interventions (McMurtry et al. 2015). Table 12.1 provides an overview of common fear assessment measures (see Chapter 6 for details on pain assessment methods).

> **PRACTICE POINT**
>
> - Understanding pain and fear are important for understanding the child's experience, guiding treatment and facilitating future procedures. Child self-report needs to be developmentally appropriate.
> - Numerous tools have been developed and are freely available for assessing pain and fear in CYP. Guidelines exist on the best-practice tools for different populations.

Additional Assessment Considerations

Screening for High Levels of Needle Fear

In the context of needle procedures, screening for high levels of needle fear is recommended as

Table 12.1 Recommended guidelines for the assessment of procedure-related fear.

Measure	Type	Description	Scoring details	Originally intended age range
Children's Fear Scale (McMurtry et al. 2011)	Self-report	One item measure of fear	Score range: 0–4	5–10 years
	Caregiver/proxy	Children (or caregivers) choose between one of five sex-neutral faces ranging from a neutral face showing no fear to a face showing extreme fear		
Verbal Descriptor Scale (Taddio et al. 2015)	Self-report	■ One item measure of fear ■ Children report level of fear: not at all, a little bit, a medium amount, a lot, or very much/ most possible	Score range: 0–4	5–12 years
Numerical Rating Scale of Fear (Taddio et al. 2015)	Self-report	One item measure of fear	Score range: 0–10	8 years and older
	Caregiver/proxy	0–10 Numerical Rating Scale (NRS), where 0 means no fear/not scared at all and 10 is most fear/most scared possible		

high levels of needle fear interfere with the implementation and success of pain management strategies (McMurtry et al. 2015). CYP identified as having high levels of needle fear should be treated by a professional with mental health expertise before the procedure, unless it is urgently required, or sedation can be used. Table 12.2 lists questions that can be posed to screen for high levels of needle fear (see Taddio et al. 2015 for full guideline).

Fears Related to Needle Procedures

Identifying the needle fear focus (i.e. what the child is afraid of) is needed to treat the fear and/ or modify the procedural context to facilitate

care. Fear is complex and may involve worry related to any of the following:

■ fear of the unknown (what will happen)
■ experiencing pain
■ feeling sick/dizzy before, during or after getting a needle procedure
■ fainting
■ seeing blood
■ travelling to and/or waiting at the hospital/ clinic/lab
■ hearing and seeing other children screaming or crying
■ seeing the needle
■ seeing the needle in their arm

Table 12.2 Questions to screen for high needle fear.

Age	Questions

Young children (5–10 years)
 	
(Caregivers can be asked these questions about their child, if the child is unable to respond)
	▪ How scared of needles are you?
	  ▪ Not at all scared
	  ▪ A little bit
	  ▪ Medium amount
	  ▪ A lot
	  ▪ Very, very much/most possible
	▪ Do you try really hard to miss getting the needle because you are so scared?

Older children (> 10 years)
 	
(Caregivers can be asked these questions about their CYP, if the CYP is unable to respond)
	▪ How afraid of needles are you?
	  ▪ Not afraid
	  ▪ A little bit
	  ▪ Medium/moderate amount
	  ▪ A lot
	  ▪ Most afraid possible
	▪ Do you think this is higher than you want it to be? Or than it should be?
	▪ Do you avoid getting needles because you are afraid?

▪ being 'poked' multiple times
▪ being held down for the needle.

Referral sources for CYP with high needle fear include anxiety clinics and programmes, and licensed practitioners of psychology, social work and psychiatry with knowledge of the treatment of anxiety disorders.

Screening for a History of Vasovagal Syncope (Fainting)

Fainting during a procedure carries a risk of injury. Risk factors for fainting include high levels of needle fear, adolescence, low body mass and female sex (Yamada and Yanagimoto 2017). The following are screening questions for vasovagal syncope (Taddio et al. 2015). A positive response to any of them may trigger a pre-emptive intervention (see Box 12.2 for more details):

▪ 'Have you ever felt quite dizzy, light-headed, nauseated/like you are going to throw up, and/or sweaty when getting a needle?' These represent prodromal signs of vasovagal syncope.

▪ 'Have you ever fainted, that is, lost consciousness or passed out during a needle procedure?'
▪ Caregivers can be asked analogous questions about their child.

BOX 12.2 USEFUL TECHNIQUE FOR MINIMISING THE RISK OF FAINTING IN CYP OVER SEVEN YEARS OF AGE

Muscle tension: steps

A. Before, during and after the procedure, the CYP tenses major muscle groups (e.g. legs, abdomen, arms) other than the body part where the needle will be inserted.

B. Tension is held for around 10–15 seconds or until a warm feeling ('flush') is felt in the face.

C. Tension is released back to baseline (not fully relaxed) for around 20–30 seconds.

D. Steps B and C are repeated until the procedure is over and/or the symptoms pass.

Caregiver Distress

Medical procedures can be distressing for both CYP and caregivers (McMurtry et al. 2015). Assessing caregiver distress is relevant as (i) caregiver responses play a significant role in shaping CYP's procedural pain, and (ii) distress may interfere with their ability to support their child effectively (Martin et al. 2013; McMurtry et al. 2015). Caregiver distress can be assessed using an 11-point numeric rating scale:

> *How distressed are you about your child's procedure on a scale from 0 to 10, where 0 = not distressed at all and 10 = extremely distressed?*

CASE STUDY: PART 1

Charlotte is an eight-year-old girl with type 1 diabetes who arrived at the clinic with her caregivers for routine blood work. Charlotte says she does not feel good and her stomach feels weird. She hates coming to the clinic and recalled how last time it took several attempts to complete the procedure. Her caregivers respond by saying she will be fine, and that the procedure is quick.

1. What do you need to know?
2. What assessment tools would you use with Charlotte?

Managing Procedural Pain

General Overview and Considerations

It is important that each procedure is necessary and the least painful or least invasive procedure is used to reach the objective (Association of Paediatric Anaesthetists of Great Britain and Ireland [APA] 2012). Sufficient time to implement the relevant interventions should be observed, unless it is an emergency (APA 2012). Interventions can be grouped into categories (Taddio et al. 2015), but there is overlap and a multicomponent approach is recommended, as described at the end of this chapter (see Table 12.9).

Physical Interventions

Environmental Considerations

Use of procedure rooms or other designated places for hospitalised CYP is recommended so that beds and play areas stay safe spaces (Young 2005). The environment should be as quiet and calm as possible (APA 2012). Advising an individual to look away from the needle is commonly used to direct an individual's visual attention away from pain and fear cues and is believed to reduce pain and fear during needle procedures (Höfle et al. 2012). Current evidence is mixed, and therefore more work is needed to ascertain for whom this intervention is most effective (Vijayan et al. 2015; Mithal et al. 2018). Asking the child about their preference (e.g. 'Do you prefer to look towards or away from the needle') and proceeding according to their preference is recommended.

Positioning

Positioning is an important physical intervention for all ages (e.g. 'comfort positioning'). The procedure should be completed in a position that gives CYP a sense of control (e.g. sitting or upright rather than lying down with staff looming over them; Taddio et al. 2015; Friedrichsdorf and Goubert 2020). Children should not be restrained as this increases fear and pain experience (Taddio et al. 2015; Friedrichsdorf and Goubert 2020).

Tactile Stimulation

The Buzzy® (MMJ Labs, Atlanta, GA, USA) is a vibrating device in the shape of a bee that also incorporates cold (via ice 'wings') and distraction. It is placed near the site where a needle will enter approximately 30–60 seconds before the procedure, and kept there for the duration. A recent systematic review of nine trials concluded that the Buzzy is a promising intervention for reducing pain and 'anxiety' from needle procedures (Ballard et al. 2019; note that these authors use 'anxiety' to refer to distress, fear, and/or stress). Manual tactile stimulation (e.g. rubbing, stroking) is not recommended in a practice guideline for vaccinations due to lack of observed benefit (Taddio et al. 2015).

PRACTICE POINT

Physical interventions include body position and activity (e.g. upright positioning, breastfeeding) and consideration of the broader environment that together reduce pain and related symptoms.

Additional Considerations: Fainting

If screening shows a risk for fainting, muscle tension could be helpful for young people aged over seven years (Öst and Sterner 1987; Taddio et al. 2015; McMurtry et al. 2016). This technique is designed to avoid a sudden drop in blood pressure and heart rate that can lead to fainting (see Box 12.2 and https://pphc.uoguelph.ca/needle-fear-resources/).

Procedural Interventions

Procedural interventions that have been found to effectively reduce pain across all ages include (Taddio et al. 2015; Trottier et al. 2019):

- central catheter rather than peripheral catheter for long-term vascular access
- performing venepuncture rather than heel lance for newborn screening test
- eliminating the use of aspiration during intramuscular vaccine injections
- injecting the most painful vaccine last during vaccine injections
- injecting vaccines quickly
- buffering and warming local anaesthetic solutions before subcutaneous injections.

CASE STUDY: PART 2

1. Is there any information you could obtain from Charlotte that could help determine the procedural and physical strategies that would be helpful?
2. What physical strategies could you use to manage Charlotte's pain related to her procedure?

Psychological Interventions

Psychological interventions often take a cognitive behavioural therapy (CBT) approach and focus on providing CYP with strategies to change the way they think, feel and/or respond to the procedure. Psychological interventions are appealing given that they rely on a child's coping tendencies and require minimal or widely available resources (Birnie et al. 2018). Psychological interventions can be implemented as described below.

- In preparation for the visit: preparatory information, modelling, creating positive self-statements.

■ On the day of the visit: communication, distraction, relaxation, hypnosis, applying positive self-statements.

Preparatory Information

Medical procedures and the setting in which they occur are often unfamiliar, including the people and equipment involved (Bray et al. 2019). Preparing CYP for the procedure involves explaining in advance what the procedure will entail. This can help reduce anxiety and uncertainty and is recommended for children aged three years and older (Taddio et al. 2015). The level of detail provided should be tailored to the CYP's developmental stage, temperament and individual coping styles (Table 12.3). Optimal timing will differ based on age and procedure (Jaaniste et al. 2007).

General guidance is available for caregivers and health professionals on how they can help CYP prepare for the procedure (Jaaniste et al. 2007; Reid et al. 2013; Pillai Riddell et al. 2015; Bray et al. 2019; see section Relevant web resources).

■ Describe the procedure by breaking down the steps involved. This should include sensory information, such as what they will see, hear and feel (e.g. 'The nurse will tie a rubber band around your arm').

■ Show where the procedure will take place and the equipment that will be used.

■ Use medical play or developmentally appropriate procedure preparation kits to increase familiarity of equipment, which can enhance a CYP's understanding of the procedure, allow them to express their feelings towards the procedure, and clarify misconceptions.

■ Provide opportunities to ask questions.

■ Provide coping strategies. Give choices whenever possible. Avoid providing an option that results in not having to complete the procedure.

■ Avoid saying it will not hurt or that it will definitely hurt. Instead, you might say 'Some kids say it hurts, others say it doesn't

Table 12.3 Information needs of CYP.

Age/developmental stage	Type of information
Preschool age and young children	■ What they will see, hear, smell and feel during the procedure (e.g. it will feel cold when their skin is cleaned, when the needle is inserted it 'will pinch for a little while but this will go away')
School-aged children	■ Clear concrete explanations related to the details of the procedure and what the child might feel (e.g. 'It may tingle', 'You might notice a cold feeling when the medicine goes in') ■ Why the procedure is necessary and how long it will take ■ Analogies to explain things (e.g. describing a cannula as being 'like a soft bendy tube like a straw that is in your hand') ■ Function and operation of medical equipment in concrete terms ■ Strategies for self-regulation and coping (see the Comfort, Ask, Relax, Distract or CARD system at https://www.aboutkidshealth.ca/CARD)
Adolescents	■ Why the procedure is necessary and how the results will be used ■ How the procedure may affect appearance (e.g. scar) and what can be done to minimise this ■ Any physical benefits of the procedure ■ Models or computer images to aid understanding

Source: Adapted from Reid et al. (2013).

bother them. I'll check in with you after and you can tell me how it was for you'.

- Avoid providing new information immediately before and during the procedure. However, information on pain management should be provided on the day of the procedure.
- Modelling and rehearsing adaptive coping strategies by an adult or another CYP undergoing the procedure may be completed by viewing video demonstrations with a clinician (e.g. child life specialist) or by coaching a caregiver. However, it is often most beneficial for the CYP to be actively engaged in the process.

Communication

CYP's experience of pain and fear related to procedures can be shaped by what their caregiver and health professionals say to them (Martin et al. 2013). Caregivers and clinicians should aim to stay calm, confident and comforting. Communication strategies to use and avoid are listed in Table 12.4.

Distraction

This involves shifting the child's attention away from the pain and towards stimuli that are more pleasant or engaging (Birnie et al. 2017; see Table 12.5 for examples). The distractor should be engaging and developmentally appropriate, stimulate the senses, and sustain a child's interest.

Caregivers may act as distraction coaches to help young children use distraction effectively (McCarthy et al. 2010). Empirically, distraction has been found to effectively reduce needle-related pain and distress (Birnie et al. 2014). However, not all CYP want to be distracted during procedures and some like to focus on the procedure as this helps them to cope.

Relaxation Techniques

These aim to create a calm, relaxed, peaceful state that is incompatible with intense pain perceptions (Logan et al. 2013). CYP may be taught to practice any of the following.

- Deep breathing is a common relaxation strategy that can be used with children as young as two and three years old, with or without props, for example:
  - Blowing bubbles slowly and carefully.
  - Stuffed animals: CYP lie down on their back with the animal on their stomach, moving upwards as they breathe in, and downwards as they breathe out.
- Guided imagery or visualisation involves creating images in the mind, such as imagining a peaceful setting (e.g. beach, forest). Teach the CYP to imagine what they would experience through taste, smell, sound, sight and touch. Young children may enjoy listening to a simplified version, while older CYP may want to take part in co-creating a detailed scene.
- Progressive muscle relaxation (PMR): systematically tense and relax different muscle groups. This is *not* the same as muscle tension for a fainting response. In PMR, muscles are tensed for around five seconds and then relaxed, and suggestions for relaxation are provided. Children as young as four and five years old can be taught PMR. For younger children, a visualisation component may be helpful. For example, to illustrate how a child might tense their fist, you may say, 'Pretend you are holding a lemon in your hand. You are making lemonade, so you squeeze the lemon hard in your hand. Squeeze all the juice out'.

Hypnosis

Hypnosis is an altered state of awareness in which suggestibility and receptiveness to ideas is enhanced by guiding attention towards an

Table 12.4 Statements for health professionals to use and avoid before, during and after medical procedures.

Statements to use	
Using neutral descriptions and prompts to explain the procedure	'I am going to start now' '1, 2, 3'
Humorous statements that are light-hearted in tone	Jokes: 'Why should you not give Elsa a balloon? She will Let It Go' Outrageous ideas: 'I saw a picture of a dog riding a bicycle today!'
Talk unrelated to the procedure	Questions related to the child's interests, plans, desires: 'What activities do you like to do after school?' Conversations about the child's family, school, pets, etc. 'Do you think we should take Pebbles for a walk when we get home?'
Prompts for child to use a coping strategy, generally immediately before the procedure	Suggestions to direct the child to engage in a coping behaviour: 'You can take a deep breath in through your nose, and out through your mouth' 'You can imagine you are [superhero] and this will test your power'
Give child acceptable choices; ask about their preferences	'Do you want to look at the needle or look away?' 'Do you want me to count down 3, 2, 1 then do it? Or from 5?'
Statements to avoid	
Avoid the use of unnecessarily negative language and threatening words to describe the procedure	'Here comes the bee sting'
Repetitive reassuring comments	'You are OK. It's OK' 'Don't worry, it's almost over. Almost done'
Apologising	'I'm sorry you have to go through this' 'I wish it didn't have to hurt you'
Empathy focusing on the distress	'I know it hurts' 'This must be difficult for you'
Criticism	'Jamie is in a bad mood today' 'Don't be a baby'

Sources: Blount et al. (1997); Taddio et al. (2015).

imaginative experience that is viewed as safe or fun (Liossi et al. 2013; Twycross and Stinson 2013). Suggestions to relax often accompany hypnosis (Liossi et al. 2013).

Coping Statements

These can be used to change the CYP's distressing thoughts about the procedure. The first step is to identify distressing thoughts and then replace

Table 12.5 Potential distractors by developmental stage.

Developmental stage	Possible distractors
Toddlers	■ Blowing bubbles, party blowers ■ Playing with novel toys that engage the senses ■ Singing, music, counting ■ Pop-up picture books ■ Watching a video clip ■ Favourite object
Preschool age	■ Playing with novel toys that engage the senses ■ Singing, music, counting ■ Humour/joke books ■ Kaleidoscope ■ I Spy games ■ Pop-up picture books, read a story ■ Blowing bubbles or party blowers ■ Guided imagery ■ Watching a video clip ■ Favourite object
School age	■ Playing an interactive game/video game ■ Listening to music ■ Kaleidoscope ■ Reading a story or novel ■ Guided imagery/visualisation ■ Non-procedural talk focused conversation (see Table 12.4) ■ Non-procedural tasks (e.g. naming objects in the room) ■ Humour/joke books ■ Virtual reality technology
Adolescence	■ Playing an interactive game/video game ■ Humour/joke books ■ Watching a video clip ■ Listen to music ■ Relaxation (deep breathing, guided imagery/visualisation)

Sources: Cohen et al. (2013); Taddio et al. (2015); Twycross and Stinson (2013).

them with statements that emphasise the CYP's ability to cope with the procedure (see Box 12.3 for examples).

Coping statements should be generated in preparation for the procedure and used before, during and/or after the procedure, and may help reduce negative memories associated with the procedure (Logan et al. 2013).

Additional Considerations

High Needle Fear   Managing high levels of needle fear requires the use of exposure-based psychological and physical intervention strategies before the CYP will fully benefit from pain management strategies. See McMurtry et al. (2016) for details.

Special Populations   CYP with developmental and learning (intellectual) disabilities may benefit from some of the strategies explored in the sections above; see Genik et al. (2019) for more guidance. For psychological strategies, it is important to consider an intervention that fits with cognitive capacity (e.g. detailed preparation script vs. social story). Harnessing the knowledge of caregivers is important.

Pharmacological Interventions

Pharmacological interventions are an integral part of procedural pain management and can reduce pain, fear and anxiety, facilitate successful completion of procedures, and reduce negative memories of the event. Some pharmacological interventions require a significant amount of time and expertise to implement. Since most medical procedures are planned and resources are available to incorporate pharmacological interventions, their use should be part of routine practice.

Medications administered for the purpose of sedation for procedural pain should be administered by clinicians with appropriate training and access to equipment and monitoring. There is a distinction between sedation and analgesia, as a sedative does not necessarily provide analgesic benefit (see Chapter 5 for details on the pharmacology of analgesic drugs).

Choice of agents must consider the following:

- patient demographics (age, weight)
- medical conditions that may impact sedation and its effects
- availability of trained clinicians and equipment
- required time of onset and duration of sedation
- patient needs, acceptance and preferences (e.g. willingness to swallow certain sedative medications; some patients may have strong fear of a mask and not be able to tolerate having one covering their face).

Local Anaesthetics

Local anaesthetics are effective for a variety of skin-breaking needle procedures, including:

- intramuscular injections
- venepuncture
- venous cannulation
- Port-a-Cath puncture
- laceration repair
- they can also be combined with other pharmacological interventions (e.g. procedural sedation) for more painful procedures (e.g. lumbar puncture, bone marrow aspiration).

Local anaesthetics can be administered by intradermal injection with a needle and topical application. For both approaches, lidocaine is the most common anaesthetic used. Other anaesthetics include tetracaine (amethocaine) and prilocaine, applied alone or in combination.

Intradermal Injection   Injection of local anaesthetics bypasses the stratum corneum barrier, with a rapid onset of activity of about two minutes. The added pain from injection can be diminished if lidocaine is buffered with sodium bicarbonate (Cepeda et al. 2010), warmed to body temperature (Hogan et al. 2011) and injected slowly with a small gauge needle (Fein et al. 2012).

Topical Application for Open Skin Wounds
Anaesthetic agents have also been combined with vasoconstrictive drugs and applied topically to anaesthetise open skin wounds before their repair. The most common preparation is lidocaine–epinephrine (adrenaline)–tetracaine (LET) with an onset of action of 20–30 minutes (Fein et al. 2012; Tayeb et al. 2017).

- The two anaesthetics are combined to maximise their advantages; lidocaine has a more rapid onset of action while tetracaine has longer duration.
- Adrenaline (epinephrine), a vasoconstrictor, adds a dual benefit. Firstly, it reduces the amount of blood in the working field, making it easier to perform the repair, and secondly, it increases the duration of effect of the anaesthetics by slowing their removal from the bloodstream.
- When treating minor lacerations, LET solution can be applied into the wound before wound closure with tissue adhesives (Harman et al. 2013).
- For laceration repairs that require suturing, the wound can be premedicated with LET or a combination of LET followed by injection of local anaesthetics (Fein et al. 2012).
- These preparations can be compounded by the hospital pharmacy (Fein et al. 2012).

Topical Application for Needle Procedures
Topical anaesthetic formulations can passively diffuse through intact skin, forgoing the need

for injection. Their application avoids fear and pain associated with the additional needle puncture as well as potential tissue distortion that can occur following injection of anaesthetic liquids.

Topical anaesthetics are recommended for reducing pain from any cutaneous procedure involving a needle. However, they are associated with an onset of action of 20–60 minutes depending on the specific product, owing to the time that is required for diffusion into the skin (Table 12.6). To facilitate absorption and minimise risk of accidental ingestion or being wiped off, they are routinely covered with an occlusive dressing (e.g. Tegaderm, Opsite, or plastic wrap). Some products do not require an occlusive dressing (e.g. liposomal lidocaine, Maxilene) or are available in a patch dosage form that is impregnated with the drug (e.g. lidocaine–prilocaine, EMLA). A self-heating lidocaine and tetracaine patch is also available to accelerate absorption (lidocaine–tetracaine, Synera). Topical anaesthetics commonly cause transient skin pallor and/or redness. Vasoactive effects have not been demonstrated to interfere with the success of needle procedures (Taddio et al. 2005).

Access to Topical Anaesthetics Depending on the country, topical anaesthetics can be purchased with or without a prescription. Clinicians or caregivers can apply them to the procedure site for the requisite waiting time.

Considerations for Timing While lengthening the duration of application can improve effectiveness, application times should not extend beyond one to two hours. One systematic review reported that amethocaine is superior to lidocaine–prilocaine for reducing pain when applied for short or long durations, or when applied according to the manufacturer's recommended length of time (Lander et al. 2006), suggesting that different topical anaesthetic preparations are not equianalgesic. However, no differences have been observed in procedural success rate among various preparations (Arendts et al. 2008).

Needleless Injection Needleless injection device technology is also now available that achieves superficial skin anaesthesia without a prolonged application time. One such device, called the J-Tip™, uses carbon dioxide to instantly drive liquid lidocaine through the skin and into the subcutaneous tissue. This delivery system is feasible for more emergent procedures as it has an onset of action similar to that of injectable local anaesthetic. However, it can be associated with discomfort during application.

Local Anaesthetic Safety Considerations Systemic side effects from local anaesthetics are rare. The risk of toxicity is higher in newborn preterm infants, and in overdose situations (i.e. large injection dose or application surface area and/or application duration), and can include cardiac dysrhythmias and methaemoglobinaemia.

Table 12.6 Onset of action of topical anaesthetics used for needle procedures.

Topical agents	Onset of action (minutes)
Lidocaine/prilocaine	45–60
Amethocaine/tetracaine	30–40
Liposomal lidocaine	20–30
Lidocaine/tetracaine self-warming	10–20
Needle-free injection (J-Tip™) lidocaine	1–2

> **PRACTICE POINT**
>
> Local anaesthetics are effective for superficial skin procedures. They are available in different formulations and delivery systems, allowing for flexibility in mode of administration and onset of action (Zempsky 2008).

Vapocoolants/Refrigerants

Vapocoolants are volatile chemicals that, when applied to the skin, rapidly and temporarily induce a cooling sensation. They are believed to work by slowing conduction of nociceptive input in sensory nerves. They are applied immediately before an impending needle procedure and are therefore feasible for emergent procedures. However, to date, their effectiveness has not been reliably demonstrated in CYP undergoing needle procedures (Hogan et al. 2014; Shah et al. 2015). This lack of benefit may be partially due to discomfort associated with their application. They are currently not recommended for routine use during needle procedures in CYP.

Sweet-tasting Solutions

Orally administered sweet-tasting solutions (e.g. sucrose in water) have calming and analgesic effects in infants undergoing medical procedures. Their effectiveness has been demonstrated across a variety of procedures (Stevens et al. 2016; McNair et al. 2019) and they are recommended in clinical practice guidelines (Taddio et al. 2015). While the underlying mechanism of effect is not known, it is speculated to involve activation of endogenous opioids and/or distraction effects.

Dosage   The optimum dose has not been determined (Stevens et al. 2016). A typical single dose varies from 0.5 to 2 mL of 12% or 24% sucrose solution (weight/volume). Smaller doses have been used in preterm infants (e.g. 0.05 mL of 24% sucrose solution) and larger doses in older infants (e.g. 10 mL of 25% sucrose solution; McNair et al. 2019). A dose–response effect has been demonstrated in infants premedicated with sucrose solutions during vaccine injections, with higher concentrations (i.e. 50–75%) being more effective (Shah et al. 2015).

Onset of Action and Duration of Effects
Sweet-tasting solutions have a fast onset of action (within two minutes) and short duration of action (5–10 minutes). Calming effects have been noted well beyond the painful procedure to non-painful but distressing handling procedures carried out for an hour afterwards (Taddio et al. 2009).

Administration and Access   They are administered in the infant's mouth using a syringe, medicine cup or pacifier two minutes before a procedure. The effects are augmented by concomitant use of a pacifier (Stevens et al. 2016). Sucrose solutions are commercially available, can be compounded by hospital pharmacies, or easily made by mixing table sugar with water immediately before needle procedures (Taddio et al. 2015).

Side Effects   Sucrose solutions are well tolerated by infants. Side effects are uncommon and transient, and include oxygen desaturation, choking and bradycardia (McNair et al. 2019). The analgesic effects of sweet-tasting solutions appear to wane over time with a dampening of effect with increasing postnatal age (Harrison et al. 2015).

> **PRACTICE POINT**
>
> Sweet-tasting solutions are effective for procedural pain management in young infants and should be used in combination with other pain-reducing strategies (Shah et al. 2015; Stevens et al. 2016).

Oral Analgesics: Paracetamol (Acetaminophen) and Ibuprofen

Paracetamol and ibuprofen are commonly used to treat pain and fever in CYP. However, there is no evidence of their effectiveness for reducing acute pain during needle procedures and they are not recommended for this purpose (Taddio et al. 2015). Moreover, paracetamol may interfere with the immune response after vaccine injections (Prymula et al. 2009). At present, both paracetamol and ibuprofen are recommended for delayed pain reactions and fever that occur after, not during, vaccine injections.

CASE STUDY: PART 4

Charlotte is due for her yearly influenza vaccination. Her parents would like to know what they can do to mitigate pain in addition to physical and psychological interventions.

1. What pharmacological interventions might be appropriate for Charlotte?
2. When are these interventions administered relative to the vaccination and why?

Procedural Sedation

Procedural sedation is increasingly used to minimise discomfort and facilitate successful completion of procedures. Sedation is typically employed for procedures that are more painful, that are long-lasting and/or that require stasis (minimal movement) and cooperation (Table 12.7).

Table 12.7 Overview of procedural sedation.

Examples of procedures for which sedation is administered	▪ Lumbar puncture ▪ Bone marrow aspiration/biopsy ▪ Wound care ▪ Fracture reduction ▪ Laceration repair
Most common drugs used for procedural sedation (administered individually or combined together, with or without therapeutically related compounds)	▪ Nitrous oxide ▪ Ketamine ▪ Midazolam ▪ Propofol ▪ Dexmedetomidine ▪ Fentanyl
Routes of administration	▪ Oral ▪ Intranasal ▪ Inhalation ▪ Injection

Fear of needles or face masks can hinder administration by injection or inhalation respectively, and requires that additional interventions be employed to mitigate fear (e.g. topical anaesthetics, preparation).

Sedation in children ranges from mild to deep sedation and may even enter the realm of general anaesthesia (at which point even painful stimulation will not arouse the CYP). It is imperative that appropriately trained clinicians be involved when higher levels of sedation are required, specifically those with airway management skills and appropriate equipment available.

Depth of Sedation   Mild sedation is useful for interventions which are of short duration, without prolonged pain afterwards, e.g. insertion of peripheral intravenous lines or accessing indwelling venous ports (Port-a-Caths), and for highly fearful CYP. Sedative agents may be administered using non-parenteral routes, including oral or intranasal (with the use of child-specific atomisers). Commonly used medications include midazolam, ketamine or dexmedetomidine. Lorazepam is available in a sublingual formulation. Intranasal and sublingual administration results in rapid effects.

Moderate to deep sedation is often necessary for more painful or invasive procedures that may require more than one agent to provide sedation as well as analgesia. For example:

▪ topical local anaesthetic application to the proposed site of lumbar puncture followed by nitrous oxide sedation at the time of needle puncture
▪ fracture reduction, a quick but intensely painful procedure, could be facilitated with a combination of an opioid and a sedative medication e.g. ketamine.

The goal with moderate to deep sedation is to maintain spontaneous ventilation and the clinicians administering medications should be prepared to intervene if there are significant changes to ventilation. Given this risk, close monitoring including heart rate, blood pressure and oxygen saturation should be available, with the patient receiving supplemental oxygen during the administration of medications.

Procedural sedation can be effectively and safely administered by non-anaesthetists when safeguards and protocols are in place, as demonstrated in a large study including various provider specialties (Couloures et al. 2011).

Guidelines for Sedation in Children and Young People

Before Sedation

Assessment by the clinician including:

- pre-sedation vital signs and weight
- medical history including medication history, allergies and comorbidities
- fasting status (standard nil-by-mouth guidelines if patient will be receiving moderate/deep sedation)
- relevant physical examination.

During the Procedure

- monitoring of vital signs (heart rate and rhythm, blood pressure, oxygen saturation, capnography).

After the Procedure

- interval monitoring of vital signs until child is back to baseline level of consciousness.
- duration of monitoring will be impacted by medications that were administered during the procedure.

Currently Accepted Practice   Currently, many invasive procedures that previously would have been performed under light sedation, now involve sedation or anaesthesia teams. This is particularly beneficial for certain patient populations who require repeated procedures and who therefore are at risk of harm from inadequately managed fear and pain, including patients with burns or cancer.

Most paediatric centres with robust oncology departments will have an anaesthetist involved for lumbar punctures, central port placements (Port-a-Cath, Hickman lines) and bone marrow aspirations. These procedures occur soon after cancer diagnosis and, given the emotional toll at such a time, addressing sedation and pain needs is imperative to avoid further trauma.

The availability of medications e.g. propofol (an intravenous general anaesthetic agent) that deliver deep sedation with a short duration of action has simplified sedation:

- propofol can be administered without anaesthetic machines, gas lines or scavenging systems
- however, given propofol's ability to induce general anaesthesia and apnoea, its use is limited to clinicians with advanced airway skills, such as anaesthetists and intensive care physicians.

ADDITIONAL INFORMATION

- Coté, C.J., Wilson, S., American Academy of Pediatrics and American Academy of Pediatric Dentistry. (2016) Guidelines for monitoring and management of pediatric patients before, during, and after sedation for diagnostic and therapeutic procedures: update 2016. *Pediatrics* 138(1). Available at https://pubmed.ncbi.nlm.nih.gov/27354454/

■ Hartling, L. et al. (2016) What works and what's safe in pediatric emergency procedural sedation: an overview of reviews. *Academic Emergency Medicine* 23(5), 519–530. `https://doi.org/10.1111/acem.12938`

Nitrous Oxide   Nitrous oxide (N_2O) is a well-known colourless, odourless, anaesthetic gas that may be used for procedural pain, most often administered by inhalation through a mask (face or nasal).

Onset, Duration and Administration

■ Nitrous oxide is colloquially referred to as 'laughing gas' due to its euphoric effects.
■ It is advantageous in its rapid onset and offset, both being within minutes.
■ It has an unclear mechanism of action.
■ NO can be self-administered or administered by clinicians. Self-administration limits the level of sedation as the child will let go of the mask if they fall asleep.
■ It requires a concentration of 50–70% (mixed with oxygen) to provide adequate/reliable sedation.

Nitrous oxide is a weak analgesic and, on its own, is probably not sufficient to provide appropriate conditions for painful procedures like bone marrow aspiration or chest tube insertions. It is therefore imperative that other analgesics be administered concurrently when significant pain is anticipated.

Side Effects and Contraindications

Nitrous oxide has a very low incidence of side effects. It does have an impact on ventilatory drive, which is advantageous as a means of self-limiting the level of sedation, as the CYP will inhale less gas as level of sedation increases.

The side effects of nitrous oxide sedation include:

■ nausea and vomiting
■ hallucinations and confusion
■ respiratory depression.

Despite its widespread use, nitrous oxide is contraindicated in specific medical situations (mainly due to its expansion of air-filled cavities):

■ pneumothorax
■ bowel obstruction
■ head injury or raised intracranial pressure
■ chronic respiratory disease or acute asthma
■ certain cardiac conditions e.g. pulmonary hypertension.

Other Considerations

■ Prolonged or repeated exposure to nitrous oxide is associated with impairment of vitamin B_{12} metabolism, with potential alterations in bone marrow function and subsequent neurological dysfunction.
■ Increased incidence of early pregnancy loss in health professionals involved with administration of nitrous oxide.
■ Nitrous oxide, along with other inhaled anaesthetics, carries a heavy carbon footprint and has a significant impact on ozone depletion and greenhouse gas accumulation.

Other Sedative Medications   Details on other common medications used for procedural sedation are included in Table 12.8.

ADDITIONAL INFORMATION

For further details on sedative drugs, see Barash, P.G. et al. (2017) *Clinical Anesthesia*. Lippincott Williams & Wilkins, Philadelphia.

Table 12.8 Other sedative medications.

Medication	Description	Routes of administration	Advantages	Possible side effects
Ketamine	Anaesthetic drug with analgesic and dissociative properties via antagonistic action on the NMDA receptor, historically known for its strong sedative action. Increasingly used for its properties as an analgesic and sedative	Intravenous Intramuscular Intranasal Enteral	Sedation without impacting respiratory drive or haemodynamic stability. Useful when sedation is required for highly fearful CYP	Nausea, vomiting, hallucinogenic effects Duration of action is over 20 minutes, making it a less ideal sedative in some circumstances Given its hallucinogenic properties and risk of delirium, often combined with other anaesthetics e.g. benzodiazepines
Midazolam	Benzodiazepine useful for sedative purposes	Intravenous Intramuscular Intranasal Enteral	Anxiolytic and amnestic properties may be particularly useful for highly fearful CYP or those with difficulty cooperating with the procedure	Intranasal administration is associated with irritation and pain
Propofol	Anaesthetic that does not have analgesic effects and is combined with other agents when used for painful procedures	Intravenous	Fast onset of action and offset of action and is titratable to effect	Respiratory depression and hypotension are more frequent than with other sedatives
Dexmedeto-midine	Newer medication that elicits its action as an α_2-adrenergic agonist. Unlikely to provide adequate sedation for painful procedures on its own unless combined with stronger medications (e.g. propofol)	Oral Intranasal Intramuscular Intravenous	Analgesic and sedative properties without causing respiratory depression	Haemodynamic actions (bradycardia, hypotension), so patients should be closely monitored, and comorbidities reviewed before selecting it as a sedative
Fentanyl	Synthetic opioid that binds 50–100 times stronger than morphine to opioid receptors. Should not be used as a sedative on its own but can supplement other sedatives to provide pain control	Intranasal Intravenous	Excellent analgesic for painful procedures given its quick onset of action and short duration	Significant respiratory depression, possible apnoea. Must be dosed and administered based on a CYP's weight and titrated to effect

Source: Barash et al. (2017).

CASE STUDY: PART 5

Charlotte fell while in the school park and sustained a laceration over her right eyebrow. The laceration was sutured in the emergency department after Charlotte was given one dose of intranasal fentanyl. Charlotte cried during the procedure and afterwards reported being very scared while her laceration was repaired.

Unfortunately, two weeks later Charlotte developed an abscess at the site of the cut due to infection. She was seen by a surgeon and her parents were told she would need to have the abscess incised and drained in the operating room. To prepare her for the operating room, the surgical team asks the emergency department to place a peripheral intravenous line. Charlotte immediately begins to cry uncontrollably upon hearing this.

1. What pharmacological interventions might be appropriate for Charlotte and why?
2. What monitoring advice would you recommend?

Summary

- CYP's pain and fear related to procedural pain can be managed using psychological, physical, procedural and pharmacological components.
- Current evidence suggests that the most effective interventions are those that offer a combination of the strategies listed above.
- Recommended bundles of interventions based on developmental stage are highlighted.

- It is important that caregivers are involved in managing CYP's pain and fear. Guidelines and recommendations are provided. Also, the techniques listed include guidance and recommendations for caregivers, highlighting the importance of caregiver involvement in managing CYP pain and fear.

ADDITIONAL INFORMATION

Guidelines for treating procedural pain and associated symptoms (e.g. fear)

- American Academy of Pediatrics, Committee on Pediatric Emergency Medicine, American College of Emergency Physicians, Pediatric Committee and Emergency Nurses Association (2013) Guidelines for care of children in the emergency department. Available at https://pediatrics.aappublications.org/content/124/4/1233
- ENA Clinical Practice Guideline Committee (2019) Clinical practice guideline: needle-related or minor procedural pain in pediatric patients. Available at https://www.ncbi.nlm.nih.gov/pubmed/31280767

- Schug, S.A. et al. (2020) *Acute Pain Management: Scientific Evidence*, 5th edn. Available at https://www.anzca.edu.au/resources/college-publications/acute-pain-management/apmse5.pdf
- Taddio, A. et al. (2015) Reducing pain during vaccine injections: clinical practice guideline. Available at https://www.cmaj.ca/content/187/13/975
- Trottier, E.D. et al. (2019) Managing pain and distress in children undergoing brief diagnostic and therapeutic procedures. Available at https://www.cps.ca/en/documents/position/managing-pain-and-distress

Guideline for needle fear

- McMurtry, C.M. et al. (2016) Exposure-based interventions for the management of individuals with high levels of needle fear across the lifespan: a clinical practice guideline and call for further research. Available at https://www.ncbi.nlm.nih.gov/pmc/articles/PMC4867871/

Key to Case Study

Part 1

1. Assess Charlotte's level of pain (see Chapter 6), fear, and history of fainting via self-report and caregiver ratings using the recommended screening questions. Assessing parents' level of distress can also inform treatment.

2. If possible, screen for Charlotte's level of fear before the procedure (see Table 12.2). As a typically developing eight year old, any of the measures listed in Table 12.1 would be appropriate. These scales are also acceptable for obtaining caregiver perceptions of Charlotte's fear. Charlotte's parents may complete an 11-point numeric rating scale of distress.

Part 2

1. If Charlotte and her family endorse needle fear, find out the focus/foci of her fear. If she is fearful of seeing blood, the procedure could occur in such a way that she wouldn't see it. If she is developing a very high fear of venepuncture, then referral to a mental health specialist may be necessary. Consider asking whether she has experienced any of the prodromal signs of fainting today or historically.

2. The room should be as quiet and calm as possible. Seat Charlotte in a position that feels comfortable for her (e.g. on her own or on a caregiver's lap). The Buzzy could be offered. If Charlotte endorsed a vasovagal reaction in your screening, then consider teaching her muscle tension and conducting the venepuncture in a reclined position.

Part 3

1. Ask Charlotte what type of information she would like to know, with examples provided about what other children

Table 12.9 Key intervention bundles for needle pain.

Age range	Physical strategies	Psychological strategies	Pharmacological strategies
0–3 years	▪ Injections: no aspiration ▪ Injections: most painful last *and/or* simultaneous injection (<1 year) ▪ Breastfeeding before, during and after procedure *or* ▪ Skin-to-skin (<1 month), rocking, or holding (0–3 years) before, during and after ▪ Sucking/pacifier before, during and after procedure (0–2 years)	▪ Distraction ▪ Interaction/wording: 　▪ Use: neutral words 　▪ Avoid: repeated reassurance, suggesting it will not hurt ▪ Education about pain management for caregivers	▪ Sweet-tasting solution: sucrose or glucose before procedure (0–2 years) ▪ Topical anaesthetics 20–60 minutes before procedure ▪ Topical combination anaesthetic–vasoconstrictive agents 10–20 minutes before procedure, *and/or* ▪ Injectable anaesthetics 5 minutes before procedure ▪ Inhalational/systemic analgesics and sedation for more invasive or long procedures and for highly fearful CYP and/or those having difficulty coping and cooperating
3–12 years	▪ Sitting upright position ▪ Buzzy tactile stimulation with distraction ▪ Muscle tension (for history of fainting) ▪ Injections: no aspiration ▪ Injections: most painful last	▪ Distraction ▪ Interaction/wording (as above) ▪ Education about pain management for caregivers and CYP	▪ Topical anaesthetics 20–60 minutes before procedure ▪ Needleless injection device delivery 1–2 minutes before procedure ▪ Topical combination anaesthetic–vasoconstrictive agents 10–20 minutes before procedure, *and/or* ▪ Injectable anaesthetics 5 minutes before procedure ▪ Inhalational/systemic analgesics and sedation for more invasive or long procedures and for highly fearful CYP and/or CYP having difficulty coping and cooperating
12–17 years	▪ Sitting upright position ▪ Tactile stimulation with distraction (e.g. Buzzy) ▪ Muscle tension (for history of fainting) ▪ Injections: no aspiration ▪ Injections: most painful last	▪ Interaction/wording and education about pain management (as above).	▪ Topical anaesthetics 20–60 minutes before procedure ▪ Topical combination anaesthetic–vasoconstrictive agents 10–20 minutes before procedure, *and/or* ▪ Injectable anaesthetics 5 minutes before procedure ▪ Inhaled/systemic analgesics and sedation for more invasive or long procedures and for highly fearful CYP and/or CYP having difficulty coping and cooperating

Source: Adapted from Taddio et al. (2015).

typically ask (e.g. What will happen? How will it feel? What strategies will she and others use to make the procedure comfortable?). Support her choice of what she wants to hear about *and* facilitate her understanding as she may not know what she needs to know. Explain the procedural steps for a blood test, including placing a rubber band around her arm and wiping the area clean. The needle will be inserted into her arm and attached to a container which will fill with her blood, so the needle has to be in her arm for up to a minute. It might hurt for a little bit. The procedure will check how her medicines are working and how her blood sugars have been lately. Explain the types of pain management strategies available as per below. Allow time for questions.

2. Charlotte would benefit from distraction, e.g. guided imagery, reading a book, listening to music, watching a video, or conversation unrelated to the procedure. Deep breathing using a toy or object can help with relaxation and distraction. Consider providing parents with psychoeducation on pain and fear, and management strategies.

3. Additional information that would be relevant to gather includes screening for Charlotte's level of needle fear (see Part 1.2 above) and a history of fainting, previous pain management strategies, previous experience with needles, and possibly caregiver presence of fear and anxiety related to the procedure.

Part 4

1. Charlotte can be offered topical local anaesthetics. These need to be organised ahead of time. Depending on the setting of the vaccination, parents may have to purchase the anaesthetics before the procedure or they may be available via the healthcare provider/institution. Institutional settings may also have needleless injection delivery systems.

2. Depending on which anaesthetic is used, a waiting time is required before the drug is active. This ranges from one to two minutes (needleless injection) to 20–60 minutes (various topical local anaesthetic products).

Part 5

1. Charlotte's previous negative experience related to a medical procedure contributed to significant fear and anxiety after hearing that she must undergo further medical treatment. Consider administering topical local anaesthetics and light sedation (intranasal or orally) before inserting the peripheral intravenous line. An ideal pharmacological agent would be midazolam, given orally to provide light sedation and an amnestic effect that will be beneficial when she is separated from her parents for surgery.

2. Appropriately dosed oral midazolam would require minimal monitoring, mainly pulse oximetry.

PRACTICE POINT

Bundled interventions tailored to the CYP's developmental level, needs and preferences are recommended (see Table 12.9).

Multiple Choice Questions

1. Unmanaged pain and fear related to painful procedures can lead to which of the following?
   a. The development of fearful memories related to pain
   b. Greater pain, fear and distress at future procedures
   c. Avoidance of preventive healthcare in adulthood
   d. Longer procedure time
   e. All of the above

2. Which of the following is a recommended treatment bundle to manage school-aged children's pain and fear during needle procedures?
   a. Distraction, use an empathetic and reassuring tone, topical anaesthetics, comfortable position
   b. Inform the child of the steps involved in the procedure, distraction, use neutral wording, provide paracetamol
   c. Education about pain and fear management, neutral wording, topical anaesthetics, distraction, sitting upright
   d. Provide the child with as few details as possible, use neutral wording, distraction, comfortable position, and ibuprofen

3. Which pharmacological intervention is most appropriate for vaccine injections?
   a. Vapocoolants
   b. Paracetamol
   c. Topical local anaesthetics
   d. Nitrous oxide

4. Which of the following is *not* a recommended way to prepare a CYP for an upcoming painful procedure?
   a. Explain the procedure to the CYP in detail, tailored to their developmental level
   b. Provide the CYP with relevant new information immediately before the procedure
   c. Allow the CYP opportunities to ask questions
   d. Acknowledge variability in experience ('some kids say it hurts, others don't')

5. Which of the following is the next recommended course of action if a child is crying inconsolably and refuses to receive a vaccination or complete a venepuncture?
   a. Restrain the child to complete the procedure and explain why it was necessary
   b. Tell the child to look away from the needle and take deep breaths
   c. Reassure them repeatedly that it will be over soon
   d. Assess the child's level of fear and refer the child to an appropriate practitioner or programme if needed to manage their fear before completing the procedure

Relevant Web Resources

Pain management resources for families and healthcare professionals: https://itdoesnthavetohurt.ca

Solutions for Kids in Pain (SKIP) knowledge mobilization network: https://www.kidsinpain.ca

Help Eliminate Pain in Kids and Adults provides resources, systematic reviews, and clinical practice guidelines related to vaccination pain and fear management: http://phm.utoronto.ca/helpinkids/index.html

The CARD system provides resources for students, caregivers and teachers to prepare students for a vaccination: https://www.aboutkidshealth.ca/CARD

Comfort Promise information hub on evidence-based approaches to reduce children's needle-related pain: https://www.aboutkidshealth.ca/comfortpromise

References

American Academy of Pediatrics, Committee on Pediatric Emergency Medicine, American College of Emergency Physicians and Emergency Nurses Association (2013) Joint policy statement: guidelines for care of children in the emergency department. *Journal of Emergency Nursing* 39(2), 116–131.

Arendts, G., Stevens, M. and Fry, M. (2008) Topical anaesthesia and intravenous cannulation success in paediatric patients: a randomized double-blind trial. *British Journal of Anaesthesia* 100, 521–524.

Association of Paediatric Anaesthetists of Great Britain and Ireland (APA) (2012) Good practice in postoperative and procedural pain, 2nd edition. *Pediatric Anaesthesia* 22(Suppl. 1), 1–79.

Ballard, A., Khadra, C., Samara, A., Trottier, E. and Le May, S. (2019) Efficacy of the Buzzy device for pain management during needle-related procedures: a systematic review and meta-analysis. *Clinical Journal of Pain* 35(6), 532–543.

Barash, P.G., Cullen, B.F., Stoelting, R.K., et al. (2017) *Clinical Anesthesia*, 8th edn. Lippincott Williams & Wilkins, Philadelphia.

Birnie, K.A., Chambers C.T., Fernandez C.V., et al. (2014) Hospitalized children continue to report undertreated and preventable pain. *Pain Research and Management* 19, 198–204.

Birnie, K.A., Chambers, C.T. and Spellman, C.M. (2017) Mechanisms of distraction in acute pain perception and modulation. *Pain* 158(6), 1012–1013.

Birnie, K.A., Noel, M., Chambers, C.T., Uman, L.S. and Parker, J.A. (2018) Psychological interventions for needle-related procedural pain and distress in children and adolescents. *Cochrane Database of Systematic Reviews* (10), CD005179.

Blount, R.L., Cohen, L.L., Frank, N.C., et al. (1997) The Child–Adult Medical Procedure Interaction Scale-Revised: an assessment of validity. *Journal of Pediatric Psychology* 22, 73–88.

Bray, L., Appleton, V. and Sharpe, A. (2019) The information needs of children having clinical procedures in hospital: Will it hurt ? Will I feel scared ? What can I do to stay calm ? *Child Care Health Development* 45, 737–743.

Cepeda, M.S., Tzortzopoulou, A., Thackrey, M., Hudcova, J., Arora Gandhi, P. and Schumann, R. (2010) Adjusting the pH of lidocaine for reducing pain on injection. *Cochrane Database of Systematic Reviews* (8), CD006581.

Cohen, L.L., Cousins, L.A. and Martin, S.R. (2013) Procedural pain distraction. In *Oxford Textbook of Paediatric Pain* (eds P.J. McGrath, B.J. Stevens, S.M. Walker and W.T. Zempsky), pp. 519–530. Oxford University Press, Oxford.

Coté, C.J., Wilson, S., American Academy of Pediatrics and American Academy of Pediatric Dentistry (2016) Guidelines for monitoring and management of pediatric patients before, during, and after sedation for diagnostic and therapeutic procedures: update 2016. *Pediatrics* 138(1), e20161212.

Couloures, K.G., Beach, M., Cravero, J.P., Monroe, K.K. and Hertzog, J.H. (2011) Impact of provider specialty on pediatric procedural sedation complication rates. *Pediatrics* 127(5), 1154–1160.

ENA Clinical Practice Guideline Committee (2019) Clinical practice guideline: needle-related or minor procedural pain in pediatric patients. *Journal of Emergency Nursing* 45(4), 437.e1–437.e32.

Fein, J.A., Zempsky, W.T., Cravero, J.P. and Committee on Pediatric Emergency Medicine (2012) Relief of pain and anxiety in pediatric patients in emergency medical systems. *Pediatrics* 130(5), 1391–1405.

Friedrichsdorf, S.J. and Goubert, L. (2020) Pediatric pain treatment and prevention for hospitalized children. *Pain Reports* 5(1), e804.

Friedrichsdorf, S.J., Postier, A., Eull, D., et al. (2015) Pain outcomes in a US children's hospital: a prospective cross-sectional survey. *Hospital Pediatrics* 5(1), 18–26.

Genik, L.M., Constantin, K., Symons, F. and McMurtry, C.M. (2019) Pain. In *Handbook of Intellectual Disabilities: Integrating Theory, Research, and Practice* (ed. J.L. Matson), pp. 1011–1036. Springer, New York.

Harman, S., Zemek, R., Duncan, M.J., Ying, Y. and Petrcich, W. (2013) Efficacy of pain control with topical lidocaine–epinephrine–tetracaine during laceration repair with tissue adhesive in children: a randomized controlled trial. *Canadian Medical Association Journal* 185(13), E629–E634.

Harrison, D., Yamada, J., Adams-Webber, T., Ohlsson, A., Beyene, J. and Stevens, B. (2015) Sweet tasting solutions for reduction of needle-related procedural pain in children aged one to 16 years. *Cochrane Database of Systematic Reviews* (5), CD008408.

Hartling, L., Milne, A., Foisy, M., et al. (2016) What works and what's safe in pediatric emergency procedural sedation: an overview of reviews. *Academic Emergency Medicine* 23(5), 519–530.

Höfle, M., Hauck, M., Engel, A.K. and Senkowski, D. (2012) Viewing a needle pricking a hand that you perceive as yours enhances unpleasantness of pain. *Pain* 153(5), 1074–1081.

Hogan, M.E., Vandervaart, S., Perampaladas, K., Machado, M., Einarson, T. R. and Taddio, A. (2011) Systematic review and meta-analysis of the effect of warming local anesthetics on injection pain. *Annals of Emergency Medicine* 58(1), 86–98.

Hogan, M.E., Smart, S., Shah, V. and Taddio, A. (2014) A systematic review of vapocoolants for reducing pain from venipuncture and venous cannulation in children and adults. *Journal of Emergency Medicine* 47(6), 736–745.

Jaaniste, T., Hayes, B. and von Baeyer, C.L. (2007) Providing children with information about forthcoming medical procedures: a review and synthesis. *Clinical Psychology: Science and Practice* 14(2), 124–143.

Jibb, L.A., Nathan, P.C., Stevens, B.J., et al. (2015) Psychological and physical interventions for the management of cancer-related pain in pediatric and young adult patients: an integrative review. *Oncology Nursing Forum* 42(6), E339–E357.

Lander, J.A., Weltman, B.J. and So, S.S. (2006) EMLA and amethocaine for reduction of children's pain associated with needle insertion. *Cochrane Database of Systematic Reviews* (3), CD004236.

Liossi, C., Kuttner, L., Wood, C. and Zeltzer, L.K. (2013) Hypnosis and relaxation. In *Oxford Textbook of Paediatric Pain* (eds P.J. McGrath, B.J. Stevens, S.M. Walker and W.T. Zempsky), pp. 560–568. Oxford University Press, Oxford.

Logan, D.E., Coakley, R.M. and Barber Garcia, B.N. (2013). Cognitive-behavioural interventions. In *Oxford Textbook of Paediatric Pain* (eds P.J. McGrath, B.J. Stevens, S.M. Walker and W.T. Zempsky), pp. 519–530. Oxford University Press, Oxford.

McCarthy, A.M., Kleiber, C., Hanrahan, K., Zimmerman, M.B., Westhus, N. and Allen, S. (2010) Factors explaining children's responses to intravenous needle insertions. *Nursing Research* 59(6), 407.

McMurtry, C.M., Noel, M., Chambers, C.T. and McGrath, P.J. (2011) Children's fear during procedural pain: preliminary investigation of the Children's Fear Scale. *Health Psychology* 30(6), 780–788.

McMurtry, C.M., Riddell, R.P., Taddio, A., et al. (2015) Far from 'just a poke': common painful needle procedures and the development of needle fear. *Clinical Journal of Pain* 31(10), 3–11.

McMurtry, C.M., Taddio, A., Noel, M., et al. (2016) Exposure-based interventions for the management of individuals with high levels of needle fear across the lifespan: a clinical practice guideline and call for further research. *Cognitive Behaviour Therapy* 45(3), 217–235.

McNair, C., Campbell Yeo, M., Johnston, C. and Taddio, A. (2019) Non-pharmacological management of pain during common needle puncture procedures in infants: current research evidence and practical considerations. An update. *Clinics in Perinatology* 46(4), 709–730.

Martin, S.R., Chorney, J.M., Cohen, L.L. and Kain, Z.N. (2013) Sequential analysis of mothers' and fathers' reassurance and children's postoperative distress. *Journal of Pediatric Psychology* 38(10), 1121–1129.

Mithal, P., Simmons, P., Cornelissen, T., et al. (2018) To look or not to look during vaccination: a pilot randomized trial. *Canadian Journal of Pain* 2(1), 1–8.

Öst, L.G. and Sterner, U. (1987) Applied tension. A specific behavioral method for treatment of blood phobia. *Behavioural Research and Therapy* 25, 25–29.

Pillai Riddell, R.P., Taddio, A., McMurtry, C.M., et al. (2015) Process interventions for vaccine injections: systematic review of randomized controlled trials and quasi-randomized controlled trials. *Clinical Journal of Pain* 31(10 Suppl.), S99–S108.

Prymula, R., Siegrist, C.A., Chlibek, R., et al. (2009) Effect of prophylactic paracetamol administration at time of vaccination on febrile reactions and antibody responses in children: two open-label, randomized controlled trials. *Lancet* 374(9698), 1339–1350.

Public Health Agency of Canada (2023) Canadian immunization guide. Available at http://www.

phac-aspc.gc.ca/publicat/cig-gci/index-eng.php (accessed 28 February 2020).

Reid, K., Twycross, A. and Tuterra, D. (2013) Management of painful procedures. In *Managing Pain in Children: A Clinical Guide for Nurses and Healthcare Professionals*, 2nd edn (eds A. Twycross, S. Dowden and J. Stinson), pp. 246–270. Wiley Blackwell, Oxford.

Schug, S.A., Palmer, G., Scott, D., Alcock, M., Halliwell, R. and Mott, J.F. (eds) (2020) *Acute Pain Management: Scientific Evidence*, 5th edn. Australian and New Zealand College of Anaesthetists and Faculty of Pain Medicine, Melbourne. Available at https://www.anzca.edu.au/resources/college-publications/acute-pain-management/apmse5.pdf

Shah, V., Taddio, A., McMurtry, C.M., et al. (2015) Pharmacological and combined interventions to reduce vaccine injection pain in children and adults: systematic review and meta-analysis. *Clinical Journal of Pain* 31(10 Suppl.), S38–S63.

Stevens, B., Abbott, L.K., Yamada, J., et al. (2011) Epidemiology and management of painful procedures in children in Canadian hospitals. *Canadian Medical Association Journal* 183(7), e403–e410.

Stevens, B., Yamada, J., Ohlsson, A., Haliburton, S. and Shorkey, A. (2016) Sucrose for analgesia in newborn infants undergoing painful procedures. *Cochrane Database of Systematic Reviews* (7), CD001069.

Taddio, A., Soin, H., Schuh, S., Koren, G. and Scolnik, D. (2005) A randomized controlled trial of liposomal lidocaine to improve procedural success rates and reduce procedural pain in children. *Canadian Medical Association Journal* 172(13), 1691–1695.

Taddio, A., Shah, V. and Katz, J. (2009) Reduced infant response to a routine care procedure after sucrose analgesia. *Pediatrics* 123(3), e425–e429.

Taddio, A., Ipp, M., Thivakaran, S., et al. (2012) Survey of the prevalence of immunization non-compliance due to needle fears in children and adults. *Vaccine* 30(32), 4807–4812.

Taddio, A., McMurtry, C.M., Shah, V., et al. (2015) Reducing pain during vaccine injections: clinical practice guideline. *Canadian Medical Association Journal* 187(13), 975–982.

Tayeb, B.O., Eidelman, A., Eidelman, C.L., McNicol, E.D. and Carr, D.B. (2017) Topical anaesthetics for pain control during repair of dermal laceration. *Cochrane Database of Systematic Reviews* (2), CD005364.

Trottier, E.D., Doré-Bergeron, M.J., Chauvin-Kimoff, L., Baerg, K. and Ali, S. (2019) Managing pain and distress in children undergoing brief diagnostic and therapeutic procedures. *Paediatrics and Child Health* 24(8), 509–521.

Twycross, A. and Collis, S. (2013) How well is acute pain in children managed? A snapshot in one English hospital. *Pain Management Nursing* 14(4), e204–e215.

Twycross, A. and Stinson, J. (2013) Physical and psychological methods of pain relief in children. In *Managing Pain in Children: A Clinical Guide for Nurses and Healthcare Professionals*, 2nd edn (eds A. Twycross, S. Dowden and J. Stinson), pp. 86–110. Wiley Blackwell, Oxford.

Vijayan, R., Scott, G. and Brownlie, W. (2015) Out of sight, but not out of mind? Greater reported pain in patients who spontaneously look away during venepuncture. *European Journal of Pain* 19(1), 97–102.

Yamada, T. and Yanagimoto, S. (2017) Dose–response relationship between the risk of vasovagal syncope and body mass index or systolic blood pressure in young adults undergoing blood tests. *Neuroepidemiology* 49(1–2), 31–33.

Young, K.D. (2005) Pediatric procedural pain. *Annals of Emergency Medicine* 45(2), 160–171.

Zempsky, W.T. (2008) Pharmacologic approaches for reducing venous access pain in children. *Pediatrics* 122(Suppl. 3), S140–S153.

13 Pain in the Neonate

Marsha Campbell-Yeo, Mats Eriksson, and Britney Benoit

This chapter provides an overview of the epidemiology and adverse outcomes associated with untreated pain in neonates, in addition to current best evidence regarding the assessment, prevention and management of neonatal pain.

Causes, Prevalence and Consequences of Neonatal Pain

Exposure to nociceptive pain is inevitable for all newborns, typically experienced by most within the initial hour as well as the first day(s) after birth as part of recommended medical care (Box 13.1) (World Health Organization 2022).

For newborns delivered preterm or those who are critically ill and require neonatal intensive care, pain exposure is even higher. A review including 18 studies examining pain exposure and analgesic practices across numerous countries reported that hospitalised neonates underwent 7–17 painful procedures per day, the most common being:

- heel lancing
- nasotracheal and endotracheal suctioning
- venepuncture
- insertion of peripheral venous catheter.

> **BOX 13.1   ROUTINE PAINFUL MEDICAL PROCEDURES AFTER BIRTH**
>
> - Routine intramuscular injection of vitamin K to prevent bleeding (Ng and Loewy 2018)
> - A heel lance to collect blood for metabolic testing (Therrell et al. 2015)
> - Routine total serum bilirubin screening (Barrington and Sankaran 2018)
> - Routine glucose monitoring (Narvey and Marks 2019)
> - Upwards of 20 intramuscular injections for immunisations both shortly after birth and between 2 and 18 months of age (Centers for Disease Control and Prevention 2021)

Additional routinely performed painful procedures related to neonatal intensive care include:

- intubation
- chest tube placement
- lumbar puncture
- insertion of arterial and venous umbilical catheters and peripheral arterial catheters
- intramuscular and subcutaneous injections
- retinopathy of prematurity eye examinations.

Managing Pain in Children and Young People: A Clinical Guide, Third Edition. Edited by Alison Twycross, Jennifer Stinson, William T. Zempsky, and Abbie Jordan.
© 2024 John Wiley & Sons Ltd. Published 2024 by John Wiley & Sons Ltd.

Despite the frequency of painful procedures, infants were not provided with any form of analgesia during painful procedures 42–100% of the time (Cruz et al. 2016). Predictors of the use of pharmacological interventions (e.g. opioids) during tissue-breaking procedures include being less ill at birth and receiving high-frequency ventilator support, whereas parental presence significantly predicted the use of sweet taste or non-pharmacological interventions, namely non-nutritive sucking, swaddling, rocking, positioning, skin-to-skin contact (SSC) and breast-feeding (Johnston et al. 2011a).

Exposure to unmanaged pain has been associated with multiple consequences in both full-term and preterm infants. While most research regarding the impact of pain in early life has focused on preterm infants, there is some evidence demonstrating that pain exposure may be associated with heightened pain responses to later painful stimuli in full-term infants after major surgery (Schmelzle-Lubiecki et al. 2007), circumcision (Taddio et al. 1997), burns (Wollgarten-Hadamek et al. 2009) and repeated nociceptive pain (Ozawa et al. 2011).

For infants delivered very preterm, there is now compelling evidence that early pain-related distress is associated with both immediate physiological instability and pain sensitivity as well as long-lasting deleterious effects including:

- reduced cognition and altered behaviour (Vinall and Grunau 2014; Walker 2019)
- poor executive function and visual abilities (Doesburg et al. 2013)
- blunting of behavioural responses, increases in physiological response, changes to pain thresholds and alterations in hypothalamic–pituitary–adrenal axis development (Fitzgerald et al. 1989; Grunau et al. 2005, 2006, 2007; Fitzgerald and Walker 2009; Walker 2019)

- altered brain growth (Smith et al. 2011; Brummelte et al. 2012; Ranger et al. 2015; Duerden et al. 2018)
- epigenetic changes (Chau et al. 2014; Provenzi et al. 2016).

Assessing Pain in the Neonate

Most guidelines on neonatal pain management declare pain assessment to be essential for achieving optimal pain and stress management (AAP Committee on Fetus and Newborn and Section on Anesthesiology and Pain Medicine 2016; Balice-Bourgois et al. 2020; Guo et al. 2020). Carrying out a pain assessment allows situations when the newborn infant may experience pain to be identified and treated, therefore avoiding analgesic under- or over-treatment. However, a study of 243 European neonatal units showed that the link between assessment of continuous pain and the use of analgesic drugs was weak (Anand et al. 2017). In other words, there was no guarantee the neonates received appropriate treatment for their pain.

While the subjective and complex nature of pain makes pain assessment challenging for all patients, it is particularly challenging in non-verbal infants unable to self-report. Instead, health professionals must learn to recognise and observe signs or indicators of pain in infants and determine when pain-relieving strategies need to be used (Table 13.1).

Indicators of neonatal pain are reactions to stimuli in the nociceptive system. Such indicators can be seen in the behavioural, physiological, hormonal or neurophysiological domains, and can either be observed individually or, preferably, in combination for better accuracy. To capture both the intensity of the painful stimulus and on how it is processed and interpreted, a multi-dimensional approach to pain assessment is recommended (Eriksson and Campbell-Yeo 2019).

Table 13.1 Indicators of neonatal pain.

Category	Description	Example of inclusion in pain assessment scales
Behavioural signs		
Alertness and sleep–wake state	■ A hyperalert state is often seen during ongoing or prolonged pain ■ Younger or sicker infants can need more time to comfort themselves and get back to rest after a painful event	BIIP, BPSN, N-PASS
Body movements and muscle tension	■ Full-term infants withdraw limbs from pain, but in preterm infants these responses are more diffuse and harder to control ■ Strong infants can react with increased muscle tension in arms and legs ■ Younger or sicker infants can turn flaccid	COMFORT neo, DAN, MBPS
Crying	■ Healthy, awake and full-term newborn infants react with moaning or crying that gets more intense and with longer duration with increasing discomfort ■ Infants of lower gestational age, sick or in a sleeping state or sedated will have difficulties showing a vocal reaction so the absence of crying must not be taken for absence of pain. Crying can often be noted as a weaker moaning sound	FLACC, CRIES
Facial activity, grimacing	■ Among the most studied and used signs to assess pain ■ Facial expressions that are indicators of pain: 　■ brow bulge 　■ squeezed eyes 　■ distinct furrows from the nose to ends of the mouth 　■ tense and stretched mouth and tongue 　■ raised cheeks	NFCS, PIPP/PIPP-R, BIIP, COMFORT neo, ALPS-neo, EDIN
Physiological signs		
Heart rate and heart rate variability	■ In healthy full-term infants, pain triggers an increased heart rate which leads to increased blood pressure and a red skin colour ■ Younger and sicker infants may react with an increase or decrease in heart rate or even bradycardia ■ Pain reduces heart rate variability (HRV) ■ HRV is best suited for assessing prolonged pain	PIPP/PIPP-R, PAT, NIAPAS
Respiration rate	■ In robust infants, respiration rate will increase as a result of acute pain, whereas the opposite, and even apnoea, can be seen in infants who do not have the energy to trigger the fight-or-flight system ■ Pain in the thorax region, from a chest tube or a surgical wound for example, can lead to impaired breathing	PAT, NIAPAS, NIPS

Table 13.1 (Continued)

Category	Description	Example of inclusion in pain assessment scales
Oxygen saturation	▇ Changes in oxygen saturation follow pain-associated changes in respiration and heart rate ▇ Both an increase and decrease in oxygen saturation can be seen, depending on the context	N-PASS, NIAPAS, PIPP/PIPP-R

Hormonal and metabolic signs

Cortisol	▇ A steroid hormone involved in the body's fight-or-flight system ▇ Increased levels can be seen after surgery (Franck et al. 2011) and painful procedures (Mörelius et al. 2009) ▇ Measured in plasma, saliva or urine ▇ High variability, more useful in research than clinically	

Neurophysiological signs

Cerebral oxygenation	▇ Pain measured with near-infrared spectroscopy (NIRS) associated with cerebral activation and changes in oxygenated and deoxygenated haemoglobin concentration in the brain ▇ An increase in oxygenated haemoglobin is assumed to reflect neuronal activation caused by pain ▇ NIRS is sensitive to movement artefacts (Bembich et al. 2013; Pettersson et al. 2019)	
Electroencephalogram (EEG) evoked potentials	▇ Multichannel EEG used as a proxy for neuronal activity, with most studies reporting on pain-related event-related potentials during acute painful procedures (Fabrizi et al. 2011; Jones et al. 2021) ▇ Primarily used in research, no standard clinical pain assessment method/tool	
Functional magnetic resonance imaging	▇ Has shown which areas in the infant brain are activated by pain (Goksan et al. 2015; Hartley et al. 2017) ▇ Not relevant as a bedside pain assessment tool ▇ Can help in developing and validating other measures	

ALPS-neo, Astrid Lindgren and Lund Children's Hospital's Pain and Stress Assessment Scale for Preterm and Sick Newborn Infants; BIIP, Behavioral Indicators of Infant Pain; BPSN, Bernese Pain Scale for Neonates; CRIES, Crying Requires oxygen Increased vital signs Expression Sleep; DAN, Douleur Aiguë Nouveau-né (Newborn Acute Pain); EDIN, Échelle Douleur Inconfort Nouveau-né; FLACC, Face, Legs, Activity, Cry, Consolability scale; MBPS, Modified Behavioural Pain Scale; NFCS, Neonatal Facial Coding System; NIAPAS, Neonatal Infant Acute Pain Assessment Scale; NIPS, Neonatal Infant Pain Scale; N-PASS, Neonatal Pain, Agitation and Sedation Scale; PAT, Pain Assessment Tool; PIPP/PIPP-R, Premature Infant Pain Profile–Revised.

Pain reactions can be dampened by analgesic or sedative drugs, or by illness. Other sources of non-pain-related stress or discomfort can cause similar reactions, so a combination of pain signs should increase the specificity of pain assessment (Ranger et al. 2013). It should be noted that, in many cases, how pain indicators are expressed depends on the gestational age, illness and alertness of the infant. Full-term, healthy and awake infants will react with an upregulation of the fight-or-flight system, whereas younger sicker infants or infants in a deep sleep might instead react with dampened signs.

Observational Pain Assessment Scales

There are over 40 neonatal pain assessment scales published and even more constructed and used locally (Eriksson and Campbell-Yeo 2019; Olsson et al. 2021). This chapter presents scales published in the last two decades (after 2000), indicating their recentness and clinical utility (Tables 13.2–13.4). Additional details about some other commonly used neonatal pain assessment tools can be found in Chapter 6.

Table 13.2 Pain assessment scales for acute procedural pain in term and preterm infants.

Acronym/name	Items
ABC (Bellieni et al. 2007)	Acuteness, rhythmicity and continuity of crying
BIIP: Behavioral Indicators of Infant Pain (Holsti and Grunau 2007)	Behavioral state, brow bulge, eye squeeze, nasolabial furrow, horizontal mouth stretch, taut tongue, finger splay, fisting
BPSN: Bernese Pain Scale for Neonates (Cignacco et al. 2004)	Alertness, duration of crying, time to calm, skin colour, eyebrow bulge with eye squeeze, posture, breathing pattern
FANS: Faceless Acute Neonatal Pain Scale (Milesi et al. 2010)	Heart rate variation, acute discomfort, limb movements, vocal expressions
FLACC: Face, Legs, Activity, Cry, Consolability scale (validated birth to adolescence) (Merkel et al. 1997)	Face, legs, activity, cry, consolability
MBPS: Modified Behavioural Pain Scale (validated 2–6 months) (Taddio et al. 1995)	Facial expression, cry, body movement
NFCS: Neonatal Facial Coding System (some validation for postoperative pain) (Grunau and Craig 1987)	Brow bulge, eye squeeze, nasolabial furrow, open lips, horizontal mouth stretch, vertical mouth stretch, lip purse, taut tongue, chin quiver
NIPS: Neonatal Infant Pain Scale (Lawrence et al. 1993)	Facial expression, cry, breathing patterns, arms, legs, state of arousal
NIAPAS: Neonatal Infant Acute Pain Assessment Scale (Pölkki et al. 2014)	Gestational age, alertness, facial expressions, crying, muscle tension, breathing, respirator/CPAP, reaction to handling, heart rate, oxygen saturation
PIPP, PIPP-R: Premature Infant Pain Profile–Revised (Gibbins et al. 2014; Stevens et al. 1996)	Gestational age, behavioural state, heart rate, oxygen saturation, brow bulge, eye squeeze, nasolabial furrow

Table 13.3 Pain assessment scales for postoperative pain in term and preterm infants.

Acronym/name	Items
N-PASS: Neonatal Pain, Agitation and Sedation Scale (some validation for acute procedural pain) (Hummel et al. 2008)	Crying/irritability, behaviour state, facial expression, extremities tone, vital signs
PAT: Pain Assessment Tool (Hodgkinson et al. 1994)	Posture/tone, sleep pattern, expression, colour, cry, respirations, heart rate, oxygen saturation, blood pressure, nurse's perception

Table 13.4 Pain assessment scales for prolonged pain in term and preterm infants.

Acronym/name	Items
ALPS-Neo: Astrid Lindgren and Lund Children's Hospital's Pain and Stress Assessment Scale for Preterm and Sick Newborn Infants (Lundqvist et al. 2014)	Facial expression, breathing pattern, tone of extremities, hand/foot activity, level of activity
COMFORT neo (also validated for sedated infants) (van Dijk et al. 2009)	Alertness, calmness/agitation, respiratory response, crying, body movement, facial tension, body muscle tone
EDIN: Échelle Douleur Inconfort Nouveau-né (Debillon et al. 2001)	Facial activity, body movements, quality of sleep, quality of contact with nurses, consolability
MAPS: Multidimensional Assessment of Pain Scale (validated birth to 31 months) (Ramelet et al. 2007)	Vital signs, breathing pattern, facial expressions, body movement, state of arousal

What Are the Most Sensitive and Specific Pain Assessment Tools?

A review of 352 clinical trials on neonatal pain revealed that 16% of the included studies used pain scales that were not validated for the studied specific neonatal population or pain type (Olsson et al. 2020), which raises concern about the validity of the study results. Pain scales considered valid and reliable for assessing infant pain most commonly used in clinical studies are the PIPP and PIPP-R (154 studies), followed by NIPS (84), NFCS (33) and DAN (20) (Olsson et al. 2020). In both clinical and research settings, the choice of tools should consider validity for the population and the type of pain being assessed.

An optimal pain assessment tool should (Meesters et al. 2019):

1. detect all painful situations (high sensitivity)
2. discriminate from non-painful situations (high specificity)
3. measure the type of pain they are supposed to measure (good validity)
4. give the same results when used repetitively or by different observers (good reliability)
5. measure if a pain-relieving intervention is effective (good responsiveness).

Automated Pain Assessment

Investigations into the efficacy of using machine learning automated techniques to accurately analyse signals from infants and evaluate if they indicate pain are ongoing. Currently, there is no system that is ready for clinical use (Gholami et al. 2010; Roué et al. 2021).

Pain Assessment by Parents

Modern neonatal care is family-centred and supports parental presence in the neonatal unit and parental involvement in care procedures, including pain management with proper counselling and information (McNair et al. 2020; Pierrat et al. 2020). Studies show that parents can recognise their infant's pain. While there is some evidence that parents may underestimate their infant's pain compared with health professionals (Tannous Elias et al. 2014; Olsson et al. 2019), parent assessment skills become more accurate over time with greater exposure to their child undergoing medical procedures and improved collaboration with health professionals (Axelin et al. 2015).

Using Pain Assessment to Deliver Adequate Pain Relief

In the clinical context there is a need for clear guidelines on how and when to assess pain and, above all, what to do with the results. We recommend following an algorithm, or pathway, with different actions for different pain scores, e.g. assess more often, use comfort measures, or give analgesic medication (Hummel and van Dijk 2006; Spence et al. 2010).

Physical Pain-relieving Interventions

Breastfeeding and Breast Milk

While the underlying pain-reducing mechanisms of direct breastfeeding are unknown, it is hypothesised that the effectiveness of breastfeeding as a multimodality intervention may be due to the synergistic benefits of maternal closeness and SSC (Johnston et al. 2017), maternal odour (Baudesson de Chanville et al. 2017),

auditory recognition (Lee and Kisilevsky 2014) and sucking (Pillai Riddell et al. 2015).

Direct breastfeeding (latching at the breast with active sucking and swallowing) for at least two minutes before a painful procedure has consistently been found to be more effective than comparator interventions, such as:

- swaddling (Shah et al. 2012; Yilmaz and Inal 2020)
- maternal holding or SSC (Thomas et al. 2011; Marín Gabriel et al. 2013; Modarres et al. 2013; Obeidat and Shuriquie 2015; Fallah et al. 2017)
- topical anaesthetics and cooling sprays (Boroumandfar et al 2013; Gupta et al. 2013)
- non-nutritive sucking (Lima et al. 2013)
- heel warming (Aydin and İnal 2019)
- music therapy (Zhu et al. 2015)
- placebo or no treatment (Dar et al. 2019; Erkul and Efe 2017; Shah et al. 2012).

When compared with sweet-tasting solutions, results are mixed. However, direct breastfeeding has been found to be as or more effective (Bembich et al. 2013; Goswani et al. 2013; Roué et al. 2014; Chiabi et al. 2016; Rioualen et al. 2018; Benoit et al. 2021). Studies on the feeding of expressed breast milk alone report mixed results (Benoit et al. 2017). Sucking maturity (Holsti et al. 2011) and combination of breast milk with other known pain-reducing strategies (Rosali et al. 2015; Peng et al. 2018) have been identified as factors that may contribute to the pain-reducing benefit.

Skin-to-skin Contact

SSC between a neonate and care provider is commonly referred to as kangaroo care. In the most recent Cochrane systematic review on SSC for procedural pain in neonates, all 25 studies ($n = 2001$) report favourable findings for SSC (Johnston et al. 2017). Of the 17 studies ($n = 801$) that compared SSC to standard care, significant reductions in heart rate, crying time,

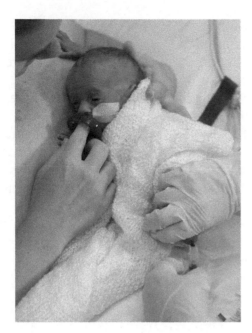

Figure 13.1 Capillary blood collection during maternal–infant skin-to-skin contact.

Source: Scott Munn.

and composite behavioural and biobehavioural pain scores were found in meta-analyses (Johnston et al. 2017).

There is evidence that:

- SSC is as or more effective than sweet-tasting solutions (Shukla et al. 2018; Nimbalkar et al. 2020; Sen and Manav 2020)
- SSC provides the same pain-reducing efficacy as sucrose (Campbell-Yeo et al. 2019) and control (Gao et al. 2015) over repeated heel lance procedures for preterm infants.

Figure 13.1 shows capillary blood collection during maternal infant SSC.

Studies comparing maternal SSC with alternative provider (father, alternative female) SSC have demonstrated that mothers are marginally more effective than fathers (Johnston et al. 2011b) and not significantly different from alternative female providers (Johnston et al. 2012). No significant difference in neurodevelopment outcomes measured at discharge were reported in the one study that compared the use of maternal SSC versus sucrose provided during repeated painful procedures across neonatal intensive care unit (NICU) hospitalisation for preterm infants (Campbell-Yeo et al. 2019).

Facilitated Tucking and Containment Interventions

Facilitated tucking is a physical containment intervention that involves placing hands on the head and limbs of an infant undergoing a painful procedure to maintain them in a side-lying flexed fetal position (Axelin et al. 2006). Figure 13.2 illustrates facilitated tucking.

Non-nutritive Sucking

A Cochrane systematic review and meta-analysis demonstrated that non-nutritive sucking improved regulation after painful procedures

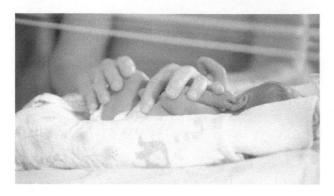

Figure 13.2 Facilitated tucking.

in both full-term and preterm neonates, and also improved pain reactivity in full-term neonates (Pillai Riddell et al. 2015). The combination of non-nutritive sucking with containment interventions (Peng et al. 2018) and oral sucrose (Stevens et al. 2016) may improve pain reactivity and regulation after acute needle procedures.

Oral Sucrose

Orally administered sucrose is the most extensively studied treatment for the management of neonatal procedural pain, with 74 randomised controlled trials ($n = 7049$) being included in the most recent Cochrane systematic review and meta-analysis examining its efficacy (Stevens et al. 2016). While various concentrations of sucrose have been tested, the strongest evidence for the pain-reducing effect of 24% sucrose solution is when combined with non-nutritive sucking (Stevens et al. 2016). Combining sucrose with adjuvant interventions (e.g. non-nutritive sucking and swaddling) appears to provide added pain-reducing benefit (Leng et al. 2016).

Despite the overwhelming evidence for the efficacy of sucrose in reducing biobehavioural pain response during single procedures, some concern regarding the sedative versus analgesic effect of sucrose has been raised in the

literature based on data derived using neonatal electroencephalographic recording (Slater et al. 2010; Benoit et al. 2021). A systematic review of eight studies examining the efficacy and safety of repeated oral sucrose for procedural pain provides evidence supportive of the safety and efficacy of repeated sucrose administration. However, results were mixed (Gao et al. 2016). Data on appropriate dosing of sucrose are limited. However, there is evidence to suggest that smaller volumes (e.g. 0.1 mL, 0.2 mL) provide the same benefit in reducing pain measured using composite pain measures as larger volumes (e.g. 0.5–1.0 mL) (Stevens et al. 2018; Tanyeri-Bayraktar et al. 2019).

Pharmacological Interventions for Neonatal Pain

Despite significant progress over the past three decades addressing the prevention, assessment and management of neonatal pain, many questions remain regarding optimal use of pharmacological agents to manage pain in neonates. Lack of efficacy data and uncertainty regarding long-term outcomes are two of the primary research gaps that clinicians face when attempting to manage neonatal pain (McPherson et al. 2020). Further, the optimal approach to the management of pain-related distress remains unclear. Despite these uncertainties, recognition of the significant adverse effects of untreated pain in early life and some existing evidence have led to the consistent inclusion of pharmacological agents in pain prevention and management guidelines for neonates (AAP Committee on Fetus and Newborn and Section on Anesthesiology and Pain Medicine 2016; Lago et al. 2017). See Chapter 5 for a detailed discussion of the pharmacology of analgesic drugs. Tables detailing relevant drug dosages can be found in Appendix 1.

Non-opioid Analgesics

Paracetamol

Paracetamol (acetaminophen) is one of the most commonly used analgesic drugs in the NICU. Interestingly, given paracetamol has not been reported to provide effective pain relief for infants undergoing procedural pain (Allegaert 2020; Ohlsson and Shah 2016), its use to relieve acute procedural pain is not recommended. However, there is some evidence that paracetamol has opioid-sparing effects for major pain and post-operative conditions and is effective in treating minor to moderate pain conditions (McPherson et al. 2020). A recent consensus statement from the Enhanced Recovery After Surgery (ERAS) Society recommends that, unless contraindicated, regular dosing (i.e. not on an as-needed or PRN basis) with paracetamol after neonatal intestinal surgery during the early postoperative period (to minimise but not replace opioid use) should be used (Brindle et al. 2020).

Other Non-opioid Analgesic Drugs

Non-steroidal anti-inflammatory drugs (NSAIDs), dexmedetomidine and gabapentin are also used to prevent/manage pain in neonates. Despite the widespread use of NSAIDs to treat pain in older children, their use for neonatal populations is less common. Given the risk associated with renal injury and gastrointestinal bleeding, most NSAIDs are not approved for reducing pain in infants less than six months of age, with greatest risk reported in infants less than three weeks of age and those delivered preterm (Aldrink et al. 2011).

Given the benefits of pain relief and opioid sparing in older children and adults, there is increasing interest in the off-label use of dexmedetomidine and gabapentin to treat postoperative pain and pain-related distress in neonates. Dexmedetomidine has been associated with less respiratory depression or gastrointestinal dysmotility compared with fentanyl (O'Mara et al. 2012) and has potential neuroprotective effects (Laudenbach et al. 2002).

Gabapentin, a gamma-aminobutyric acid analogue, has been reported to be potentially beneficial in treating irritability and refractory pain-related distress in neonates (Sacha et al. 2017). Despite these promising findings, further study regarding its efficacy and safety are warranted before routine use can be recommended.

Local Anaesthetics

Regional Anaesthetics

Local agents such as bupivacaine, lidocaine or ropivacaine can be administered as regional anaesthesia in infants not requiring a general anaesthetic for minor surgeries (e.g. inguinal hernia repair and circumcision) or for procedures such as chest tube placement (Bosenberg and Flick 2013; Jones et al. 2015). The use of regional anaesthesia has been associated with:

- reduced apnoea and bradycardia postoperatively but no reduction in postoperative opioid use (Jones et al. 2015)
- underuse due to the variability in available skilled practitioners (Marhofer et al. 2015).

Topical Anaesthetics

Considerable variation in degree of efficacy regarding the use of topical anaesthetics in neonates has been reported across different painful procedures (Foster et al. 2017). There is some evidence that the use of topical anaesthetic eye drops reduces pain associated with routine eye examinations conducted in the NICU for screening of retinopathy of prematurity, although its use alone does not provide optimal pain relief (Disher et al. 2018).

Topical agents, such as EMLA, a eutectic mixture of 2.5% prilocaine and 2.5% lidocaine, have been shown to reduce the pain associated with lumbar puncture at the time of needle insertion (Kaur et al. 2003), although caution regarding the application is required particularly in very preterm infants (Foster et al. 2017). While topical anaesthetics have demonstrated some effectiveness for reducing circumcision-related pain, a recent review of 29 randomised trials demonstrated that topical anaesthetics used as a single agent provided insufficient pain relief (Labban et al. 2020). There is also strong evidence that topical anaesthetics are ineffective in reducing the pain associated with routinely performed procedures, e.g. heel lance, venepuncture and insertion of intravenous or arterial lines (Foster et al. 2017) and frenotomy (Shavit et al. 2017).

Opioids

Opioids are the mainstay for the effective treatment of moderate to severe pain across all age groups, including neonates. The most commonly used agents for neonates are morphine and fentanyl. Despite the benefits, safe and effective dosing of opioids for pain relief in neonates is challenging as their neurodevelopmental stage makes them highly sensitive to drug effects and they can demonstrate slow drug clearance (Völler et al. 2019). Higher exposure to morphine when compared with lower morphine exposure has been associated with:

- higher incidence of death, intraventricular haemorrhage or periventricular leukomalacia, hypotension, and prolonged ventilation (Anand et al. 2004)
- feeding intolerance (Hall et al. 2005)
- reduced cerebellar volume and poorer 18-month motor and cognitive scores (Ranger et al. 2015)
- no reported long-term adverse neurological effects at age five years (De Graaf et al. 2011) or at eight and nine years (De Graaf et al. 2013).

Higher dosages of continuous infusion of fentanyl in contrast to the use of lower dosing has been associated with decreased cerebellar growth (McPherson et al. 2015) and poorer neurodevelopmental outcome at two years of age (Ancora et al. 2017).

Continuous Versus Bolus Dosing

One significant question which remains unanswered relates to the optimal administration of opioids or adjuvant therapies, either as a continuous infusion or intermittent bolus, most notably to achieve effective pain reduction and reduce cumulative opioid exposure and risk for adverse outcome. In the few studies addressing this question, results are mixed (Abiramalatha et al. 2019; Mitra et al. 2020; de Tristan et al. 2021). Currently, there is no consensus on the optimal administration of opioids in neonatal populations.

Families and Pain Management

In many neonatal units parents can now stay with their hospitalised infant most of the time. This means they should be seen as the primary caregivers, being the ones who best know how the infant feels and how to comfort them. Previously many health professionals have rejected the parents' role as experts of their own child and denied them the language and tools to manage infant pain. There is now increasing recognition that parents are impacted by seeing their infant in pain, which is stressful for them (Abdelmageed et al. 2022; Gallagher and Franck 2012). Parents want to be informed and involved, and to contribute to prevent and relieve that pain, which also strengthens their parental role (Skene et al. 2012). Many non-pharmacological pain-relieving methods are best or even exclusively performed by parents, such as SSC, facilitated tucking or breastfeeding (Campbell-Yeo et al.

2011; McNair et al. 2019; Ullsten et al. 2021). The role of health professionals is to guide parents, provide them with tools and knowledge and strengthen their self-esteem, so they can be advocates and pain relievers for their newborn infant (Axelin et al. 2015; Gates et al. 2018). Despite being an area of high concern for parents of newborns, there are few studies that address parent-targeted education regarding infant pain. Future research examining the impact and efficacy of parent-targeted education is essential (Richardson et al. 2020).

Summary

- Neonates are highly vulnerable to untreated pain in early life, given an immature pain-processing system, high exposure to pain and inability to verbalise their pain. This exposure to pain is associated with immediate and significant long-lasting consequences.
- Pain assessment using validated age-appropriate multidimensional pain assessment tools should be regularly conducted, and all painful procedures should be associated with the use of the most effective pain-reducing interventions.
- Parent-led non-pharmacological interventions (e.g. breastfeeding and SSC) should be considered first-line approaches for needle-related procedures. Sweet-tasting solutions should be offered if parent-led interventions are not available.
- Additional adjuvant non-pharmacological interventions may be offered in addition to breastfeeding, SSC or sweet-tasting solutions.
- More invasive procedures should be associated with the provision of pharmacological analgesics including topical and regional anaesthetics or intravenous opioids.
- Despite strong evidence regarding effective pain-reducing interventions, inconsistent use in clinical practice remains a significant concern.
- Ongoing advocacy, education and quality improvement initiatives for care providers, and greater inclusion of parents as active participants in pain care, is essential to ensure optimal pain assessment and management in neonatal populations.

Key to Case Study

1. Keisha held Kay in skin-to-skin contact (SSC) immediately after birth and during a routine intramuscular vitamin K injection. She noticed that Kay did not cry or grimace during the injection when being held, so she asked the nurse in the neonatal unit if she could hold Kay during the heel-lance procedure. Her nurse notes that holding preterm babies in SSC during blood work reduces their pain and agrees to help Keisha hold Kay in SSC before and during the procedure. Ten minutes before the heel-lance procedure, Keisha holds Kay in SSC in a ventral position, wearing only a nappy (diaper), on her bare chest. The nurse places a blanket over Keisha and Kay so only Kay's foot is exposed. The nurse sits beside Keisha on a low stool to complete the heel lance. Kay displays no facial response to the heel lance and remains settled throughout the procedure. Both Keisha and the nurse agree that

Kay appeared comforted throughout the heel-lance procedure. Keisha indicates she would like to use SSC for Kay's immunisations and the nurse suggests she can also consider breastfeeding Kay for additional pain-reducing benefit during immunisations.

2. You could ask Keisha if someone else in the family can come and stay with Kay and provide pain alleviation when needed. Evidence suggests that another parent or family member providing SSC is able to effectively provide pain relief. If this is not possible, you should use other measures to reduce pain, for example sweet solution (oral sucrose) combined with non-nutritive sucking.

3. Studies suggest that venepuncture is less painful than heel lancing. Blood can also be drawn from indwelling umbilical or arterial catheters, and there are instruments for transcutaneous measurement of bilirubin or levels of oxygen and carbon dioxide in the blood.

Multiple Choice Questions

1. What should optimal pain assessment in neonates involve?
   a. Routinely performed and documented with a regular frequency and with any painful procedure
   b. Using tools that include one indicator of pain such as physiological signs
   c. Performed by nursing staff only
2. Which two of the following statements about needle pain-relieving interventions in neonates are true?
   a. Direct breastfeeding is more effective than swaddling or non-nutritive sucking
   b. Opioids are safe and should be used for all needle-related procedures in neonates
   c. The pain-relieving effect of non-nutritive sucking can be enhanced when combined with other physical methods
   d. Skin-to-skin contact is less effective for pain relief than sweet-tasting solutions like sucrose
3. Which one of the following statements regarding the administration of sweet-tasting solutions such as sucrose is true?
   a. It is important to use sufficient volume, at least 0.5 mL sucrose
   b. It is important to use a sufficient concentration, at least 0.24% sucrose
   c. There is no effect of adding adjuvant interventions to enhance the pain-relieving effect of sucrose
4. Which two of the following statements about pain signs are correct?
   a. You should choose between using either physiological or behavioural signs for pain assessment
   b. The pain reactions of full-term healthy infants are usually more robust than those of preterm or sick infants
   c. Many pain assessment scales combine signs from more than one dimension, e.g. physiological and behavioural signs
   d. All neonates cry when they are in pain
5. Which one of the following statements is most correct?
   a. To realise that their newborn infant is subjected to pain can be frightening to many parents. Health professionals should protect them by doing

painful procedures when parents are not present

b. Breastfeeding, facilitated tucking and regional anaesthesia are examples of pain-relieving interventions that parents can provide to their newborn infant

c. Many non-pharmacological pain-relieving methods, such as skin-to-skin contact or breastfeeding, are best performed by parents

Additional Online Resources

In addition to the chapter content, the current best-practice guidelines for neonatal pain can be accessed using the hyperlinks below:

American Academy of Pediatrics Committee on Fetus and Newborn. Prevention and management of pain in the neonate: an update. https://pubmed.ncbi.nlm.nih.gov/17079598/

Ancora, G. et al. Evidence-based clinical guidelines on analgesia and sedation in newborn infants undergoing assisted ventilation and endotracheal intubation. https://pubmed.ncbi.nlm.nih.gov/30290021/

Balice-Bourgois, C. et al. A systematic review of clinical practice guidelines for acute procedural pain on neonates. https://pubmed.ncbi.nlm.nih.gov/31977372/

Lago, P. et al. Systematic review of nonpharmacological analgesic interventions for common needle-related procedure in newborn infants and development of evidence-based clinical guidelines. https://pubmed.ncbi.nlm.nih.gov/28295585/

Pirelli, A. et al. Literature review informs clinical guidelines for pain management during screening and laser photocoagulation for retinopathy of prematurity. https://pubmed.ncbi.nlm.nih.gov/30054933/

References

AAP Committee on Fetus and Newborn and Section on Anesthesiology and Pain Medicine (2016) Prevention and management of procedural pain in the neonate: an update. *Pediatrics* 137(2), e20154271.

Abdelmageed, R.I., Youssef, A.M., El-Farrash, R.A., Mohamed, H.M. and Abdelaziz, A.W. (2022) Measurement of cumulative preterm neonatal and maternal stressors during neonatal intensive care unit admission. *Journal of Pediatric Psychology* 47(5), 595–605.

Abiramalatha, T., Mathew, S.K., Mathew, B.S., et al. (2019) Continuous infusion versus intermittent bolus doses of fentanyl for analgesia and sedation in neonates: an open-label randomised controlled trial. *Archives of Disease in Childhood* 104(4), F433–F439.

Aldrink, J.H., Ma, M., Wang, W., Caniano, D.A., Wispe, J. and Puthoff, T. (2011) Safety of ketorolac in surgical neonates and infants 0 to 3 months old. *Journal of Pediatric Surgery* 46(6), 1081–1085.

Allegaert, K. (2020) A critical review on the relevance of paracetamol for procedural pain management in neonates. *Frontiers in Pediatrics* 8, 89.

Anand, K.J., Hall, R.W., Desai, N., et al. (2004) Effects of morphine analgesia in ventilated preterm neonates: primary outcomes from the NEOPAIN randomised trial. *Lancet* 363(9422), 1673–1682.

Anand, K.J., Eriksson, M., Boyle, E., et al. (2017) Assessment of continuous pain in newborns admitted to NICUs in 18 European Countries. *Acta Paediatrica* 106(8), 1248–1259.

Ancora, G., Lago, P., Garetti, E., et al. (2017) Follow-up at the corrected age of 24 months of preterm newborns receiving continuous infusion of fentanyl for pain control during mechanical ventilation. *Pain* 158(5), 840–845.

Axelin, A., Salantera, S. and Lehtonen, L. (2006) 'Facilitated tucking by parents' in pain management of preterm infants: a randomized crossover trial. *Early Human Development* 82(4), 241–247.

Axelin, A., Anderzén-Carlsson, A., Eriksson, M., Pölkki, T., Korhonen, A. and Franck, L.S. (2015) Neonatal intensive care nurses' perceptions of parental participation in infant pain management: a comparative focus group study. *Journal of Perinatal and Neonatal Nursing* 29(4), 363–374.

Aydin, D. and İnal, S. (2019) Effects of breastfeeding and heel warming on pain levels during heel stick in neonates. *International Journal of Nursing Practice* 25(3), e12734.

Balice-Bourgois, C., Zumstein-Shaha, M., Vanoni, F., Jaques, C., Newman, C.J. and Simonetti, G.D. (2020) A systematic review of clinical practice guidelines for acute procedural pain on neonates. *Clinical Journal of Pain* 36(5), 390–398.

Barrington, K. and Sankaran, K. (2018) Guidelines for detection, management and prevention of hyperbilirubinemia in term and late preterm newborn infants. *Paediatrics and Child Health* 12(Suppl. B), 1B–12B.

Baudesson de Chanville, A., Brevaut-Malaty, V., Garbi, A., Tosello, B., Baumstarck, K. and Gire, C. (2017) Analgesic effect of maternal human milk odor on premature neonates: a randomized controlled trial. *Journal of Human Lactation* 33(2), 300–308.

Bellieni, C.V, Bagnoli, F., Sisto, R., Neri, L., Cordelli, D. and Buonocore, G. (2007) Development and validation of the ABC pain scale for healthy full-term babies. *Acta Paediatrica* 94(10), 1432–1436.

Bembich, S., Davanzo, R., Brovedani, P., Clarici, A., Massaccesi, S. and Demarini, S. (2013) Functional neuroimaging of breastfeeding analgesia by multichannel near-infrared spectroscopy. *Neonatology* 104(4), 255–259.

Benoit, B., Martin-Misener, R., Latimer, M. and Campbell-Yeo, M. (2017) Breast-feeding analgesia in infants: an update on the current state of evidence. *Journal of Perinatal and Neonatal Nursing* 31(2), 145–159.

Benoit, B., Newman, A., Martin-Misener, R., Latimer, M. and Campbell-Yeo, M. (2021) The influence of breastfeeding on cortical and bio-behavioural indicators of procedural pain in newborns: findings of a randomized controlled trial. *Early Human Development* 154, 105308.

Boroumandfar, K., Khodaei, F., Abdeyazdan, Z. and Maroufi, M. (2013) Comparison of vaccination-related pain in infants who receive vapocoolant spray and breastfeeding during injection. *Iranian Journal of Nursing and Midwifery Research* 18(1), 33–37.

Bosenberg, A. and Flick, R. (2013) Regional anesthesia in neonates and infants. *Clinics in Perinatology* 40(3), 525–538.

Brindle, M.E., McDiarmid, C., Short, K., et al. (2020) Consensus guidelines for perioperative care in neonatal intestinal surgery: Enhanced Recovery After Surgery (ERAS®) Society recommendations. *World Journal of Surgery* 44(8), 2482–2492.

Brummelte, S., Grunau, R.E., Chau, V., et al. (2012) Procedural pain and brain development in premature newborns. *Annals of Neurology* 71(3), 385–396.

Campbell-Yeo, M., Fernandes, A. and Johnston, C. (2011) Procedural pain management for neonates using nonpharmacological strategies. Part 2: Mother-driven interventions. *Advances in Neonatal Care* 11(5), 312–320.

Campbell-Yeo, M., Johnston, C.C., Benoit, B., et al. (2019) Sustained efficacy of kangaroo care for repeated painful procedures over neonatal intensive care unit hospitalization: a single-blind randomized controlled trial. *Pain* 160(11), 2580–2588.

Centers for Disease Control and Prevention (2021) Child and adolescent immunization schedule by age. https://www.cdc.gov/vaccines/schedules/hcp/imz/child-adolescent.html

Chau, C.M.Y., Ranger, M., Sulistyoningrum, D., Devlin, A.M., Oberlander, T.F. and Grunau, R.E. (2014) Neonatal pain and COMT Val158Met genotype in relation to serotonin transporter (SLC6A4) promoter methylation in very preterm children at school age. *Frontiers in Behavioral Neuroscience* 8, 409.

Chiabi, A., Eloundou, E., Mah, E., Nguefack, S., Mekone, I. and Mbonda, E. (2016) Evaluation of breastfeeding and 30% glucose solution as analgesic measures in indigenous African term neonates. *Journal of Clinical Neonatology* 5(1), 46–50.

Cignacco, E., Mueller, R., Hamers, J.P. and Gessler, P. (2004) Pain assessment in the neonate using the Bernese Pain Scale for neonates. *Early Human Development* 78(2), 125–131.

Cruz, M.D., Fernandes, A.M. and Oliveira, C.R. (2016) Epidemiology of painful procedures performed in neonates: a systematic review of observational studies. *European Journal of Pain* 20(4), 489–498.

Dar, J.Y., Goheer, L. and Shah, S.A. (2019) Analgesic effect of direct breastfeeding during BCG vaccination in healthy neonates. *Journal of Ayub Medical College, Abbottabad* 31(3), 379–382.

Debillon, T., Zupan, V., Ravault, N., Magny, J.F. and Dehan, M. (2001) Development and initial validation of the EDIN scale, a new tool for assessing prolonged pain in preterm infants. *Archives of Disease in Childhood* 85(1), F36–F41.

De Graaf, J., van Lingen, R.A., Simons, S.H.P., et al. (2011) Long-term effects of routine morphine infusion in mechanically ventilated neonates on children's functioning: five-year follow-up of a randomized controlled trial. *Pain* 152(6), 1391–1397.

De Graaf, J., van Lingen, R.A., Valkenburg, A.J., et al. (2013) Does neonatal morphine use affect neuropsychological outcomes at 8 to 9 years of age? *Pain* 154(3), 449–458.

de Tristan, M.A., Martin-Marchand, L., Roué, J.M., et al. (2021) Association of continuous opioids and/or midazolam during early mechanical ventilation with survival and sensorimotor outcomes at age 2 years in premature infants: results from the French Prospective National EPIPAGE 2 Cohort. *Journal of Pediatrics* 232, 38–47.e8.

Disher, T., Gullickson, C., Singh, B., et al. (2018) Pharmacological treatments for neonatal abstinence syndrome: a systematic review and network meta-analysis. *JAMA Pediatrics* 173(3), 234–243.

Doesburg, S.M., Chau, C.M., Cheung, T.P.L., et al. (2013) Neonatal pain-related stress, functional cortical activity and visual-perceptual abilities in school-age children born at extremely low gestational age. *Pain* 154(10), 1946–1952.

Duerden, E.G., Grunau, R.E., Guo, T., et al. (2018) Early procedural pain is associated with regionally-specific alterations in thalamic development in preterm neonates. *Journal of Neuroscience* 38(4), 878–886.

Eriksson, M. and Campbell-Yeo, M. (2019) Assessment of pain in newborn infants. *Seminars in Fetal and Neonatal Medicine* 24(4), 101003.

Erkul, M. and Efe, E. (2017) Efficacy of breastfeeding on babies' pain during vaccinations. *Breastfeeding Medicine* 12(2), 110–115.

Fabrizi, L., Worley, A., Patten, D., et al. (2011) Electrophysiological measurements and analysis of nociception in human infants. *Journal of Visualized Experiments* (58), e3118.

Fallah, R., Naserzadeh, N., Ferdosian, F. and Binesh, F. (2017) Comparison of effect of kangaroo mother care, breastfeeding and swaddling on Bacillus Calmette–Guerin vaccination pain score in healthy term neonates by a clinical trial. *Journal of Maternal-Fetal and Neonatal Medicine* 30(10), 1147–1150.

Fitzgerald, M. and Walker, S.M. (2009) Infant pain management: a developmental neurobiological approach. *Nature Clinical Practice Neurology* 5(1), 35–50.

Fitzgerald, M., Millard, C. and McIntosh, N. (1989) Cutaneous hypersensitivity following peripheral tissue damage in newborn infants and its reversal with topical anaesthesia. *Pain* 39(1), 31–36.

Foster, J.P., Taylor, C. and Spence, K. (2017) Topical anaesthesia for needle-related pain in newborn infants. *Cochrane Database of Systematic Reviews* (2), CD010331.

Franck, L.S., Ridout, D., Howard, R., Peters, J. and Honour, J.W. (2011) A comparison of pain measures in newborn infants after cardiac surgery. *Pain* 152(8), 1758–1765.

Gallagher, K. and Franck, L. (2012) Ten lessons from 10 years of research into parental involvement in infant pain management. *Infant* 8(3), 78–80.

Gao, H., Xu, G., Gao, H., et al. (2015) Effect of repeated kangaroo mother care on repeated procedural pain in preterm infants: a randomized controlled trial. *International Journal of Nursing Studies* 52(7), 1157–1165.

Gao, H., Gao, H., Xu, G., et al. (2016) Efficacy and safety of repeated oral sucrose for repeated procedural pain in neonates: a systematic review. *International Journal of Nursing Studies* 62, 118–125.

Gates, A., Shave, K., Featherstone, R., et al. (2018) Procedural pain: systematic review of parent experiences and information needs. *Clinical Pediatrics* 57(6), 672–688.

Gholami, B., Haddad, W.M.M. and Tannenbaum, A.R.R. (2010) Relevance vector machine learning for neonate pain intensity assessment using digital imaging. *IEEE Transactions on Bio-Medical Engineering* 57(6), 1457–1466.

Gibbins, S., Stevens, B.J., Yamada, J., et al. (2014) Validation of the Premature Infant Pain Profile-Revised (PIPP-R). *Early Human Development* 90(4), 189–193.

Goksan, S., Hartley, C., Emery, F., et al. (2015) FMRI reveals neural activity overlap between adult and infant pain. *ELife* 4, e06356.

Goswani, G., Upadhyay, A., Gupta, N., Chaudhry, R., Chawla, D. and Sceenivas, V. (2013) Comparison of analgesic effect of direct breastfeeding, oral 25% dextrose solution, and placebo during first DPT vaccination in health term infants: a randomized placebo contolled trial. *Indian Pediatrics* 50(4), 649–653.

Grunau, R.E. and Craig, K.D. (1987) Pain expression in neonates: facial action and cry. *Pain* 28(3), 395–410.

Grunau, R.E., Holsti, L., Haley, D.W., et al. (2005) Neonatal procedural pain exposure predicts lower cortisol and behavioral reactivity in preterm infants in the NICU. *Pain* 113(3), 293–300.

Grunau, R.E., Holsti, L. and Peters, J.W.B. (2006) Long-term consequences of pain in human neonates. *Seminars in Fetal and Neonatal Medicine* 11(4), 268–275.

Grunau, R.E., Haley, D.W., Whitfield, M.F., Weinberg, J., Yu, W. and Thiessen, P. (2007) Altered basal cortisol levels at 3, 6, 8 and 18 months in infants born at extremely low gestational age. *Journal of Pediatrics* 150(2), 151–156.

Guo, W., Lui, X., Zhou, X., Wu, T. and Sun, J. (2020) Efficacy and safety of combined nonpharmacological interventions for repeated procedural pain in preterm neonates: a systematic review of randomized controlled trials. *International Journal of Nursing Studies* 102, 103471.

Gupta, N.K., Upadhyay, A., Agarwal, A., Goswami, G., Kumar, J. and Sreenivas, V. (2013) Randomized controlled trial of topical EMLA and breastfeeding for reducing pain during wDPT vaccination. *European Journal of Pediatrics* 172(11), 1527–1533.

Hall, R.W., Kronsberg, S.S., Barton, B.A., Kaiser, J.R., Anand, K.J. and Group, N.T.I. (2005) Morphine, hypotension, and adverse outcomes among preterm neonates: who's to blame? Secondary results from the NEOPAIN trial. *Pediatrics* 115(5), 1351–1359.

Hartley, C., Duff, E.P., Green, G., et al. (2017) Nociceptive brain activity as a measure of analgesic efficacy in infants. *Science Translational Medicine* 9(388), eaah6122.

Hodgkinson, K., Bear, M., Thorn, J. and van Blaricum, S. (1994) Measuring pain in neonates: evaluating an instrument and developing a common language. *Australian Journal of Advanced Nursing* 12(1), 17–22.

Holsti, L. and Grunau, R.E. (2007) Initial validation of the Behavioral Indicators of Infant Pain (BIIP). *Pain* 132(3), 264–272.

Holsti, L., Oberlander, T.F. and Brant, R. (2011) Does breastfeeding reduce acute procedural pain in preterm infants in the neonatal intensive care unit? A randomized clinical trial. *Pain* 152(11), 2575–2581.

Hummel, P. and van Dijk, M. (2006) Pain assessment: current status and challenges. *Seminars in Fetal and Neonatal Medicine* 11(4), 237–245.

Hummel, P., Puchalski, M., Creech, S.D. and Weiss, M.G. (2008) Clinical reliability and validity of the N-PASS : neonatal pain, agitation and sedation scale with prolonged pain. *Journal of Perinatology* 28(1), 55–60.

Johnston, C., Barrington, K.J., Taddio, A., Carbajal, R. and Filion, F. (2011a) Pain in Canadian NICUs: have we improved over the past 12 years? *Clinical Journal of Pain* 27(3), 225–232.

Johnston, C., Campbell-Yeo, M. and Filion, F. (2011b) Paternal vs maternal kangaroo care for procedural pain in preterm neonates: a randomized crossover trial. *Archives of Pediatrics and Adolescent Medicine* 165(9), 792–796.

Johnston, C., Byron, J., Filion, F., Campbell-Yeo, M., Gibbins, S. and Ng, E. (2012) Alternative female kangaroo care for procedural pain in preterm neonates: a pilot study. *Acta Paediatrica* 101(11), 1147–1150.

Johnston, C., Campbell-Yeo, M., Disher, T., et al. (2017) Skin-to-skin care for procedural pain in neonates. *Cochrane Database of Systematic Reviews* (2), CD008435.

Jones, L.J., Craven, P.D., Lakkundi, A., Foster, J.P. and Badawi, N. (2015) Regional (spinal, epidural, caudal) versus general anaesthesia in preterm infants undergoing inguinal herniorrhaphy in early infancy. *Cochrane Database of Systematic Reviews* (6), CD003669.

Jones, L., Laudiano-Dray, M.P., Whitehead, K., et al. (2021) The impact of parental contact upon cortical noxious-related activity in human neonates. *European Journal of Pain* 25(1), 149–159.

Kaur, G., Gupta, P. and Kumar, A. (2003) A randomized trial of eutectic mixture of local anesthetics during lumbar puncture in newborns. *Archives of Pediatrics and Adolescent Medicine* 157(11), 1065–1070.

Labban, M., Menhem, Z., Bandali, T., Hneiny, L. and Zaghal, A. (2020) Pain control in neonatal male circumcision: a best evidence review. *Journal of Pediatric Urology* 17(1), 3–8.

Lago, P., Garetti, E., Bellieni, C.V., et al. (2017) Systematic review of nonpharmacological analgesic interventions for common needle-related procedure in newborn infants and development of evidence-based clinical guidelines. *Acta Paediatrica* 106(6), 864–870.

Laudenbach, V., Mantz, J., Lagercrantz, H., Desmonts, J.M., Evrard, P. and Gressens, P. (2002) Effects of α_2-adrenoceptor agonists on perinatal excitotoxic brain injury: comparison of clonidine and dexmedetomidine. *Anesthesiology* 96(1), 134–141.

Lawrence, J., Alcock, D., McGrath, P., Kay, J., MacMurray, S.B. and Dulberg, C. (1993) The development of a tool to assess neonatal pain. *Neonatal Network* 12(6), 59–66.

Lee, G.Y. and Kisilevsky, B.S. (2014) Fetuses respond to father's voice but prefer mother's voice after birth. *Developmental Psychobiology* 56(1), 1–11.

Leng, H.Y., Zheng, X.-L., Zhang, X.-H., et al. (2016) Combined non-pharmacological interventions for newborn pain relief in two degrees of pain procedures: a randomized clinical trial. *European Journal of Pain* 20(6), 989–997.

Lima, A.H., Hermont, A.P. and Friche, A.A.D.L. (2013) Analgesia in newborns: a case-control study of the efficacy of nutritive and non-nutritive sucking stimuli. *CoDAS* 25(4), 365–368.

Lundqvist, P., Kleberg, A., Edberg, A.-K., Larsson, B.A., Hellström-Westas, L. and Norman, E. (2014)

Development and psychometric properties of the Swedish ALPS-Neo pain and stress assessment scale for newborn infants. *Acta Paediatrica* 103(8), 833–839.

McNair, C., Campbell-Yeo, M., Johnston, C. and Taddio, A. (2019) Nonpharmacologic management of pain during common needle puncture procedures in infants: current research evidence and practical considerations. An update. *Clinics in Perinatology* 46(4), 709–730.

McNair, C., Chinian, N., Shah, V., et al. (2020) Meta-synthesis of factors that influence parents' participation in pain management for their infants in the NICU. *Journal of Obstetric, Gynecologic, and Neonatal Nursing* 49(3), 263–271.

McPherson, C., Haslam, M., Pineda, R., Rogers, C., Neil, J.J. and Inder, T.E. (2015) Brain injury and development in preterm infants exposed to fentanyl. *Annals of Pharmacotherapy* 49(12), 1291–1297.

McPherson, C., Ortinau, C.M. and Vesoulis, Z. (2020) Practical approaches to sedation and analgesia in the newborn. *Journal of Perinatology* 41(3), 383–395.

Marhofer, P., Keplinger, M., Klug, W. and Metzelder, M.L. (2015) Awake caudals and epidurals should be used more frequently in neonates and infants. *Paediatric Anaesthesia* 25(1), 93–99.

Marín Gabriel, M.Á., del Rey Hurtado de Mendoza, B., Jiménez Figueroa, L., et al. (2013) Analgesia with breastfeeding in addition to skin-to-skin contact during heel prick. *Archives of Disease in Childhood* 98(6), F499–F503.

Meesters, N., Dilles, T., Simons, S. and van Dijk, M. (2019) Do pain measurement instruments detect the effect of pain-reducing interventions in neonates? A systematic review on responsiveness. *Journal of Pain* 20(7), 760–770.

Merkel, F., Voepel, S.I., Lewis, T., Shayevitz, J.R. and Malviya, S. (1997) The FLACC: a behavioral scale for scoring postoperative pain in young children. *Pediatric Nursing* 23(3), 293–297.

Milesi, C., Cambonie, G., Jacquot, A., et al. (2010) Validation of a neonatal pain scale adapted to the new practices in caring for preterm newborns. *Archives of Disease in Childhood* 95(4), F263–F266.

Mitra, S., Babadagli, M.E., Hatfield, T., et al. (2020) Effect of fentanyl boluses on cerebral oxygenation and hemodynamics in preterm infants: a prospective observational study. *Neonatology* 117(4), 480–487.

Modarres, M., Jazayeri, A., Rahnama, P. and Montazeri, A. (2013) Breastfeeding and pain relief in full-term neonates during immunization injections: a clinical randomized trial. *BMC Anesthesiology* 13(1), 22.

Mörelius, E., Theodorsson, E. and Nelson, N. (2009) Stress at three-month immunization: parents' and infants' salivary cortisol response in relation to the use of pacifier and oral glucose. *European Journal of Pain* 13(2), 202–208.

Narvey, M. and Marks, S. (2019) The screening and management of newborns at risk for low blood glucose. *Paediatrics and Child Health* 24(8), 536–544.

Ng, E. and Loewy, A.D. (2018) Guidelines for vitamin K prophylaxis in newborns. *Paediatrics and Child Health* 23(6), 394–397.

Nimbalkar, S., Shukla, V.V., Chauhan, V., et al. (2020) Blinded randomized crossover trial: skin-to-skin care vs. sucrose for preterm neonatal pain. *Journal of Perinatology* 40(6), 896–901.

Obeidat, H.M. and Shuriquie, M.A. (2015) Effect of breast-feeding and maternal holding in relieving painful responses in full-term neonates. *Journal of Perinatal and Neonatal Nursing* 29(3), 248–254.

Ohlsson, A. and Shah, P.S. (2016) Paracetamol (acetaminophen) for prevention or treatment of pain in newborns. *Cochrane Database of Systematic Reviews* (6), CD011219.

Olsson, E., Pettersson, M., Eriksson, M. and Ohlin, A. (2019) Oral sweet solution to prevent pain during neonatal hip examination: a randomised controlled trial. *Acta Paediatrica* 108(4), 626–629.

Olsson, E., Ahl, H., Bengtsson, K., et al. (2021) The use and reporting of neonatal pain scales: a systematic review of randomized trials. *Pain* 162(2), 353–360.

O'Mara, K., Gal, P., Wimmer, J., et al. (2012) Dexmedetomidine versus standard therapy with fentanyl for sedation in mechanically ventilated premature neonates. *Journal of Pediatric Pharmacology and Therapeutics* 17(3), 252–262.

Ozawa, M., Kanda, K., Hirata, M., Kusakawa, I. and Suzuki, C. (2011) Influence of repeated painful procedures on prefrontal cortical pain responses in newborns. *Acta Paediatrica* 100(2), 198–203.

Peng, H.F., Yin, T., Yang, L., et al. (2018) Non-nutritive sucking, oral breast milk, and facilitated tucking relieve preterm infant pain during heel-stick procedures: a prospective, randomized controlled trial. *International Journal of Nursing Studies* 77, 162–170.

Pettersson, M., Olsson, E., Ohlin, A. and Eriksson, M. (2019) Neurophysiological and behavioral measures of pain during neonatal hip examination. *Paediatric and Neonatal Pain* 1(1), 15–20.

Pierrat, V., Marchand-Martin, L., Durrmeyer, X., et al. (2020) Perceived maternal information on premature infant's pain during hospitalization: the French EPIPAGE-2 national cohort study. *Pediatric Research* 87(1), 153–162.

Pillai Riddell, R.R., Racine, N.M., Gennis, H.G., et al. (2015) Non-pharmacological management of infant and young child procedural pain. *Cochrane Database of Systematic Reviews* (12), CD006275.

Pölkki, T., Korhonen, A., Axelin, A., Saarela, T. and Laukkala, H. (2014) Development and preliminary validation of the Neonatal Infant Acute Pain Assessment Scale (NIAPAS). *International Journal of Nursing Studies* 51(12), 1585–1594.

Provenzi, L., Giusti, L., Fumagalli, M., et al. (2016) Pain-related stress in the neonatal intensive care unit and salivary cortisol reactivity to socio-emotional stress in 3-month-old very preterm infants. *Psychoneuroendocrinology* 72, 161–165.

Ramelet, A.S., Rees, N., McDonald, S., Bulsara, M. and Abu-Saad, H.H. (2007) Development and preliminary psychometric testing of the Multidimensional Assessment of Pain Scale: MAPS. *Paediatric Anaesthesia* 17(4), 333–340.

Ranger, M., Johnston, C., Rennick, J.E., Limperopoulos, C., Heldt, T. and du Plessis, A.J. (2013) A multidimensional approach to pain assessment in critically ill infants during painful procedure. *Clinical Journal of Pain* 29(7), 613–620.

Ranger, M., Zwicker, J.G., Chau, C.M.Y., et al. (2015) Neonatal pain and infection relate to smaller cerebellum in very preterm children at school age. *Journal of Pediatrics* 167(2), 292–298.

Richardson, B., Falconer, A., Shrestha, J., Cassidy, C., Campbell-Yeo, M. and Curran, J.A. (2020) Parent-targeted education regarding infant pain management delivered during the perinatal period: a scoping review. *Journal of Perinatal and Neonatal Nursing* 34(4), 56–65.

Rioualen, S., Durier, V., Herve, D., Misery, L., Sizun, J. and Roué, J.-M. (2018) Cortical pain response of newborn infants to venepuncture: a randomized controlled trial comparing analgesic effects of sucrose versus breastfeeding. *Clinical Journal of Pain* 34(7), 650–656.

Rosali, L., Nesargi, S., Mathew, S., Vasu, U., Rao, S.P. and Bhat, S. (2015) Efficacy of expressed breast milk in reducing pain during ROP screening: a randomized controlled trial. *Journal of Tropical Pediatrics* 61(2), 135–138.

Roué, J., Rioualen, S., Nowak, E., Roudaut, S. and Sizun, J. (2014) PS-195 sucrose versus breastfeeding for venipuncture in term infants: a randomised, prospective, controlled study with analysis of the specific cortical response. *Archives of Disease in Childhood* 99(Suppl. 2), A183.

Roué, J.M., Morag, I., Haddad, W.M., Gholami, B. and Anand, K.J.S. (2021) Using sensor-fusion and machine-learning algorithms to assess acute pain in non-verbal infants: a study protocol. *BMJ Open* 11(1), e039292.

Sacha, G.L., Foreman, M.G., Kyllonen, K. and Rodriguez, R.J. (2017) The use of gabapentin for pain and agitation in neonates and infants in a neonatal ICU. *Journal of Pediatric Pharmacology and Therapeutics* 22(3), 207–211.

Schmelzle-Lubiecki, B.M., Campbell, K.A.A., Howard, R.H., Franck, L. and Fitzgerald, M. (2007) Long-term consequences of early infant injury and trauma upon somatosensory processing. *European Journal of Pain* 11(7), 799–809.

Sen, E. and Manav, G. (2020) Effect of kangaroo care and oral sucrose on pain in premature infants: a randomized controlled trial. *Pain Management Nursing* 21(6), 556–564.

Shah, P.S., Herbozo, C., Aliwalas, L.L. and Shah, V.S. (2012) Breastfeeding or breast milk for procedural pain in neonates. *Cochrane Database of Systematic Reviews* (12), CD004950.

Shavit, I., Peri-Front, Y., Rosen-Walther, A., et al. (2017) A randomized trial to evaluate the effect of two topical anesthetics on pain response during frenotomy in young infants. *Pain Medicine* 18(2), 356–362.

Shukla, V., Chapla, A., Uperiya, J., Nimbalkar, A., Phatak, A. and Nimbalkar, S. (2018) Sucrose vs. skin to skin care for preterm neonatal pain control: a randomized control trial. *Journal of Perinatology* 38(10), 1365–1369.

Skene, C., Franck, L., Curtis, P. and Gerrish, K. (2012) Parental involvement in neonatal comfort care. *Journal of Obstetric, Gynecologic, and Neonatal Nursing* 41(6), 786–797.

Slater, R., Cornelissen, L., Fabrizi, L., et al. (2010) Oral sucrose as an analgesic drug for procedural pain in newborn infants: a randomised controlled trial. *Lancet* 376(9748), 1225–1232.

Smith, G.C., Gutovich, J., Smyser, C., et al. (2011) Neonatal intensive care unit stress is associated with brain development in preterm infants. *Annals of Neurology* 70(4), 541–549.

Spence, K., Henderson-Smart, D., New, K., Evans, C., Whitelaw, J. and Woolnough, R. (2010) Evidenced-based clinical practice guideline for management of newborn pain. *Journal of Paediatrics and Child Health* 46(4), 184–192.

Stevens, B., Johnston, C., Petryshen, P. and Taddio, A. (1996) Premature Infant Pain Profile: development and initial validation. *Clinical Journal of Pain* 12(1), 13–22.

Stevens, B., Yamada, J., Gy, L. and Ohlsson, A. (2016) Sucrose for analgesia in newborn infants undergoing painful procedures. *Cochrane Database of Systematic Reviews* (7), CD001069.

Stevens, B., Yamada, J., Campbell-Yeo, M., et al. (2018) The minimally effective dose of sucrose for procedural pain relief in neonates: a randomized controlled trial. *BMC Pediatrics* 18(1), 85.

Taddio, A., Nulman, I., Koren, B.S., Stevens, B. and Koren, G. (1995) A revised measure of acute pain in infants. *Journal of Pain and Symptom Management* 10(6), 456–463.

Taddio, A., Katz, J., Ilersich, A.L. and Koren, G. (1997) Effect of neonatal circumcision on pain response during subsequent routine vaccination. *Lancet* 349(9052), 599–603.

Tannous Elias, L.S.D., dos Santos, A.M.N. and Guinsburg, R. (2014) Perception of pain and distress in intubated and mechanically ventilated newborn infants by parents and health professionals. *BMC Pediatrics* 14(1), 44.

Tanyeri-Bayraktar, B., Bayraktar, S., Hepokur, M. and Güzel Kıran, G. (2019) Comparison of two different doses of sucrose in pain relief. *Pediatrics International* 61(8), 797–801.

Therrell, B.L., Padilla, C.D., Loeber, J.G., et al. (2015) Current status of newborn screening worldwide: 2015. *Seminars in Perinatology* 39(3), 171–187.

Thomas, T., Shetty, A.P. and Bagali, P.V. (2011) Role of breastfeeding in pain response during injectable immunisation among infants. *Nursing Journal of India* 102(8), 3p.

Ullsten, A., Andreasson, M. and Eriksson, M. (2021) State of the art in parent-delivered pain-relieving interventions in neonatal care: a scoping review. *Frontiers in Pediatrics* 9, 651846.

Van Dijk, M., Roofthooft, D.W.E., Anand, K.J.S., Guldemond, F., de Graaf, J. and Simons, S. (2009) Taking up the challenge of measuring prolonged pain in (premature) neonates: the COMFORTneo Scale seems promising. *Clinical Journal of Pain* 25(7), 607–616.

Vinall, J. and Grunau, R.E. (2014) Impact of repeated procedural pain-related stress in infants born very preterm. *Pediatric Research* 75(5), 584–587.

Völler, S., Flint, R.B., Andriessen, P., et al. (2019) Rapidly maturing fentanyl clearance in preterm neonates. *Archives of Disease in Childhood* 104(6), F598–F603.

Walker, S.M. (2019) Long-term effects of neonatal pain. *Seminars in Fetal and Neonatal Medicine* 24(4), 101005.

Wollgarten-Hadamek, I., Hohmeister, J., Demirakça, S., Zohsel, K., Flor, H. and Hermann, C. (2009) Do burn injuries during infancy affect pain and sensory sensitivity in later childhood? *Pain* 141 (1–2), 165–172.

World Health Organization (2022) *WHO Recommendations on Maternal and Newborn Care for a Positive Postnatal Experience.* Available at https://www.who.int/publications/i/item/9789240045989

Yilmaz, D. and Inal, S. (2020) Effects of three different methods used during heel lance procedures on pain level in term neonates. *Japan Journal of Nursing Science* 17(4), e12338.

Zhu, J., He, H.-G., Zhou, X., et al. (2015) Pain relief effect of breast feeding and music therapy during heel lance for healthy-term neonates in China: a randomized controlled trial. *Midwifery* 31(3), 365–372.

14 Palliative Care in Children and Young People

Poh Heng Chong and Hwee Hsiang Liow

In this chapter, we discuss the approach to children and young people (CYP) with pain and related issues in the context of palliative care, using examples from two patient populations: advanced incurable cancer and severe neurological impairment (SNI). Each group is expected to have different pain experiences, with concomitant implications for assessment and management.

The chapter begins by defining paediatric palliative care (PPC), highlighting its unique features and where it may differ from adult palliative care. Then, the different types of pain and their assessment, pharmacological management, psychological interventions and physical approaches that together constitute a multimodal strategy to pain relief (World Health Organization (WHO) 2020) are outlined in relation to the two distinct populations of CYP. Case examples are provided, where appropriate, to facilitate reader understanding and translation to clinical practice. In closing, ethical considerations in the context of PPC and end-of-life symptom management to optimise overall comfort are shared.

What is Paediatric Palliative Care?

The definition and features of PPC are provided in Box 14.1. The aim of PPC is to *reduce suffering* and *improve quality of life* for CYP and their family (Benini et al. 2022). PPC is always multimodal in delivery, using pharmacological, psychological and physical interventions, attending to myriad needs of the CYP and their families across different dimensions. PPC can be provided in the community (at home), in hospital and in hospices. Depending on the resources available, it can be delivered by a specialised team or individual health professionals (WHO 2018a).

Four groups of life-limiting and life-threatening conditions that are eligible for palliative care have been identified (Table 14.1).

While the underlying philosophy to safeguard quality of life in the face of life-threatening or life-limiting illness is similar, PPC differs from adult palliative care in many ways (Fraser et al. 2020). PPC cares for CYP from neonates to young adults; and

Managing Pain in Children and Young People: A Clinical Guide, Third Edition. Edited by Alison Twycross, Jennifer Stinson, William T. Zempsky, and Abbie Jordan.

BOX 14.1   DEFINITION AND FEATURES OF PAEDIATRIC PALLIATIVE CARE

Definition

The prevention and relief of suffering of paediatric patients and their families facing the problems associated with life-threatening illness.

Features

- Attending to the physical, psychological, social and spiritual suffering of patients, and the psychological, social and spiritual suffering of family members.
- The early identification and impeccable assessment and treatment of problems.
- Application early in the course of illness in conjunction with other therapies intended to prolong life.
- Accompanying bereaved family members after the patient's death.

Source: WHO (2018a)

Table 14.1 Categories of conditions eligible for PPC.

Category	Description	Examples
1	Life-threatening conditions for which curative treatment may be feasible but can fail	Cancer, cardiac anomalies with failure
2	Where premature death is inevitable; involving long periods of intensive disease-directed treatment aimed at prolonging life, and allowing participation in normal activities	Cystic fibrosis, Duchenne muscular dystrophy
3	Progressive conditions without curative treatment options	Mitochondrial disorders, mucopolysaccharidoses
4	Irreversible but non-progressive conditions causing severe disability, predisposing to health complications and likelihood of premature death	Cerebral palsy, hypoxic ischaemic encephalopathy

Source: Chambers (2018).

at different levels of neurocognitive development, not always defined by an individual's chronological age. To the professional provider, this has many implications, particularly around sharing medical information and eliciting treatment preferences from the seriously ill young patient.

CYP as a group present with heterogeneous conditions:

- some may be so rare that trajectories are unclear

- others may be genetic in origin, resulting in multiple young family members afflicted, with parents often bearing a nagging sense of guilt
- with a preponderance of non-cancer diagnoses observed in clinical practice, physical disabilities and dependencies are common, including frequent use of technology or devices like ventilators and gastrostomy tubes (Horridge et al. 2016).

Rapidly advancing medical interventions and pursuit of aggressive life-sustaining therapies in the context of childhood serious illness have led to proportionately longer and more uncertain prognoses compared with adult counterparts. Providing opportunities for respite to family caregivers therefore becomes instrumental in PPC (Benini et al. 2022). On top of the disease-related considerations outlined above, often CYP continue to grow older through illness, with normal developmental needs for play, school and friends (Benini et al. 2017). Owing to mental capacity issues in the immature or cognitively impaired sick CYP, and a highly technical medical environment, ethical dilemmas are prevalent in PPC (Feudtner and Nathanson 2014; Rapoport and Morrison 2016; Marty and Carter 2018); an important consideration that is discussed later in the chapter. It is also worth noting that the bereavement experience, both anticipated and after a CYP dies, compared to when an adult dies, is more likely to be complicated. This may require extended follow-up, and even supportive counselling in some cases (Van der Geest et al. 2014; Snaman et al. 2020; Wiener et al. 2020).

In light of the above, PPC adopts a biopsychosocial and spiritual model in assessment, care planning and delivery. With multidimensional symptoms and anticipated patient diversity, a variety of skillsets and competencies is needed and hence a care team comprising different professionals is ideal (Sisk et al. 2020).

Access to the much needed whole-person and family-focused support that PPC provides is often hampered by its strong association with end-of-life care, leading to late referrals (Harrop and Edwards 2013; Twamley et al. 2014; Weaver et al. 2016). This is most pronounced in paediatric oncology, with informal caregivers and health professionals alike holding these misconceptions (Friedrichsdorf 2017; Friedrichsdorf and Bruera 2018). Opportunities for deep conversations on goals of care and treatment preferences to minimise CYP suffering and parental regrets may be lost because of this. Despite expansion of its geographical footprint in terms of service development, persistent conflation of PPC with end-of-life care signals unfinished work that PPC as a growing global movement needs to advocate for (WHO 2018a; Benini et al. 2022).

More than 21 million CYP worldwide live with a condition that can benefit from a palliative care approach by their normal healthcare providers (e.g. paediatric subspecialty oncologists or cardiologists) and 8.1 million are estimated to require specialist PPC (Connor et al. 2017). Most of these CYP live in low- and middle-income countries (LMIC) where access to services and support is minimal, while PPC is fairly established in high-income countries (Arias-Casais et al. 2020; Knaul et al. 2020). Lack of access to PPC in LMIC is further compounded by gaps in availability of essential medicines (Knaul et al. 2018). See Chapter 15 for additional information about preventing and treating CYP's pain in LMIC.

The WHO believes that, with creative planning, PPC can still be provided where resources are limited; e.g., support may be obtained through tapping community resources (WHO 2018a). Moderate success in service development has been reported in LMIC (Downing et al. 2016).

In England, the prevalence of CYP aged 0–19 years with life-limiting conditions rose from 26.7 to 63.2 per 10 000 population between 2001/2 and 2017/18 (Fraser et al. 2020). In the USA, more than 40 children with complex chronic conditions aged 0–19 years die each day (Friebert and Williams 2015; Osterman et al. 2015).

In summary, though developing worldwide and evidently impactful in some areas, PPC continues to face significant barriers to its uptake and administration. However, where available, its holistic and flexible approaches rendered by a team of diverse professionals address unique needs around the seriously ill CYP, with the ultimate goal being to prevent and reduce suffering among all types of stakeholders involved.

Treating and Preventing Pain in Children and Young People with Advanced Incurable Cancer

Types and Sources of Pain in CYP with Advanced Incurable Cancer

Regardless of diagnosis, pain is the most common symptom experienced by this group of CYP on palliative care (Friedrichsdorf et al. 2015; Wolfe et al. 2015), and suboptimal pain management at end of life has a lasting impact on the family (Snaman et al. 2016; Greenfield et al. 2022). Pain may be characterised by its pathophysiology (nociceptive, neuropathic or mixed), acute or chronic, intensity, temporality and location (Beecham et al. 2015; Fink and Gallagher 2019). The different types of pain encountered in oncology PPC are identified in Table 14.2.

Assessing Pain in CYP with Advanced Incurable Cancer

The first step in managing pain is its assessment. Pain assessment is discussed in detail in Chapter 6. A thorough pain history minimally includes the quality of the pain, its intensity and temporality. The process of assessment should also consider:

- triggers that provoke, contribute to or exacerbate pain, such as fear and anxiety (Harrop et al. 2017)
- previous pain experiences, including responses to past treatments (Downing et al. 2015; Lathrop 2016)
- the impact of pain on function (Thomas et al. 2018; Fink and Gallagher 2019).

As part of good practice, use of validated pain assessment tools is encouraged. The choice of pain assessment tool will depend on several factors, including the CYP's age, level of cognitive development and communication skills (Lathrop 2016; Cascella et al. 2019; Carter 2020). After clinical examination, and

Table 14.2 Typologies of pain in oncology palliative care.

Pain typologies	Characteristics	Considerations
Breakthrough pain	Transient exacerbation of pain on background of persistent but well-controlled pain	Increase background analgesia. Addition of adjuvants for synergistic effects
Incident pain	Episodic pain provoked by physical action (e.g. bowel movements) or bodily movement (e.g. changing posture)	Anticipate or avoid triggers if possible. Use rapid-acting but short-lasting medication to manage these episodes. Explore interventional strategies early
End-of-dose failure pain	Recurrence of pain just before next dose of scheduled analgesic drug is due	Dose of existing regular analgesics may need to be increased to prevent systemic analgesic levels from dropping below threshold

Sources: Komatz and Carter (2015); Fink and Gallagher (2019); Løhre et al. (2020).

further investigations (if indicated and setting permits), the underlying cause(s) of the pain will become clearer. This guides formulation of a preliminary management plan. After treatment has been started, frequent assessment of pain at regular intervals is required to monitor effectiveness in order to allow changes in the care plan if needed.

PRACTICE POINT

The PQRST model described by Neale (2012) provides a useful way of remembering the elements of a pain assessment in this patient group.

Palliating/provoking: What makes your pain better, or worse?

Quality: How would you rate your pain? What does it feel like?

Radiation: Does your pain stay in one location or does it travel?

Site/symptoms: Where is your pain located? Are there associated symptoms?

Timing/triggers: Is the pain new? When did your pain begin? How long does it last? Is it worse during different times of the day? Any precipitating factors? Does it wake you up from sleep?

Pharmacological Interventions in CYP with Advanced Incurable Cancer

As discussed in Chapter 1, when deciding on appropriate pharmacological pain-relieving interventions the WHO two-step ladder (Box 14.2) is a useful guide (WHO 2020). Table 14.3 details different considerations when deciding on the most appropriate pharmacological interventions. The aim of drug treatment for pain in the context of palliative care is to

BOX 14.2   THE WHO TWO-STEP LADDER

Step 1: Mild pain

Non-opioids (e.g. paracetamol and NSAIDs[a]) +/− adjuvants[b]

Step 2: Severe pain

Strong opioids (e.g. morphine and fentanyl) +/− non-opioids +/− adjuvants

[a] Non-steroidal anti-inflammatory drugs (discussed later under CYP with non-cancer diagnoses)
[b] Also called co-analgesics, with alternative indications but additional analgesic properties

Table 14.3 Factors to consider during drug therapy using the WHO two-step ladder.

By the ladder	Moderate to severe pain requires stronger medications, using opioids like morphine in calibrated doses
By the clock	Scheduling regular doses of medications to reduce 'peaks and troughs' over the course of the day
By appropriate route	Administering the drug by the least invasive route, picked by the child wherever possible
By the child	Select drugs based on the individual child, to adjust accordingly in subsequent reviews

bring prompt and meaningful pain relief safely, without excessive accompanying adverse effects.

Using Opioids to Manage Pain in CYP with Advanced Incurable Cancer

In PPC there is no one right dose of opioids. The optimal dose is determined by careful titration to pain relief, or when adverse effects appear. The effective dose varies between CYP and even for the same CYP at different times. This may mean prescribing doses higher than those in dosage tables. Given the anticipated dose-limiting adverse effects of opioid use (discussed below), the CYP needs to be engaged where feasible to locate the right balance between, comfort (benefit of treatment) and sedation (as adverse effect). Physiological tolerance that develops over time should also be taken into consideration during the process of drug titration (Wood et al. 2018). Additional factors involved in deciding the most appropriate drugs, doses and routes include the following (Snaman et al. 2016):

1. Disease severity: response to disease-modifying treatments or disease progression.
2. Comorbidities: worsening liver or renal function.
3. Other medications: drug–drug interactions or additive effects.
4. Pathophysiology of pain: visceral or neuropathic pain may not be as responsive to opioids.
5. Drug pharmacokinetics: vary according to age or genetic expression of receptor types.

There are a number of other issues to consider when managing pain in CYP with advanced incurable cancer.

- In a *pain crisis*, rapid titration may be indicated, administering strong opioids through oral or parenteral routes or, where available, using a patient-controlled analgesia (PCA) device (Nijland et al. 2019).
- The use of PCA is also recommended for prompt relief of *incident pain*, particularly in the inpatient ward setting where processes to obtain controlled drugs may prevent timely breakthrough drug administration (Henderson et al. 2019).
- When oral routes for drug administration are unavailable, such as at the end of life, and parenteral options are declined, *transmucosal administration* of drugs may be explored to achieve pain relief (Drolet et al. 2016; Sutherland et al. 2020).
- Common adverse effects of opioids encountered in practice, particularly when the CYP is opioid naive, include nausea, lethargy, itch, urinary retention and constipation. They are generally experienced transiently over the first few days at the start of treatment, before tolerance occurs. These may require specific treatments temporarily, but constipation generally persists and will need long-term mitigation (e.g. regular laxatives) (Wood et al. 2018).
- Where control of pain is only achieved with intolerable adverse effects, an alternative opioid can replace the existing one through *opioid rotation* (Downing et al. 2015; Friedrichsdorf and Postier 2019), where the balance of analgesic properties and adverse effects between opioids for the individual patient is leveraged to good effect.

It is important to remember that CYP receiving chemotherapy may already be experiencing a myriad of adverse effects (e.g. nausea, mucositis and neuropathy), some of which are self-limiting while others possibly long-standing. These should be managed actively alongside primary oncologists as additional drugs are introduced for pain management in order to limit overall symptom burden (including from adverse effects) while not compromising concurrent goals for cancer treatment (Dalberg et al. 2018).

Adjuvant Drugs for Treating Pain in CYP with Advanced Cancer

Adjuvant drugs are used to treat (Snaman et al. 2016):

■ bone pain using NSAIDs, steroids and bisphosphonates

■ painful bladder or bowel contractions from various causes using antispasmodics (e.g. propantheline or oxybutynin)

■ muscle spasms as a result of cancer infiltration using muscle relaxants (e.g. baclofen or benzodiazepines).

This section focuses on the use of adjuvants alongside opioids in the management of neuropathic or mixed pain for CYP with advanced cancer. Though prevalent in clinical practice, there is limited paediatric evidence to support decision-making in this context.

■ Specific scales for neuropathic pain have only been validated in the adult setting.

■ Neuropathic pain in CYP is identified by the presence of symptoms, such as allodynia, paraesthesia or hyperalgesia (Fink and Gallagher 2019).

■ There are no randomised controlled trials for treatment of neuropathic pain in CYP.

The adjuvant drugs used with this client group are listed in Table 14.4. In addition to this list of pharmacological agents, steroids and radiotherapy are commonly used to treat neuropathic pain, particularly where nerve compression is involved (WHO 2018b).

When Pain Becomes Resistant to Opioids or Adjuvants

Whatever the pathophysiology of pain, whether nociceptive, neuropathic or mixed, there may be situations where the CYP continues to experience distressing pain despite escalating opioid doses and co-administration of adjuvants. These cancer pains are commonly described as intractable or refractory (Afsharimani et al. 2015; Chong and Yeo 2021). Therapeutic options become limited and, if available, associated with much higher risks of side effects (Table 14.5).

Psychological Interventions in CYP with Advanced Incurable Cancer

Many factors can impact on CYP's perception and experience of pain (Table 14.6). As discussed in Chapter 4, pain is a biopsychosocial phenomenon. The gate control theory, outlined

Table 14.4 Adjuvant drugs commonly used in treatment of neuropathic pain in palliative care.

Adjuvant drugs	Advantages in neuropathic pain
Tricylic antidepressants	Once-a-day dosing, improves insomnia, renal friendly
Gabapentinoids	Few drug interactions, NNT in adult studies 2.9–3.9
Topical lidocaine	Where pain is localised, patch can be cut to fit
NMDA receptor blockers	Ketamine used most commonly, immediate onset of action
Parenteral lidocaine	May be considered in refractory neuropathic pain that failed first- and second-line treatments outlined above (including antidepressants, antiepileptics and NMDA antagonists). See next section
Clonidine	Given orally, transdermally or intraspinally; opioid sparing
SNRI	Some evidence for neuropathic pain in adult studies

NNT, number needed to treat; NMDA, *N*-methyl-ᴅ-aspartate; SNRI, serotonin/noradrenaline reuptake inhibitor.
Source: Friedrichsdorf and Goubert (2020); Chong and Yeo (2021).

Table 14.5 Other modalities of treatment in complex situations.

Ketamine (oral or parenteral infusions)	NMDA receptor antagonist. Used to treat intractable neuropathic pains that do not respond to high-dose opioids or added adjuvants. ***Does not cause respiratory depression*** (Jonkman et al. 2017; Sheehy et al. 2017; Fallon et al. 2018; Courade et al. 2022)
Lidocaine infusions	Decreases neuronal membrane permeability to sodium ions, blocking initiation and conduction of impulses. Modulates pain 'wind-up' (Berde et al. 2016; Gibbons et al. 2016; Chong and Yeo 2021)
Anaesthetic approaches	Regional anaesthesia (epidural or intrathecal) and neurolytic blocks. Risks include bleeding, infection and neurological complications (Berger and Goldschneider 2019; Magee et al. 2021; Le-Short et al. 2022)

NMDA, *N*-methyl-ᴅ-aspartate.

Table 14.6 Factors influencing the perception and experience of pain.

Healthcare variables	Previous healthcare encounters, prior painful or invasive procedures, disease progression and treatment, relationship between medical team and CYP parents/carers
CYP variables	Personality, temperament, chronological and developmental age, coping style, anxiety, culture, spirituality
Family variables	Parental/carer distress, their level of involvement, family composition, socioeconomic status, employment or family stressors, culture, spirituality

in Chapter 3, explains how psychological distress can increase pain sensations. Anxiety, fear of the unknown, overstimulation, depressive states, fatigue and any other negative emotion can open this 'gate'. Good communication between health professionals and the CYP and their family, particularly that aimed at enhancing adjustment or underpinned by principles of positive psychology, can help (Wechsler et al. 2014; Iddon et al. 2016).

While there is limited evidence to support the use of psychological pain-relieving interventions in CYP with cancer on palliative care, a vast evidence base exists for their use in other types of pain (Markozannes et al. 2017; Fisher et al. 2018, 2022). Different psychological interventions will suit individual CYP. Decisions on which intervention to try should be made in partnership with the CYP and their family. A sample of those that could complement pain management in the paediatric oncology setting is summarised in Table 14.7. Case illustrations to demonstrate how these psychological interventions may be utilised at the bedside are provided below. Additional information about psychological methods can be found in Chapter 1.

Table 14.7 Psychological pain management techniques for CYP with advanced cancer by developmental age.

Age	Distraction techniques	Cognitive and behavioural methods
Infants (0–1 years)	Music, massage therapy, sensory soothing measures (e.g. comforting and familiar voice)	Guide and coach parents in ways to increase infant's comfort
Toddlers and preschool children (2–5 years)	Comfort items (e.g. cuddly toys), videos, interactive stories, familiar songs, music, puppets, bubble-blowing, comfort hold, massage therapy	Therapeutic play (e.g. messy, sensory and medical play), art therapy, music therapy, relaxation games, breathing exercises, guided imagery and hypnosis, humour and jokes
School-age children (6–11 years)	Comfort items, familiar songs and music, puppets, favourite toys and games, videos, electronic handheld games, virtual reality (VR) games or stories, animal-assisted therapy, comfort hold, massage therapy	Therapeutic play, art therapy, music therapy, guided imagery and hypnosis, relaxation games, breathing exercises, progressive muscle relaxation, humour and jokes, exchanging information about disease and treatment of pain
Adolescents (12–18 years)	Favourite music or videos, electronic handheld or VR games, surfing internet, animal-assisted therapy, massage therapy	Art therapy, music therapy, visual imagery, self-regulatory and psychophysiological techniques (e.g. deep breathing, progressive muscle relaxation and hypnosis), cognitive behavioural therapy (CBT), acceptance and commitment therapy (ACT), acupuncture/acupressure, mindfulness-based stress reduction, humour and jokes, information sharing

Sources: Friedrichsdorf and Postier (2019); Kuttner (2010); Coughtrey et al. (2018); Jibb et al. (2015).

CASE ILLUSTRATIONS

Therapeutic play

Min Hui was a six-year-old girl with a terminal brain tumour. She lost the ability to walk, eat and communicate. At one home visit, she was helped to the living room in her wheelchair. Armed with water balloons, the therapist told Min Hui they were going to throw away everything nasty and demonstrated with one shot. Min Hui was amused as the balloon burst with a splash on the balcony. She was invited to have a go. She hesitantly raised her arm and lobbed the balloon placed in her hand. A smile came to her face. She would not stop till the balloons ran out!

Distraction

The parents of nine-year-old Joseph, with end-stage liver cancer, were unable to get him into any position of comfort, as he complained of pain and was restless. The therapist diverted his attention using a familiar online game. As he clicked away to 'kill the dinosaurs', the therapist continued to engage him, asking about different dinosaurs he exterminated or predicting which dinosaur would win. He became 'invested' in the game very quickly. Throughout the session and there-after, the pain was perceived by Joseph to be more tolerable, and he reported that it stayed in the background and stopped coming 'at my face'.

Music

A four-year-old boy, Kok Wei, was diagnosed with advanced neuroblastoma. At the end of life, he spent all his time lying in bed at home. There came a point when even the weight of a blanket or gentle stroking by parents caused pain. At one home visit, the therapist sat beside him and hummed familiar songs in a soft and rhythmic way. One particular song was in the tune of Rain, Rain Go Away but in the words of Pain, Pain Go Away. In less than 15 minutes, Kok Wei turned calm, relaxed and comfortable. He soon fell asleep.

Breathing

Stanley, a 10-year-old boy with leukaemia, had a low pain tolerance. He was terrified of any inva-sive procedures and would be in a state of emotional dysregulation whenever he needed to have an injection or cannula inserted. Before his next procedure, the therapist invited him to practice deep breathing together with her. She used hand gestures as visual cues to depict an inflating balloon as he breathed in deeply through the nose, and a deflating balloon as he breathed out through the mouth. When the time came, he could feel his heart beat slowing down (and see on the monitor too) as the nurses performed the procedure smoothly.

Art

Fifteen-year-old Grace suffered extensive pains from metastatic osteosarcoma. During one session, the therapist suggested she illustrate it on paper: the intensity, the sensations and triggers. Then,

Grace was guided to connect and converse with that 'pain', before being asked what she would like to do with the picture. Grace painted her favourite colour over the 'pain', symbolic that she did not want the 'pain' to take over her life. At the end of the session, the teenager felt a sense of empowerment and her mood improved. This indirectly reduced her sense of pain and the distress it caused.

Physical Pain-relieving Interventions in CYP with Advanced Incurable Cancer

Evidence for physical pain-relieving interventions in CYP with advanced cancer is similarly sparse. Nonetheless, examples include:

- rehabilitative measures including splints or specially constructed mobility devices that reduce pain at rest and during transfers, such as bed to chair (Friedrichsdorf and Postier 2019; Fisher et al. 2022)
- acupuncture, acupressure and aromatherapy are also used to complement drug treatments in the clinical setting (O'Connor et al. 2013; Friedrichsdorf and Goubert 2020)
- non-nutritive sucking for infants has increasing evidence supporting its efficacy (Carter and Brunkhorst 2017). See Chapter 11 for a discussion of physical pain-relieving methods for neonates.

When All Else Fails, and Suffering Becomes Overwhelming Close to the End of Life

Rarely, and always as a last resort, palliative sedation becomes an option, when all previous interventions fail to bring relief to the imminently dying CYP (Burns et al. 2017; Miele et al. 2019; Maeda et al. 2020). This is only considered in a very specific context of refractory pain: where intensive therapeutic efforts, short of sedation, have failed to bring relief; alternative treatments are associated with excessive or unacceptable morbidity; and remaining interventions are unlikely to stop further suffering within a reasonable time frame (Gurschick et al. 2015; Abarshi et al. 2017; Henderson et al. 2017).

Treating and Preventing Pain in Children and Young People with Severe Neurological Impairment

SNI of the central nervous system (CNS), a common description in PPC literature and practice that refers to a heterogeneous group of life-limiting conditions, results in learning (intellectual) disability and limited verbal communication, often with coexisting motor impairment (Hauer and Houtrow 2017). Contributory causes are multiple, including genetic, metabolic, neurodegenerative, CNS malformations, infections, and anoxic or other forms of traumatic brain injuries.

Prevalence of Pain in CYP with Severe Neurological Impairment

It is increasingly apparent that CYP with SNI experience significant pain, sometimes on a daily basis.

- Parents of children ($n = 275$) with incurable progressive genetic, metabolic or other neurological conditions reported pain as the most common problem faced (Steele et al. 2014).

■ Among children with all types of muco-polysaccharidosis, pain was reported in more than half in a particular cohort surveyed (Brands et al. 2015).

Providing further context to these numbers, this pain is particularly hard to identify (Carter 2020). First, compared to those with normal neurological development, CYP with SNI often behave differently when in pain. It can be hard to know if they are in pain, not to mention evaluate effects of pain-relieving interventions. Second, above idiosyncratic presentations, the inherent complexity and dynamic nature of pain in this context challenges all types of caregivers, both formal and informal. Health professionals regularly face uncertainties in pain assessment beyond those related to knowledge and skills at the bedside (Carter et al. 2016), while parents take considerable time to develop an embodied 'sense of knowing' to determine if the CYP is indeed distressed by pain (Carter et al. 2017).

Types and Sources of Pain in CYP with Severe Neurological Impairment

Nociceptive (Acute) Pain

Nociceptive pain can be related to the CYP's underlying condition, for example discomfort from malposition on a wheelchair, or a muscle spasm that becomes intense. Alternatively, nociceptive pain can result from an emerging noxious stimulus. Common sources of nociceptive pain are described in Table 14.8.

Chronic Pain

CYP with SNI often experience persistent or long-standing intermittent pain. This can be due to gastro-oesophageal reflux disease; joint dislocations or acquired spinal deformities like scoliosis; uncontrolled seizures; spasticity, spasms, dystonia (Hauer and Solodiuk 2015). Alternatively, pain can persist because of an impaired CNS. The latter may be undetectable on routine clinical tests or even high-resolution imaging. These types of pain can be characterised as *neuropathic pain* (both peripheral and central), *visceral hyperalgesia* (Asaro et al. 2017; Hauer 2018), or *autonomic dysfunction* (Freundlich and Hall 2018). The features of each type are described in Table 14.9.

Assessing Pain in CYP with Severe Neurological Impairment

The objective of assessing pain in CYP with SNI is to identify the presence of pain, put in place an early treatment plan and evaluate the effectiveness of administered interventions. As mentioned, assessing pain in CYP with SNI can

Table 14.8 Nociceptive sources that cause acute pain.

Head	Acute otitis media, dental abscess, sinusitis, corneal abrasion, ventriculo-peritoneal shunt malfunction, hair tourniquet
Chest	Aspiration pneumonia, reflux oesophagitis, cardiac ischaemia
Abdomen	Peptic ulcer disease, intussusception, appendicitis, constipation, rectal fissure, pancreatitis, cholecystitis, nephrolithiasis, urinary tract infection, inguinal hernia, testicular torsion, ovarian cyst, menstrual cramps
Skin	Pressure sore or decubitus ulcers
Limbs	Fracture, hip subluxation, osteomyelitis

Sources: Hauer (2010); Warlow and Hain (2018).

Table 14.9 Pain syndromes from an impaired CNS that cause chronic pain.

Type of pain	Features
Neuropathic pain	Symptoms include pain localised to the gastrointestinal tract (e.g. pain triggered by gastrointestinal distension). Pain can occur spontaneously and with no trigger. Attributable to impairment of the spinothalamic tract and thalamus
Visceral hyperalgesia	Altered threshold to pain generation in response to a stimulus in the gastrointestinal tract. Attributable to sensitisation of visceral afferents as well as central sensitisation in the CNS
Autonomic dysfunction	Features that suggest dysautonomia: skin flushing, hyperthermia, retching, bowel dysmotility, agitation, tachycardia, sweating. Dysautonomia can be a source of discomfort, and pain can trigger the features that occur with dysautonomia

be problematic, as they often respond differently from developmentally normal CYP who can self-report.

Pain assessment is often suboptimal among CYP with SNI. For example, of 149 children in a study cohort with progressive neurological, metabolic or chromosomally based conditions reported by parents to experience pain, up to 60% of their professional providers had no documented pain assessments or analgesic treatments in their medical records (Friedrichsdorf et al. 2017). Indeed, health professionals encounter significant uncertainty and often find themselves feeling inadequate when it comes to pain assessment in this particular group (Carter et al. 2016; Carter 2020).

Best practice related to pain assessment in CYP with SNI is set out in Box 14.3. Frequently observed pain behaviours and validated pain assessment tools for CYP with SNI are discussed in the next section.

Pain Behaviours

Observation of different pain behaviours is a legitimate approach to initial pain assessment in the CYP who cannot self-report (Herr et al. 2011). A variety of behaviours have been characterised (Stallard et al. 2002; Hauer 2012; Warlow and Hain 2018) (Table 14.10).

BOX 14.3 BEST PRACTICE IN ASSESSING PAIN IN CYP WITH SNI

Attitude

- CYP with SNI, like other patients, can feel pain.
- Avoid assuming that pain behaviours are integral to the underlying condition and missing taking further actions (see below).
- Increased tone and abnormal movements as pain behaviours could be wrongly managed as spasticity or dystonia.
- Premature diagnosis of neuro-irritability in a persistently distressed child may result in missing an acute pain trigger that is reversible.

Actions

- A careful and detailed approach. Other than severity of pain, *frequency* and *duration* of pain should be ascertained.
- Categorise type(s) of pain (nociceptive or neuropathic) causing distress and locate possible trigger.
- Process includes triad of history, examination and investigation. Basic

diagnostics are performed, leaving more invasive studies until later, if causes for pain prove elusive.

■ Empirical treatment to commence while investigations are in progress, particularly with persistent irritability from long-standing intermittent pain. Underlying pathology may never be found despite extensive work-up.

Sources: Siden (2018); Warlow and Hain (2018); Harrop et al. (2017); Hauer and Houtrow (2017)

Behavioural Pain Assessment Tools

Validated pain assessment tools that capture some of those behaviours described above aid clinicians in evaluating pain in CYP with SNI objectively. Four commonly used instruments are shown in Table 14.11 (more information about these tools can be found in Chapter 6).

The r-FLACC and INRS can be individualised by adding pain behaviours specific to each child. Customisation ensures that atypical pain behaviours like laughing are not erroneously

Table 14.10 Examples of pain behaviours.

Category	Examples
Vocalisations	Crying, whimpering, moaning, gasping, sharp intake of breath
Facial expression	Grimacing, frowning, furrowed brow, squinting, eyes wide open, clenched teeth, teeth grinding, distressed look
Consolability	Inability to be consoled and made comfortable
Interaction	Withdrawn, seeking comfort
Sleep	Disturbed sleep, increased or decreased sleep
Movement	Increased from baseline in movement of limbs, restless and fidgety, startles easily, pulls away when touched, twists or turns
Tone	Stiffening of extremities, clenching of fists, back arching, resists movement
Physiological	Tachycardia, sweating, shivering, change in colour, pallor, breath-holding, tears
Atypical features	Blunted facial expression, laughter, breath-holding, self-injurious behaviours

Table 14.11 Commonly used validated pain assessment tools.

r-FLACC	■ Revised from FLACC to include pain behaviours specific to children with cognitive impairment ■ Five-item pain assessment tool with a score ranging from 0 to 10
INRS	■ Personalised pain-assessment tool for non-verbal children with learning (intellectual) disability ■ Parents and caregivers identify behaviours that indicate no pain to the worst possible pain on a scale ranging from 0 to 10
NCCPC-R	■ 30-item pain-assessment tool designed for non-verbal children aged 3–18 years with severe cognitive impairment ■ Moderate to severe pain determined at cut-off of ≥7 of 90
PPP	■ A 20-item pain-assessment tool for children with severe to profound cognitive impairment ■ Scores of ≥14 were generally associated, by observers, with moderate or severe pain

r-FLACC, revised Face, Leg Activity, Cry, Consolability; INRS, Individualised Numeric Rating Scale; NCCPC-R, Non-Communicative Children's Pain Checklist–Revised; PPP, Paediatric Pain Profile.
Sources: Hauer and Houtrow (2017); Cascella et al. (2019).

scored. With sound psychometric properties, the NCCPC-R and PPP have been used in diverse research studies on pain in children with SNI (Cascella et al. 2019). The shorter r-FLACC is favoured among many clinicians for its ease of use at the bedside (Carter et al. 2017).

CASE STUDY: PART 1

Rick is a 16-year-old boy with quadriplegic cerebral palsy. Bed-bound and totally dependent on caregivers, his condition is complicated by oropharyngeal dysphagia, gastro-oesophageal reflux, severe scoliosis, dislocated left hip and worsening epilepsy. With global developmental delay, communication is achieved through grunting, though only his mother understands his needs. He is recently discharged after one month's stay in hospital (including intensive care) for aspiration pneumonia. He lost much weight and is deconditioned. His distraught mother now manages continuous non-invasive ventilation and frequent suction, on top of usual five times a day bolus enteral feeding via a gastrostomy tube. Despite settling down at home comfortably in the first week, his mother called to ask why Rick appears increasingly distressed, particularly after feeding.

1. What other information or findings may need to be obtained before considering further management?

Pharmacological Interventions for CYP with Severe Neurological Impairment

Pharmacological interventions to manage pain in CYP with SNI are detailed in Table 14.12. Somewhat framing the interventions listed below, a *neuro-pain ladder*, modified from the WHO pain ladder, outlines pharmacological strategies in the management of pain in children with SNI (Hauer 2012; see Table 14.13). It is also worth remembering that there are barriers to the use of analgesic drugs in CYP with SNI. Some examples are provided in Table 14.14.

Broad principles for clinician consideration as individualised pharmacological interventions include:

- previous drug trials and their responses
- starting dose of each treatment drug
- titration regimen, including routes of administration
- interactions between medications (both old and newly introduced)
- good balance between benefits and adverse effects of individual drugs.

Finer points, gleaned from anecdotal experience, include the following:

- If there is a background of recurrent or persistent neuro-irritability, an early trial of gabapentin is proposed (Friedrichsdorf and Postier 2019).
- Drug titration may involve other drugs on the neuro-pain ladder. This can take days or weeks before an effective 'cocktail' is found.
- Caregivers need clear explanations and regular updates.
- Pre-order anticipated breakthrough or as-needed drugs (Freundlich and Hall 2018). This empowers caregivers in providing timely relief and gives a sense of control.
- Success is contingent on solid partnerships between caregivers and providers, underpinned by a commitment to achieve the realistic goal of more 'good days' for the CYP.

Table 14.12 Pharmacological interventions for CYP with SNI.

Drug type	Uses and adverse effects
Paracetamol (acetaminophen) and non-steroidal anti-inflammatory drugs (NSAIDs)	▪ Mostly used to relieve mild nociceptive or transient pain ▪ If CYP continue to be distressed, reassessment and further titration using different drugs is warranted
Tramadol	▪ Dual mu-opioid agonist and noradrenaline/serotonin reuptake inhibitory activity makes tramadol a useful agent in this setting (Friedrichsdorf 2019) ▪ There have been warnings of adverse events (including death) related to its pharmacokinetic properties, curtailing use among children younger than 12 years of age (Food and Drug Administration 2017; Jin 2017; Fortenberry et al. 2019) ▪ Concurrent use with drugs that inhibit CYP3D4 and CYP2D6 such as, respectively, macrolides (e.g. clarithromycin) and antidepressants (e.g. fluoxetine, involved in tramadol metabolism) can exacerbate pre-existing seizures ▪ Combinations with drugs also associated with the serotonergic syndrome is an inherent but small risk (Hassamal et al. 2018)
Opioids	▪ Owing to differential pain mechanisms in CYP with SNI, opioids are not commonly used as first-line treatment ▪ Prescribed for acute nociceptive pain of moderate to severe intensity, breakthrough pain in CYP with recurrent or persistent pain already on baseline medications, or as adjunct management in 'autonomic storms' (see section on clonidine below) ▪ Methadone is an exception. Other than action at the mu-opioid receptor, it has antagonistic effects at the NMDA receptor associated with generation of excitatory nerve impulses in the CNS, wind-up phenomena in chronic pain, and hyperalgesia (Madden et al. 2018). Biphasic elimination characteristics, long half-life with long-term use, and significant drug–drug interactions with commonly used medications in children with SNI (antiepileptics and antibiotics in particular) mandate knowledge and experience for effective outcomes and safe application (Friedrichsdorf and Postier 2019) ▪ All opioids share similar adverse effects, respiratory depression being the most serious. Evaluation of ventilation thresholds (e.g. in hypotonia, obstructive sleep apnoea) and avoiding concurrent sedatives at initiation or escalation of opioids are recommended (Hauer and Houtrow 2017)
Gabapentinoids	▪ Gabapentin and pregabalin commonly used ▪ Evidence mainly from the adult setting (Dworkin et al. 2010; Finnerup et al. 2015) ▪ In CYP used widely (out-of-label) in neuropathic pain of both peripheral and central types, visceral hyperalgesia, autonomic dysfunction and difficult spasticity (Liow et al. 2016; Hauer and Houtrow 2017; Sacha et al. 2017) ▪ Pregabalin has a better pharmacokinetic profile with no flattening of bioavailability at higher doses (Snaman et al., 2016), but not proven in controlled studies to be superior to gabapentin in efficacy (Collins et al. 2019) ▪ Both have similar adverse effects, need dose adjustments in renal insufficiency, and share the advantage of minimal drug interactions (Asaro et al., 2017) ▪ Studies indicate children <5 years of age may need doses up to 30% higher (Haig et al. 2001) with maximal daily doses of 72 mg/kg reported (Friedrichsdorf and Goubert 2020)

Table 14.12 (Continued)

Drug type	Uses and adverse effects
Tricyclic antidepressants	■ Amitriptyline and nortriptyline are common agents studied and used in children for various indications, including management of neuropathic pain (Friedrichsdorf and Postier 2019) ■ There is inhibition of presynaptic reuptake of noradrenaline and serotonin, enhancing descending inhibitory signals acting at the dorsal horn in the spinal cord, where pain afferents feed from the periphery (Moore et al. 2012) ■ Both have anticholinergic properties (as a secondary amine, nortriptyline less so) resulting in sedation, dry mouth, postural hypertension, constipation and urinary retention ■ Amitriptyline (a tertiary amine) used advantageously for some of these properties to improve sleep and reduce secretions (Siden 2018) ■ Other minor risk factors as a class include potential for cardiac dysrhythmia and serotonergic syndrome
Clonidine	■ As an α_2-agonist, clonidine is commonly used in the management of symptomatic spasticity and autonomic dysfunction including medical crises such as 'autonomic storms' (Rasmussen and Grégoire 2015) ■ Ability to inhibit substance P release suggests intrinsic analgesic action (Hauer 2012) ■ Also reported to reduce perception of pain in gastric and colonic distension (Kuiken et al. 2005) ■ Adverse effects include hypotension and sedation. The latter may be utilised in soothing a distressed child at night, particularly if muscle spasms are troubling ■ Started slowly to minimise adverse effects and tapered gently to prevent rebound hypertension or seizures
Serotonin/noradrenaline reuptake inhibitors (SNRIs)	■ Include venlafaxine and duloxetine in clinical practice ■ Second-line agents for management of neuropathic pain in adults (Dworkin et al. 2010; Finnerup et al. 2015) ■ More evidence in peripheral pain than for central pain ■ Limited studies in CYP
Benzodiazepines	■ Used in the management of spasticity, dystonia and dysautonomia ■ Due to rapid development of tolerance, often administered as needed for acute symptoms (Rasmussen and Grégoire 2015) ■ Metabolised by P450 system in liver, with the exception of lorazepam (conjugation) ■ Clonazepam associated with increased secretions (Hauer and Houtrow 2017). Needs to be used with caution in CYP with oropharyngeal dysphagia at higher risks of aspiration ■ Should not be stopped abruptly after long-term use. Doing so risks rebound and withdrawal

NMDA, *N*-methyl-ᴅ-aspartate.

Table 14.13 The neuro-pain ladder.

Step 1	Gabapentin +/– adjuvant[b] or PRN[c]
Step 2[a]	Nortriptyline, clonidine +/– adjuvant[b] or PRN[c]
Step 3[a]	Methadone +/– adjuvant[b] or PRN[c]

[a] Pain that is unrelieved by a medication in the previous step.
[b] Cyproheptadine.
[c] As needed (includes tramadol, opioid, benzodiazepine).

Table 14.14 Barriers to the use of analgesic drugs in children with SNI.

Medication causing harm	Respiratory depression or shortening life, particularly if opioids are used
Drug addiction	Most commonly associated with opioid prescriptions
Masking new problems	Not seen in real-life practice nor substantiated by evidence
'Giving up' too soon	Particularly when palliative care leads or coordinates overall management
Lack of experience	Range of interventions, including drugs less frequently used in this setting

Source: Hauer and Houtrow (2017).

CASE STUDY: PART 2

Rick continues to be distressed a week later despite treating a new sacral bedsore, clearing impacted stools and changing the feeds to continuous mode using a pump. His mother begins to feel it is too much suffering for Rick to bear and is reminded of what was mentioned in hospital of his poor prognosis. She declines further work-up and just wants him to be comfortable at home, no matter what happens.

1. What might be helpful next?

Psychological Interventions for CYP with Severe Neurological Impairment

The management of pain in CYP with SNI requires input from multiple stakeholders for good outcomes (Siden 2018). This may include neurology, orthopaedics, gastrointestinal, rehabilitation and complex care, for multidisciplinary care planning and integrated multimodal implementation.

Given the neurocognitive disabilities associated with SNI in this group, psychological interventions proposed before for CYP suffering from cancer may not apply or be as effective. Psychological interventions in this instance are mainly directed at caregivers, who can be at the end of their tether. Helpful strategies include, disease-specific support groups for resource and relational support (Munkombwe et al. 2020) and, short-term respite, such as care sitters or hospice stays to access much-needed breaks from the often 24/7 routine care of the CYP with SNI (WHO 2018a; Benini et al. 2017).

Physical Interventions for CYP with Severe Neurological Impairment

Triggers that elicit or exacerbate pain should be minimised, for example by venting gastrostomy tubes or clearing bowels if gut distension is an issue (Harrop et al. 2017).

A range of strategies and aids are listed below, as a comprehensive and in-depth discussion is not possible here (Hauer 2010; Thrane et al. 2017; Congedi et al. 2018; Freundlich and Hall 2018; Warlow and Hain 2018).

1. Tight swaddling, cuddling, rocking, repositioning and massage.
2. Supportive pillows and customised seating systems.
3. Warm baths and weighted blankets.
4. Complementary therapies, e.g. essential oils, Reiki, acupressure and acupuncture.
5. Vibratory stimulation using special mats or devices, and transcutaneous electrical nerve stimulation (TENS).

Most of these interventions lack evidence, but all have minimal adverse effects.

Two case illustrations are provided, highlighting where physical interventions have been most helpful to CYP with SNI as well as their caregivers.

CASE ILLUSTRATIONS

Joanne

Three-year-old Joanne has an unnamed genetic syndrome associated with multiple congenital anomalies. Her condition is complicated by oropharyngeal dysphagia (fundoplication performed and gastrostomy inserted) and intermittent gastro-motility issues. The latter necessitates careful titration of her continuous feeding schedule to minimise bloated tummy and concomitant distress, manifesting with poor sleep and night cries with dystonic posturing.

Over the past year, together with the palliative care team that visited her at home, her mum managed to discover a set of standard manoeuvres to assuage the fractious girl: rocking her calmly and gently on her lap, venting air through the gastrostomy button, and triggering a bowel movement (and passing of flatus) by inserting a saline enema.

Kok Wei

Kok Wei has X-linked adrenoleukodystrophy, diagnosed when he was seven. He is now 15 years old, non-verbal and totally dependent on caregivers for all activities of daily living. In the last two years, he continued to lose weight despite adequate enteral feeding and he gradually stopped smiling. He spent most of the day sleeping. These signs of disease progression hurt his parents so much. They knew what it meant and what lay ahead.

After recovering from a chest infection the week before, he began to moan audibly and make grunting sounds frequently. Apart from cold and dusky extremities, no apparent triggers were found on careful physical assessment. The hospice nurse suggested layering downy pillows to support his cachexic frame on the hospital bed at home. She also taught his mum to administer gentle massages to a few pressure points using a blend of lavender and frankincense aroma oils. These measures thankfully proved most effective in comforting him. He died a week later in his sleep.

When All Else Fails, and Symptoms Persistently Distress CYP with SNI and Their Caregivers

- Chronic pain in children with SNI cannot always be eliminated.
- Reasons for persistent distress cannot always be identified despite extensive investigations.
- Interventions targeting underlying causes may not produce anticipated outcomes.
- Approaches such as empirical therapeutic trials, advice from other specialists and trigger minimisation may still fail.
- Even with early success, distressing pain can prove intractable.
- Medications only *modify* symptoms (e.g. heal pain behaviours) by altering the balance between excitatory and inhibitory signals within the CNS (Hauer and Houtrow 2017).
- There is diminishing benefit over time, even in non-progressive conditions like cerebral palsy; further, increasing adverse effects are observed with decreasing pain relief with escalation of pharmacological therapy.
- Commonest (and most ominous) among adverse effects is sedation. This signals a stage when goals of care need to be reviewed through advance care planning (Hauer and Wolfe 2014). Limits to life-sustaining therapy during a crisis may need clarification, including making directives or orders ahead to allow natural death.

Ethical Considerations in Paediatric Palliative Care

From the time a CYP is first diagnosed with a life-shortening condition, parents and clinicians strive to promote well-being, reduce suffering and defer death. Decisions related to medical interventions and treatment options often involve deeply held values about disability, life and death. It is at this time conflicts can arise. As the underlying disease progresses, intense emotions surrounding end-of-life care further add to prevailing tension. An ethics consult service identified quality of life, decision-making (including withholding or withdrawing life-prolonging procedures) and end-of-life issues as the top three reasons for referrals (Leland et al. 2020). Ethical concepts relevant to paediatric practice are shared in the practice point below to guide clinicians in navigating practice conundrums that may be encountered.

PRACTICE POINT

- The therapeutic relationship between patient and provider is triadic rather than dyadic, as within paediatric practice this also involves parents; a child is presumed to lack decision-making capacity while parents are presumed to be surrogates (within limits, since the state can intervene as *parens patriae* when parental actions fall below the *threshold of 'harm'*) (Ross 2015).
- The best interest standard (BIS) is established in medical ethics and law as a *guiding and limiting standard* for parental autonomy or authority in caring for the CYP (Bester 2018); parents are expected to do their best for the child *all things considered* to minimally fulfil basic needs, appreciating that these may be culturally and contextually dependent.

- The United Nations Convention on the Rights of the Child (UNCRC) with its three Ps (protection, provision and participation) provides general guidance (UN General Assembly 1989), while the Trieste Charter (Benini et al. 2017) proposes specific actions encompassing dignified care of the dying CYP in relation to BIS.
- The shared-decision model (SDM) is the other major consideration, utilised when approaching ethical dilemmas within PPC; depending on individual circumstances, it spans the spectrum between patient/parent-led (informed-choice) and expert-led (paternalistic) models when making difficult medical decisions (Streuli et al. 2021).
- Some clinical ethicists have found the concept of zone of parental discretion (ZPD) practical in reconciling confusion and conflicts around BIS during SDM; it sets up a process to define the threshold of harm in individual cases, yet preserves the moral weight of parents as decision-makers for the CYP who is seriously ill (Gillam 2016).
- Caveats exist in neonatology and in particular perinatal practice. In the former, surrogate or parental autonomy often takes precedence, and in the latter the mother's BIS are prioritised alongside those of the fetus when serious medical decisions are made (Dan 2018; Marty and Carter 2018).

Symptom Management to Optimise Comfort at the End of Life

Whether suffering from advanced incurable cancer or SNI, a CYP facing imminent death is anticipated to confront similar issues. With the ultimate goal of minimising distress in the dying CYP, principles of management are uniform across different ages and disease heterogeneity. That said, from the beginning and throughout the uncertain and unsettling journey of dying, timely recognition of the dying phase and sensitive communication with loved ones remain cornerstones of good end-of-life care (Villanueva et al. 2016).

Table 14.15 lists six non-pain symptoms commonly encountered at this final stage of illness trajectory, and their potential management (pharmacological, psychological and physical). To qualify, substantive evidence is weak in this instance. Readers can refer to drug dosage guides in other chapters or related external resources (Together for Short Lives 2017). Given the expected loss of swallow and the fact CYP may not always have feeding tubes in place, parenteral (e.g. subcutaneous injections) and other novel routes of drug administration might have to be considered (Drolet et al. 2016; Sutherland et al. 2020).

Understandably, the parents and wider family will be distraught at this time. It is imperative that the care team continues to rally around the family with prompt and honest updates throughout, while concurrently attending to their instrumental, emotional and spiritual needs towards delivering a good death (Chong et al. 2021).

Table 14.15 Management of common physical symptoms at the end of life.

Symptom	Management (pharmacological, psychological, physical)
Breathlessness	▪ Opioids, benzodiazepines (add-on) ▪ Visual imagery, hypnosis, calm and reassuring accompaniment ▪ Oxygen supplementation, pursed lip breathing, prop up in bed if appropriate, fan blowing on the face, create cool or well-ventilated environment
Secretions	▪ Hyoscine, glycopyrrolate, atropine drops ▪ Reassurance, explanation ▪ Restrict or stop hydration, repositioning, gentle suction
Terminal agitation	▪ Neuroleptics (e.g. haloperidol or olanzapine) and/or benzodiazepines (e.g. midazolam or lorazepam) ▪ Reassurance, explanation ▪ Create calm and quiet environment, minimise uncomfortable procedures and invasive stimulation, swaddling and non-nutritive sucking (in neonates)
Fever	▪ Paracetamol, NSAIDs, steroids, clonidine or propranolol (if sympathetic storms suspected) ▪ Discuss if work-up and antibiotics still appropriate, reassurance ▪ Tepid sponging, create cool or well-ventilated environment, manage diaphoresis and frequent change of clothes
Bleeding	▪ Vitamin K, crushed tranexamic acid tablets or adrenaline (1 in 1000) for direct pressure on bleeding point, parenteral midazolam for sedation (if bleeding catastrophic) ▪ Anticipate and pre-empt caregivers ▪ Platelet or blood transfusions, Gelfoam in mucosal bleeds (where appropriate), dark towels to cover and clear, pressure packing of bleeding orifices, therapeutic presence
Seizures	▪ Midazolam (buccal or parenteral), diazepam (rectal), CSCI midazolam and/or phenobarbitone ▪ Anticipate and pre-empt caregivers, seizure management plan ▪ Safe location, appropriate positioning when fits occur, oxygen supplementation (if available)

CSCI, continuous subcutaneous infusion.
Sources: Together for Short Lives (2017); Aidoo and Rajapakse (2018); Cortezzo and Meyer (2020).

Summary

▪ Paediatric palliative care is the specialised care of CYP with life-shortening illness.
▪ With a family-centred focus and expertise across different domains, a customised and multimodal approach to management of pain is provided.
▪ Whether in advanced cancer or severe neurological impairment, principles of care are similar: impeccable and holistic assessment, careful treatment planning targeted at the cause (if possible) and regular reviews after commencement of therapy.
▪ Both pharmacological and non-pharmacological interventions are utilised and, in the latter this includes psychological and physical strategies.
▪ Common ethical challenges in the context of palliative care and approaches to their resolution are shared.
▪ At the end of life, more than just preventing or relieving pain, ensuring overall

comfort and delivering a good death become critical. A brief management guide of common physical symptoms is provided.

- Even when all possible treatments fail, palliative care continues to journey alongside, offering children and families expert and compassionate guidance without fail.

Key to Case Study

Part 1

1. In this instance, suggestions include verifying method (e.g. positioning) and speed of feeding, to exclude constipation, assessment of aspirate volumes (including their nature) and associated abdominal bloatedness, colic or vomiting.

Part 2

1. It is beginning to become clear to the mother that Rick is near the end of his disease trajectory. And she has made the decision that comfort and quality of life or 'more good days' should be the overarching therapeutic goal. Pre-ordered breakthrough medication for managing pain or discomfort may be given more regularly. Changing the route of drug administration (rectal, transmucosal or subcutaneous injection) is a consideration given questionable drug bioavailability from progressive enteral dysfunction. Anticipated end-of-life symptoms like terminal secretions or worsening seizures warrant pre-emptive guidance. Despite her early insight and acceptance, Rick's mother will need psychological support throughout this period from supporting providers like the palliative care team.

Multiple Choice Questions

1. Which of the following is not a way in which paediatric palliative care differs from adult palliative care?
    a. Predominance of non-cancer conditions
    b. Short prognoses generally
    c. Concurrent need to consider developmental needs of the young patient
    d. Higher risks of complicated grief in caregiver bereavement
2. What should be considered when using opioids to manage pain in CYP with serious illness?
    a. Risk or level of adverse effects
    b. Choice of the young person
    c. Comorbidities
    d. All of the above
3. Which of the following is not an example of a psychological intervention for pain in CYP?
    a. Distraction
    b. Breathing
    c. Hypnosis
    d. Non-nutritive sucking
4. Which of the tools below is suitable for the assessment of pain in the CYP with severe neurological impairment?
    a. Numerical rating scale
    b. r-FLACC
    c. Wong–Baker FACES Pain Rating Scale
    d. Visual Analogue Scale
5. Which of the following are examples of strategies to manage pain in the CYP with severe neurological impairment?
    a. Setting the right expectations
    b. Use of drugs like gabapentin
    c. Empirical trials of therapeutic interventions
    d. All of the above

References

Abarshi, E., Rietjens, J., Robijn, L., et al. (2017) International variations in clinical practice guidelines for palliative sedation: a systematic review. *BMJ Supportive and Palliative Care* 7, 223–229.

Afsharimani, B., Kindl, K., Good, P. and Hardy, J. (2015) Pharmacological options for the management of refractory cancer pain: what is the evidence? *Supportive Care in Cancer* 23, 1473–1481.

Aidoo, E. and Rajapakse, D. (2018) End of life care for infants, children and young people with life-limiting conditions: planning and management: the NICE guideline 2016. *Archives of Disease in Childhood. Education and Practice Edition* 103(6), 296–299.

Arias-Casais, N., Garralda, E., Pons, J.J., et al. (2020) Mapping pediatric palliative care development in the WHO-European region: children living in low-to-middle-income countries are less likely to access it. *Journal of Pain and Symptom Management* 60, 746–753.

Asaro, J., Robinson, C.A. and Levy, P.T. (2017) Visceral hyperalgesia: when to consider gabapentin use in neonates. Case study and review. *Child Neurology Open* 4, 2329048X17693123.

Beecham, E., Candy, B., Howard, R., et al. (2015) Pharmacological interventions for pain in children and adolescents with life-limiting conditions. *Cochrane Database of Systematic Reviews* (3), CD010750.

Benini, F., Vecchi, R., Lazzarin, P., et al. (2017) The rights of the dying child and the duties of healthcare providers: the 'Trieste Charter'. *Tumori Journal* 103, 33–39.

Benini, F., Pappadatou, D., Bernadá, M., et al. (2022) International standards for pediatric palliative care: from IMPaCCT to GO-PPaCS. *Journal of Pain and Symptom Management* 63(5), e529–e543.

Berde, C., Koka, A. and Donado-Rincon, C. (2016) Lidocaine infusions and other options for opioid-resistant pain due to pediatric advanced cancer. *Pediatric Blood and Cancer* 63(7), 1141–1143.

Berger, A.S. and Goldschneider, K.R. (2019) The role of neuraxial opioids in pediatric practice. *Clinical Journal of Pain* 35(6), 497–500.

Bester, J.C. (2018) The harm principle cannot replace the best interest standard: problems with using the harm principle for medical decision making for children. *American Journal of Bioethics* 18, 9–19.

Brands, M.M., Güngör, D., van den Hout, J.M., et al. (2015) Pain: a prevalent feature in patients with mucopolysaccharidosis. Results of a cross-sectional national survey. *Journal of Inherited Metabolic Disease* 38, 323–331.

Burns, J., Jackson, K., Sheehy, K.A., Finkel, J.C. and Quezado, Z.M. (2017) The use of dexmedetomidine in pediatric palliative care: a preliminary study. *Journal of Palliative Medicine* 20, 779–783.

Carter, B. (2020) Communicating pain: the challenge of pain assessment in children with profound cognitive impairment. *Comprehensive Child and Adolescent Nursing* 43, 10–14.

Carter, B., Simons, J., Bray, L. and Arnott, J. (2016) Navigating uncertainty: health professionals' knowledge, skill, and confidence in assessing and managing pain in children with profound cognitive impairment. *Pain Research and Management* 2016, 8617182.

Carter, B., Arnott, J., Simons, J. and Bray, L. (2017) Developing a sense of knowing and acquiring the skills to manage pain in children with profound cognitive impairments: mothers' perspectives. *Pain Research and Management* 2017, 2514920.

Carter, B.S. and Brunkhorst, J. (2017) Neonatal pain management. *Seminars in Perinatology* 41(2), 111–116.

Cascella, M., Bimonte, S., Saettini, F. and Muzio, M.R. (2019) The challenge of pain assessment in children with cognitive disabilities: features and clinical applicability of different observational tools. *Journal of Paediatrics and Child Health* 55, 129–135.

Chambers, L. (2018) *A Guide to Children's Palliative Care*, 4th edn. Together for Short Lives, Bristol.

Chong, P.H. and Yeo, Z.Z. (2021) Parenteral lidocaine for complex cancer pain in the home or inpatient hospice setting: a review and synthesis of the evidence. *Journal of Palliative Medicine* 24, 1154–1160.

Chong, P.H., Walshe, C. and Hughes, S. (2021) A good death in the child with life shortening illness: a qualitative multiple-case study. *Palliative Medicine* 35, 1878–1888.

Collins, A., Mannion, R., Broderick, A., Hussey, S., Devins, M. and Bourke, B. (2019) Gabapentin for the treatment of pain manifestations in children with severe neurological impairment: a single-centre retrospective review. *BMJ Paediatrics Open* 3(1), e000467.

Congedi, S., Orzalesi, M., Di Pede, C. and Benini, F. (2018) Pain in mucopolysaccharidoses: analysis of the problem and possible treatments. *International Journal of Molecular Sciences* 19, 3063.

Connor, S.R., Downing, J. and Marston, J. (2017) Estimating the global need for palliative care for children: a cross-sectional analysis. *Journal of Pain and Symptom Management* 53, 171–177.

Cortezzo, D.E. and Meyer, M. (2020) Neonatal end-of-life symptom management. *Frontiers in Pediatrics* 8, 574121.

Coughtrey, A., Millington, A., Bennett, S., et al. (2018) The effectiveness of psychosocial interventions for psychological outcomes in pediatric oncology: a systematic review. *Journal of Pain and Symptom Management* 55(3), 1004–1017.

Courade, M., Bertrand, A., Guerrini-Rousseau, L., et al. (2022) Low-dose ketamine adjuvant treatment for refractory pain in children, adolescents and young adults with cancer: a pilot study. *BMJ Supportive and Palliative Care* 12(e5), e656–e663.

Dalberg, T., McNinch, N.L. and Friebert, S. (2018) Perceptions of barriers and facilitators to early integration of pediatric palliative care: a national survey of pediatric oncology providers. *Pediatric Blood and Cancer* 65, e26996.

Dan, B. (2018) The child's best interest: ethical guide or ideology? *Developmental Medicine and Child Neurology* 60(1), 4.

Downing, J., Jassal, S.S., Mathews, L., BRITS, H. and Friedrichsdorf, S.J. (2015) Pediatric pain management in palliative care. *Pain Management* 5, 23–35.

Downing, J., Powell, R.A., Marston, J., et al. (2016) Children's palliative care in low-and middle-income countries. *Archives of Disease in Childhood* 101, 85–90.

Drolet, C., Roy, H., Laflamme, J. and Marcotte, M.-E. (2016) Feasibility of a comfort care protocol using oral transmucosal medication delivery in a palliative neonatal population. *Journal of Palliative Medicine* 19, 442–450.

Dworkin, R.H., O'Connor, A.B., Audette, J., et al. (2010) Recommendations for the pharmacological management of neuropathic pain: an overview and literature update. *Mayo Clinic Proceedings* 85(3 Suppl.), S3–S14.

Fallon, M.T., Wilcock, A., Kelly, C.A., et al. (2018) Oral ketamine vs placebo in patients with cancer-related neuropathic pain: a randomized clinical trial. *JAMA Oncology* 4(6), 870–872.

Feudtner, C. and Nathanson, P.G. (2014) Pediatric palliative care and pediatric medical ethics: opportunities and challenges. *Pediatrics* 133(Suppl. 1), S1–S7.

Fink, R.M. and Gallagher, E. (2019) Cancer pain assessment and measurement. *Seminars in Oncology Nursing* 35(3), 229–234.

Finnerup, N.B., Attal, N., Haroutounian, S., et al. (2015) Pharmacotherapy for neuropathic pain in adults: a systematic review and meta-analysis. *Lancet Neurology* 14(2), 162–173.

Fisher, E., Law, E., Dudeney, J., Palermo, T.M., Stewart, G. and Eccleston, C. (2018) Psychological therapies for the management of chronic and recurrent pain in children and adolescents. *Cochrane Database of Systematic Reviews* (9), CD003968.

Fisher, E., Villanueva, G., Henschke, N., et al. (2022) Efficacy and safety of pharmacological, physical, and psychological interventions for the management of chronic pain in children: a WHO systematic review and meta-analysis. *Pain* 163, e1–e19.

Food and Drug Administration (2017) FDA restricts use of prescription codeine pain and cough medicines and tramadol pain medicines in children. https://www.fda.gov/media/104268/download

Fortenberry, M., Crowder, J. and So, T.-Y. (2019) The use of codeine and tramadol in the pediatric population: what is the verdict now? *Journal of Pediatric Health Care* 33(1), 117–123.

Fraser, L.K., Bluebond-Langner, M. and Ling, J. (2020) Advances and challenges in European paediatric palliative care. *Medical Sciences* 8, 20.

Freundlich, K.L. and Hall, D.E. (2018) Managing the medically complex, neurologically impaired child in the inpatient setting. *Current Treatment Options in Pediatrics* 4, 300–318.

Friebert, S. and Williams, C. (2015) *Facts and Figures. Pediatric Palliative and Hospice Care in America.* National Hospice and Palliative Care Organization.

Friedrichsdorf, S. (2017) Contemporary pediatric palliative care: myths and barriers to integration into clinical care. *Current Pediatric Reviews* 13, 8–12.

Friedrichsdorf, S.J. and Bruera, E. (2018) Delivering pediatric palliative care: from denial, palliphobia, pallilalia to palliactive. *Children* 5(9), 120.

Friedrichsdorf, S.J. and Goubert, L. (2020) Pediatric pain treatment and prevention for hospitalized children. *Pain Reports* 5(1), e804.

Friedrichsdorf, S.J. and Postier, A.C. (2019) Recent advances in pain treatment for children with serious illness. *Pain Management* 9, 583–596.

Friedrichsdorf, S.J., Postier, A., Eull, D., et al. (2015) Pain outcomes in a US children's hospital: a prospective cross-sectional survey. *Hospital Pediatrics* 5, 18–26.

Friedrichsdorf, S.J., Postier, A.C., Andrews, G.S., Hamre, K.E., Steele, R. and Siden, H. (2017) Pain reporting and analgesia management in 270 children with a progressive neurologic, metabolic or chromosomally based condition with impairment of the central nervous system: cross-sectional, baseline results from an observational, longitudinal study. *Journal of Pain Research* 10, 1841–1852.

Gibbons, K., DeMonbrun, A., Beckman, E.J., et al. (2016) Continuous lidocaine infusions to manage opioid-refractory pain in a series of cancer patients in a pediatric hospital. *Pediatric Blood and Cancer* 63(7), 1168–1174.

Gillam, L. (2016) The zone of parental discretion: an ethical tool for dealing with disagreement between parents and doctors about medical treatment for a child. *Clinical Ethics* 11, 1–8.

Greenfield, K., Carter, B., Harrop, E., et al. (2022) Healthcare professionals' experiences of the barriers and facilitators to pediatric pain management in the community at end-of-life: a qualitative interview study. *Journal of Pain and Symptom Management* 63, 98–105.

Gurschick, L., Mayer, D.K. and Hanson, L.C. (2015) Palliative sedation: an analysis of international guidelines and position statements. *American Journal of Hospice and Palliative Medicine* 32, 660–671.

Haig, G.M., Bockbrader, H.N., Wesche, D.L., et al. (2001) Single-dose gabapentin pharmacokinetics and safety in healthy infants and children. *Journal of Clinical Pharmacology* 41(5), 507–514.

Harrop, E. and Edwards, C. (2013) How and when to refer a child for specialist paediatric palliative care. *Archives of Disease in Childhood* 98, 202–208.

Harrop, E.J., Brombley, K. and Boyce, K. (2017) Fifteen minute consultation: practical pain management in paediatric palliative care. *Archives of Disease in Childhood. Education and Practice Edition* 102, 239–243.

Hassamal, S., Miotto, K., Dale, W. and Danovitch, I. (2018) Tramadol: understanding the risk of serotonin syndrome and seizures. *American Journal of Medicine* 131(11), 1382.e1–1382.e6.

Hauer, J.M. (2010) Identifying and managing sources of pain and distress in children with neurological impairment. *Pediatric Annals* 39, 198–205.

Hauer, J.M. (2012) Improving comfort in children with severe neurological impairment. *Progress in Palliative Care* 20, 349–356.

Hauer, J.M. (2018) Feeding intolerance in children with severe impairment of the central nervous system: strategies for treatment and prevention. *Children* 5(1), 1.

Hauer, J.M. and Houtrow, A.J. (2017) Pain assessment and treatment in children with significant impairment of the central nervous system. *Pediatrics* 139, e20171002.

Hauer, J.M. and Solodiuk, J.C. (2015) Gabapentin for management of recurrent pain in 22 nonverbal children with severe neurological impairment: a retrospective analysis. *Journal of Palliative Medicine* 18, 453–456.

Hauer, J.M. and Wolfe, J. (2014) Supportive and palliative care of children with metabolic and neurological diseases. *Current Opinion in Supportive and Palliative Care* 8, 296–302.

Henderson, C.M., Fitzgerald, M., Hoehn, K.S. and Weidner, N. (2017) Pediatrician ambiguity in understanding palliative sedation at the end of life. *American Journal of Hospice and Palliative Medicine* 34, 5–19.

Henderson, E.M., Rajapakse, D., Kelly, P., Boggs, T. and Bluebond-Langner, M. (2019) Patient-controlled analgesia for children with life-limiting conditions in the community: results of a prospective observational study. *Journal of Pain and Symptom Management* 57, e1–e4.

Herr, K., Coyne, P. J., McCaffery, M., Manworren, R. and Merkel, S. (2011) Pain assessment in the patient unable to self-report: position statement with clinical practice recommendations. *Pain Management Nursing* 12, 230–250.

Horridge, K.A., Harvey, C., McGarry, K., et al. (2016) Quantifying multifaceted needs captured at the point of care. Development of a Disabilities Terminology Set and Disabilities Complexity Scale. *Developmental Medicine and Child Neurology* 58, 570–580.

Iddon, J.E., Dickson, J.M. and Unwin, J. (2016) Positive psychological interventions and chronic non-cancer pain: a systematic review of the literature. *International Journal of Applied Positive Psychology* 1, 133–157.

Jibb, L.A., Nathan, P.C., Stevens, B.J., et al. (2015) Psychological and physical interventions for the management of cancer-related pain in pediatric and young adult patients: an integrative review. *Oncology Nursing Forum* 42(6), E339–E357.

Jin, J. (2017) Risks of codeine and tramadol in children. *JAMA* 318(15), 1514.

Jonkman, K., van de Donk, T. and Dahan, A. (2017) Ketamine for cancer pain: what is the evidence? *Current Opinion in Supportive and Palliative Care* 11(2), 88–92.

Knaul, F.M., Farmer, P.E., Krakauer, E.L., et al. (2018) Alleviating the access abyss in palliative care and pain relief: an imperative of universal health coverage. The Lancet Commission report. *Lancet* 391, 1391–1454.

Knaul, F., Radbruch, L., Connor, S., et al. (2020) How many adults and children are in need of palliative care worldwide. In *Global Atlas of Palliative Care*, 2nd edn (ed. S.R. Connor), pp. 17–32. Worldwide Hospice and Palliative Care Alliance (WHPCA) and World Health Organization, London.

Komatz, K. and Carter, B. (2015) Pain and symptom management in pediatric palliative care. *Pediatrics in Review* 36(12), 527–534.

Kuiken, S.D., Tytgat, G.N. and Boeckxstaens, G.E. (2005) Drugs interfering with visceral sensitivity for the treatment of functional gastrointestinal disorders: the clinical evidence. *Alimentary Pharmacology and Therapeutics* 21(6), 633–651.

Kuttner, L. (2010) *A Child in Pain: What Health Professionals Can Do to Help.* Crown House Publishing, Bethel, CT.

Lathrop, E.B. (2016) Pain assessment and management in pediatric oncology patients. Thesis, University of Arizona, Tuscon.

Leland, B.D., Wocial, L.D., Drury, K., Rowan, C.M., Helft, P.R. and Torke, A.M. (2020) Development and retrospective review of a pediatric ethics consultation service at a large academic center. *HEC Forum*, 32(3), 269–281.

Le-Short, Ch., Katragadda, K., Nagda, N., Farris, D. and Halphen Gelter, M. (2022) Interventional pain management for the pediatric cancer patient: a literature review. *Children* 9(3), 389.

Liow, N.Y.-K., Gimeno, H., Lumsden, D.E., et al. (2016) Gabapentin can significantly improve dystonia severity and quality of life in children. *European Journal of Paediatric Neurology* 20(1), 100–107.

Løhre, E.T., Thronæs, M. and Klepstad, P. (2020) Breakthrough cancer pain in 2020. *Current Opinion in Supportive and Palliative Care* 14(2), 94–99.

Madden, K., Mills, S., Dibaj, S., Williams, J.L., Liu, D. and Bruera, E. (2018) Methadone as the initial long-acting opioid in children with advanced cancer. *Journal of Palliative Medicine* 21(9), 1317–1321.

Maeda, S., Kato, I., Umeda, K., et al. (2020) Continuous deep sedation at the end of life in children with cancer: experience at a single center in Japan. *Pediatric Hematology and Oncology* 37, 365–374.

Magee, D.J., Schutzer-Weissmann, J., Pereira, E.A.C. and Brown, M.R.D. (2021) Neuromodulation techniques for cancer pain management. *Current Opinion in Supportive and Palliative Care* 15(2), 77–83.

Markozannes, G., Aretouli, E., Rintou, E., et al. (2017) An umbrella review of the literature on the effectiveness of psychological interventions for pain reduction. *BMC Psychology* 5(1), 31.

Marty, C.M. and Carter, B.S. (2018) Ethics and palliative care in the perinatal world. *Seminars in Fetal and Neonatal Medicine* 23(1), 35–38.

Miele, E., Mastronuzzi, A., Cefalo, M.G., et al. (2019) Propofol-based palliative sedation in terminally ill children with solid tumors: a case series. *Medicine* 98(21), e15615.

Moore, R.A., Derry, S., Aldington, D., Cole, P. and Wiffen, P.J. (2012) Amitriptyline for neuropathic pain and fibromyalgia in adults. *Cochrane Database of Systematic Reviews* (12), CD008242.

Munkombwe, W.M., Petersson, K. and Elgán, C. (2020) Nurses' experiences of providing nonpharmacological pain management in palliative care: a qualitative study. *Journal of Clinical Nursing* 29, 1643–1652.

Neale, K.L. (2012) The fifth vital sign: chronic pain assessment of the adolescent oncology patient. *Journal of Pediatric Oncology Nursing* 29, 185–198.

Nijland, L., Schmidt, P., Frosch, M., et al. (2019) Subcutaneous or intravenous opioid administration by patient-controlled analgesia in cancer pain: a systematic literature review. *Supportive Care in Cancer* 27, 33–42.

O'Connor, N., Graham, D., O'Meara, A., et al. (2013) The use of complementary and alternative medicine by Irish pediatric cancer patients. *Journal of Pediatric Hematology/Oncology* 35, 537–542.

Osterman, M.J., Kochanek, K.D., MacDorman, M.F., Strobino, D.M. and Guyer, B. (2015) Annual summary of vital statistics: 2012–2013. *Pediatrics* 135, 1115–1125.

Rapoport, A. and Morrison, W. (2016) No child is an island: ethical considerations in end-of-life care for children and their families. *Current Opinion in Supportive and Palliative Care* 10, 196–200.

Rasmussen, L.A. and Grégoire, M.-C. (2015) Challenging neurological symptoms in paediatric palliative care: an approach to symptom evaluation and management in children with neurological impairment. *Paediatrics and Child Health* 20(3), 159–165.

Ross, L.F. (2015) Theory and practice of pediatric bioethics. *Perspectives in Biology and Medicine* 58, 267–280.

Sacha, G.L., Foreman, M.G., Kyllonen, K. and Rodriguez, R.J. (2017) The use of gabapentin for pain and agitation in neonates and infants in a neonatal ICU. *Journal of Pediatric Pharmacology and Therapeutics* 22(3), 207–211.

Sheehy, K.A., Lippold, C., Rice, A.L., Nobrega, R., Finkel, J.C. and Quezado, Z.M.N. (2017) Subanesthetic ketamine for pain management in hospitalized children, adolescents, and young adults: a single-center cohort study. *Journal of Pain Research* 10, 787–795.

Siden, H. (2018) Pediatric palliative care for children with progressive non-malignant diseases. *Children* 5, 28.

Sisk, B.A., Feudtner, C., Bluebond-Langner, M., Sourkes, B., Hinds, P.S. and Wolfe, J. (2020) Response to suffering of the seriously ill child: a history of palliative care for children. *Pediatrics* 145, e20191741.

Snaman, J.M., Baker, J.N., Ehrentraut, J.H. and Anghelescu, D.L. (2016) Pediatric oncology: managing pain at the end of life. *Pediatric Drugs* 18, 161–180.

Snaman, J., Morris, S.E., Rosenberg, A.R., Holder, R., Baker, J. and Wolfe, J. (2020) Reconsidering early parental grief following the death of a child from cancer: a new framework for future research and bereavement support. *Supportive Care in Cancer* 28, 4131–4139.

Stallard, P., Williams, L., Velleman, R., Lenton, S. and McGrath, P.J. (2002) Brief report: behaviors identified by caregivers to detect pain in noncommunicating children. *Journal of Pediatric Psychology* 27, 209–214.

Steele, R., Siden, H., Cadell, S., et al. (2014) Charting the territory: symptoms and functional assessment in children with progressive, non-curable conditions. *Archives of Disease in Childhood* 99, 754–762.

Streuli, J.C., Anderson, J., Alef-Defoe, S., et al. (2021) Combining the best interest standard with shared decision-making in paediatrics: introducing the shared optimum approach based on a qualitative study. *European Journal of Pediatrics* 180, 759–766.

Sutherland, A.E., Presland, M., Harrop, E., Carey, M., Miller, M. and Wong, I.C.K.C. (2020) Orodispersible and transmucosal alternative medications for symptom control in adults. *BMJ Supportive and Palliative Care* 12(3), 305–315.

Thomas, R., Phillips, M. and Hamilton, R.J. (2018) Pain management in the pediatric palliative care population. *Journal of Nursing Scholarship* 50, 375–382.

Thrane, S.E., Maurer, S.H., Ren, D., Danford, C.A. and Cohen, S.M. (2017) Reiki therapy for symptom management in children receiving palliative care: a pilot study. *American Journal of Hospice and Palliative Medicine* 34, 373–379.

Together for Short Lives (2017) Basic symptom control in paediatric palliative care. Available at `https://www.togetherforshortlives.org.uk/resource/basic-symptom-control-paediatric-palliative-care/` (accessed 17 April 2022).

Twamley, K., Craig, F., Kelly, P., Hollowell, D.R., Mendoza, P. and Bluebond-Langner, M. (2014) Underlying barriers to referral to paediatric palliative care services: knowledge and attitudes of health care professionals in a paediatric tertiary care centre in the United Kingdom. *Journal of Child Health Care* 18, 19–30.

UN General Assembly (1989) Convention on the Rights of the Child, 20 November, United Nations, Treaty Series, vol. 1577.

van der Geest, I.M., Darlington, A.-S.E., Streng, I.C., Michiels, E.M., Pieters, R. and van den Heuvel-Eibrink, M.M. (2014) Parents' experiences of pediatric palliative care and the impact on long-term parental grief. *Journal of Pain and Symptom Management* 47(6), 1043–1053.

Villanueva, G., Murphy, M.S., Vickers, D., Harrop, E. and Dworzynski, K. (2016) End of life care for infants, children and young people with life limiting conditions: summary of NICE guidance. *BMJ* 355, i6385.

Warlow, T.A. and Hain, R.D. (2018) 'Total Pain' in children with severe neurological impairment. *Children* 5, 13.

Weaver, M.S., Heinze, K.E., Bell, C.J., et al. (2016) Establishing psychosocial palliative care standards for children and adolescents with cancer and their families: an integrative review. *Palliative Medicine* 30, 212–223.

Wechsler, A.M., Álvarez, C.B. and Lloreda, M.J.H. (2014) Effectiveness of psychological interventions intended to promote adjustment of children with cancer and their parents: an overview. *Anales de Psicología* 30, 93–103.

Wiener, L., Tager, J., Mack, J., Battles, H., Bedoya, S.Z. and Gerhardt, C.A. (2020) Helping parents prepare for their child's end of life: a retrospective survey of cancer-bereaved parents. *Pediatric Blood and Cancer* 67, e27993.

Wolfe, J., Orellana, L., Ullrich, C., et al. (2015) Symptoms and distress in children with advanced cancer: prospective patient-reported outcomes from the PediQUEST study. *Journal of Clinical Oncology* 33, 1928.

Wood, H., Dickman, A., Star, A. and Boland, J.W. (2018) Updates in palliative care: overview and recent advancements in the pharmacological management of cancer pain. *Clinical Medicine* 18, 17–22.

World Health Organization (2018a) *Integrating Palliative Care and Symptom Relief into Paediatrics: A WHO Guide for Health Care Planners, Implementers and Managers*. WHO, Geneva.

World Health Organization (2018b) *WHO Guidelines for the Pharmacological and Radiotherapeutic Management of Cancer Pain in Adults and Adolescents*. WHO, Geneva.

World Health Organization (2020) *Guidelines on the Management of Chronic Pain in Children*. WHO, Geneva.

15 Treating and Preventing Pain in Children and Young People in Low- and Middle-Income Countries

Julia Downing, Julia Ambler, and Jennifer Hunt

Pain is a significant problem for children and young people (CYP) living in low- and middle-income countries (LMICs). However, access to pain management services for CYP is intermittent and at times non-existent in many LMICs. While within LMICs there is enormous variation in access to resources, skills and facilities, there are examples which confirm that pain can be effectively managed in CYP in LMICs. These services need to be expanded and others established to ensure good pain management for CYP living in these settings (Downing et al. 2018). Pertinent facts in this context include the following:

- approximately 80% of the world's population live in countries with little or no access to pain management (Goucke and Chaudakshetrin 2018).
- at least 26% of the global population is under 15 years of age, rising to 40% in LMICs in sub-Saharan Africa (SSA) (Population Reference Bureau 2017).
- one-third of children aged 15 or under who died in 2015 (almost 2.5 million) experienced serious health-related suffering

(SHS), including pain, and over 98% of these lived in LMICs (Knaul et al. 2018).
- a gap in need versus provision in Zimbabwe, Kenya and South Africa showed that palliative care and pain management for CYP under 19 years of age was available to less than 5% of those needing it (Connor and Sisimayi 2013).
- many health systems in LMICs have little or no access to information on pain and pain management in CYP.

In summary, too many CYP are living and dying in LMICs with needless pain. Treating and preventing pain in LMICs is crucial.

Managing Pain in CYP in LMICs

Generally, high morbidity and mortality rates due to communicable and non-communicable diseases (NCDs), injuries, violence, poverty, malnutrition and parasitic diseases are prevalent in LMICs. These all contribute to the incidence of pain in CYP. As indicated above, there are wide differences in the management of pain in CYP in LMICs. There are several reasons for these differences.

- Limited access to the range of treatments needed, such as antiretroviral therapy, chemotherapy, radiotherapy and appropriate antibiotics, impact the management of pain in a wide variety of illnesses and conditions. For example, in a significant number of SSA countries there are either no radiotherapy machines or three or less, seriously compromising management of pain through palliative radiotherapy (Zubizarreta et al. 2015).
- Often families will try to manage their child's pain themselves through traditional, herbal and self-prescribed over-the-counter medications. They may seek guidance and recommendations from friends and other non-medical practitioners, only seeking help from health services as a last resort (Friedrichsdorf and Gomez Garcia 2020).
- While the relief of pain is part of the fundamental right to the highest attainable standard of health, this can be difficult to achieve in LMICs where most people live in rural settings and where state investment in the health system is minimal.
- Healthcare is typically delivered by a network of nurse-led clinics, often without access to essential analgesic drugs or doctors.

There is an expectation that pain is inevitable, hard or impossible to manage, and an assumption that CYP, particularly young children, do not experience pain in the same way as adults. CYP's pain is often ignored or even denied, resulting in this being a public health concern of major significance in many LMICs (Downing et al. 2015a).

Recent emphasis on universal health coverage (UHC), which recognises palliative care as an essential healthcare service, has been welcomed (International Children's Palliative Care Network et al. 2018; World Health Organization (WHO) 2019). UHC cannot be achieved without access to palliative care, including pain management, for all age groups (Downing et al. 2020). This adds an ethical imperative to improving access to pain management for CYP, an essential human right.

Challenges to Treating and Preventing Pain in CYP in LMICs

While many of the principles of treating and preventing pain in CYP are the same in all countries, there are great variations in the resources available, such as trained personnel, analgesics and the health systems in which people work. Likewise, the quality of pain management training and implementation by individuals will vary and may be compromised by the lack of investment in health systems in LMICs. The Public Health Strategy for Palliative Care, developed in 2007, identified four key issues that need to be addressed to translate knowledge and skills into evidence-based and cost-effective palliative care interventions (including pain management) that can reach everyone in the population: appropriate policies; adequate availability of medicines; education of policy-makers, health professionals and the public; and the implementation of palliative care services at all levels (Stjernsward et al. 2007). This strategy was revised by the WHO in 2021 to a conceptual model of palliative care development, which includes the original core elements but expands it to include: people with palliative care needs, research, and empowered people and communities (Figure 15.1).

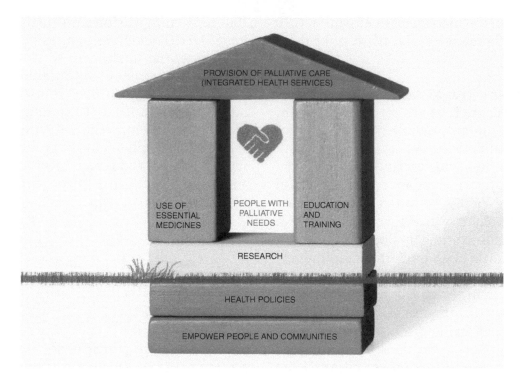

Figure 15.1 The Conceptual Model for Palliative Care Development (WHO 2021 p14. Reproduced with permission).

Empower People and Communities

It is important that CYP, families and communities are empowered in the management of pain. Often they are unaware of the availability of analgesics and that pain can be managed. Education of the public, and empowering families and communities to be more involved in decision-making about health services, their own health and pain management is key, as identified in the Declaration of Astana and the comprehensive approach for primary healthcare (WHO 2018a). An empowered and informed community will not only contribute to the improved management of pain psychologically, spiritually and socially, but will also advocate for access to essential medicines and ensure paediatric formulations are available.

Health Policies

The adoption and promotion by governments of appropriate health policies is essential for an effective healthcare system (Mwangi-Powell et al. 2015) and to ensure that CYP living in LMICs receive adequate pain relief, regardless of diagnosis. However, the following should be noted:

- In many LMICs, pain management, either as a discrete entity or as part of a wider philosophy of care such as palliative care, cancer care or HIV care, is not integrated into national policies.
- While specific policies on pain management at the national level are rare, it is essential that pain management is integrated into national-level policies relating to palliative care, NCDs, HIV, home-based care, hospital

care, maternal and child health, as well as essential medication lists for CYP.

■ As a cross-cutting issue, government policies need to include pain relief in national health plans, and should therefore implement laws and regulations to control the use of opioids and other strong analgesics, while ensuring care provision without restricting prescribing (WHO 2014).

Guidance and policy is also needed at a global level from organisations including the WHO.

■ The development of useful guidelines and policies around managing pain in CYP by the WHO has been a helpful advocacy tool for many LMICs.

■ The WHO guides for healthcare planners, implementers and managers, for children's palliative care (WHO 2018b), responses to humanitarian emergencies and crises (WHO 2018c) and primary healthcare (WHO 2018d) all recognise the importance of pain management in CYP and give guidance within the manuals.

■ Generic pain management and palliative care were included within global and national guidelines for COVID-19 (WHO 2020a).

The withdrawal of the 2012 guidelines on managing persisting pain in children with chronic illnesses (WHO 2012), and those on ensuring balance in the use of opioids (WHO 2011), left the CYP pain community without approved WHO guidelines for these issues. Revised guidelines on the management of chronic pain in children were published at the end of 2020 (WHO 2020b) and work is ongoing to develop supporting documentation, such as best-practice guidelines to inform pain management in CYP in LMICs. It is anticipated that a revision of the guidelines on ensuring balance will be published early in 2024.

Research

Generally, there has been a lack of emphasis on pain management and pain research in CYP (Milani et al 2011; WHO 2020b), particularly in LMICs. Often evidence from studies undertaken with adults and from those in high-income countries (HICs) is extrapolated to CYP in LMICs. In 2011, following the development of the WHO guidelines on managing persisting pain in children, the WHO noted (Milani et al. 2011, p. 1019):

> *There is an urgent need for research on clinical interventions for the relief of persisting pain associated with medical conditions in children.*

The gap in reliable evidence has continued to be identified in the new guidelines, which state (WHO 2020b, p. 22):

> *Importantly, research which addresses these gaps will facilitate evidence-informed guidelines as well as decision-making in Member States and at the local level.*

Research is needed in a wide variety of areas, including clinical studies on paracetamol, non-steroidal anti-inflammatory drugs (NSAIDs) and opioid analgesics, adjuvant medicines (e.g. for neuropathic pain), pharmacokinetics, pain assessment tools, and models of service delivery for pain management in CYP, particularly in LMICs, so that CYP like Doudi in Case Study Part 1 can have access to pain management.

Use of Essential Medicines

The Lancet Commission on 'Alleviating the access abyss in palliative care and pain relief: an imperative of universal health coverage' (Knaul et al. 2018) confirmed that poor availability of essential palliative care medicines offers a formidable barrier to proper pain management, with 80% of the world's population lacking adequate access. The following should also be noted:

- There are many CYP globally who are suffering needlessly due to pain and distressing symptoms because the essential medicines for palliative care are not available (WHO 2013; Knaul et al. 2018; Downing et al. 2020).
- Access to and availability of medicines for pain management, including opioids, is a challenge in many LMICs (Downing et al. 2018; Knaul et al. 2018), with the consumption of opioid analgesics in more than 100 countries classed as 'very inadequate' by the International Narcotics Control Board (Scholten et al. 2019; Ju et al. 2022).
- Ongoing barriers and challenges to the availability and accessibility of controlled medicines for pain in Africa have been identified (Mwangi-Powell et al. 2015; et al. 2018) (Table 15.1).
- Less than half of the facilities reviewed in a study in Kenya and Uganda were prescribing opioids and there were challenges with regard to supply and prescribing; with only 73% of 120 health facilities having access to non-opioid analgesics, 7% morphine, with better availability in hospitals than in health centres (Harding et al. 2014).
- It is essential that children's formulations are available, along with immediate-release liquid medications, such as oral morphine (Downing et al. 2015a).
- Even when opioids are available, they may not be where they are needed, prescribed or used appropriately due to 'opiophobia' (Box 15.1).
- Ongoing work through the Opioid Price Watch Project by the International Association for Hospice and Palliative Care (2020) has highlighted the range in availability and cost of essential medicines, both of which impact on the management of pain in CYP in LMICs (De Lima et al. 2014, 2018; Pastrana et al. 2017).
- While the cost of opioids is an issue, the Lancet Commission suggests at competitive

Table 15.1 Factors affecting opioid availability in African countries.

Policy issues	Clinical issues	Resources
Highly restrictive opioid policies and regulations	Limited time for prescription	Unreliable stocks
No national policy	Opiophobia	Few dispensers
Bureaucratic process for legislation	Lack of knowledge and skills by health professionals in assessing and managing pain	Lack of storage for opioids
Punitive regulations	Lack of education	Cost of opioids in some countries
Inadequate ability to report consumption to the narcotics board	Fear of addiction	
Lack of political will	Lack of enough prescribers	
The licenses required for pharmacies to stock opioids	Restrictions based on a patient's diagnosis	
	Cultural norms around pain and its management	

Sources: Mwangi-Powell et al. (2015); Nchako et al. (2018).

- Opiophobia leads to beliefs about:
  - the maximum doses of morphine that can be given safely
  - the fear of addiction, tolerance and respiratory depression
  - cultural issues related to the use of morphine
  - the possibility of misuse.
- There is a widely accepted myth that CYP become addicted to opioids more readily than adults and that they experience respiratory depression, thereby discouraging their use. However, there is evidence that this is not the case when opioids are given appropriately.
- Appropriate opioid use can be hindered through dysfunctional drug supply systems, the existence of unnecessarily restrictive drug control regulations and practices, poor patient compliance and unnecessarily high costs of pain medication.
- Limitations may apply as to who can prescribe strong analgesics such as morphine. In most countries only qualified doctors may prescribe, while in others this is limited to specialist practitioners. Often doctors and pharmacists are wary of the use of opioids in CYP, and in many LMICs a lack of doctors makes prescribing challenging.

Sources: African Palliative Care Association (2010); Hain and Friedrichsdorf (2012); Downing et al. (2015a); Friedrichsdorf and Gomez Garcia (2020).

international medicine prices, the cost of covering the unmet need for opioid analgesics in all children (<15 years) with SHS in LMICs is just over US$1 million per year, which is only 63 cents per child in need (Knaul et al. 2018).

The World Health Assembly (WHA) resolution on palliative care in 2014 (WHO 2014, p. 19) stressed the importance of access to essential medicines including opioids. Member states are urged to ensure that they have:

> *A medicines policy that will ensure the availability of essential medicines for the management of symptoms, including pain and psychological distress, and, in particular, opioid analgesics for relief of pain and respiratory distress.*

Education and Training

To manage pain effectively in CYP in LMIC, all health professionals should be knowledgeable in general pain management. Currently many lack education on multimodal integrative approaches to pain management in CYP that include the physical, psychological, social, spiritual and cultural components of pain; simply relying on observation and advice from colleagues (Downing et al. 2015a). Education is not only needed with regard to knowledge, but also skills and attitudes, without which improvement in pain management for CYP will not happen. There is a lack of education for all health professionals including pharmacists. However, it is essential they understand how to prevent and manage pain in CYP (Downing et al. 2015a) because:

- many health professionals in LMICs have been taught that CYP do not feel pain, opioids are dangerous and should not be given, CYP are a homogeneous group from newborn to adolescents, and pain is inevitable (Downing et al. 2015b; Friedrichsdorf and Gomez Garcia 2022)
- there is a general lack of awareness of how to manage pain both at community and

policy levels (e.g. regular round-the-clock medication is needed) and the impact it can have (Downing et al. 2018).

Education on pain management in CYP, including the myths and barriers to managing pain, is therefore essential at all levels, with a need for educational packages, guidelines and other resources as appropriate.

Provision of Palliative Care (Integrated Health Services)

In many LMICs there has been little or no access to basic practical information for managing pain in CYP and for developing services within the healthcare setting. With a lack of emphasis on pain management and inadequate resources, including staffing, medication and finances, the development of pain services is often not seen as a priority.

- While each LMIC has its own health service, and the integration of pain management for CYP will vary accordingly, it is essential that the management of pain in CYP is integrated into the services being provided.
- Many HICs have pain teams working within their children's hospitals and services, but this is not the case in most LMICs.
- Prescribing is limited to doctors and the low number of doctors available in many LMICs, particularly in rural settings, hampers pain management for CYP.
- All health professionals working with CYP should be able to assess and manage pain, and this is often not the case. Therefore, CYP being treated at home, in health centres or in hospital may not have their pain managed or receive preventive management for procedure-related pain.
- Specialist input may be required for those with more complex pain, such as CYP

with sickle-cell anaemia, cancer or HIV. This input could come from a pain team, a palliative care team or anaesthetists, depending on the system, with the aim being to ensure access to specialist expertise when required.

CASE STUDY: PART 1

Doudi is a seven-year-old boy who has a suspected rhabdomyosarcoma on his left upper leg. He lives with his family in a rural village. His mother has brought him to the regional referral hospital, which is 150 km from his home as he is in a lot of pain. She has carried him as he is unable to stand due to the pain. He is complaining of pain throughout his leg and is reluctant to move.

Bearing in mind Doudi lives in an LMIC:

1. What might be some of the barriers that would prevent Doudi from getting his pain effectively treated?
2. How might some of these barriers be overcome to provide Doudi access to pain treatment and prevention?

Overcoming Challenges to Treating and Preventing Pain in LMICs

While many barriers and challenges exist in treating and preventing pain in LMICs, CYP living in LMICs do not have to live with unnecessary pain and suffering. There are a variety of ways of overcoming such barriers and challenges, illustrated by examples from around the world. These include advocacy for pain treatment and prevention in CYP in LMICs, evaluating national policies, regional workshops, reviewing the cost of opioids, and improved access to prescribers (Table 15.2).

Table 15.2 Examples of ways to overcome barriers and challenges.

Advocacy

- Organisations have come together from around the world to strengthen advocacy efforts
- The ICPCN has led on CYP issues, working alongside the IAHPC and the Worldwide Hospice Palliative Care Alliance (WHPCA) to advocate for improving access to pain management
- Work is ongoing at the global level with the WHO, UN agencies, the INCB and other multilateral organisations to try to improve access to pain treatment and prevention for all ages, particularly with regard to LMICs

Evaluating policy

- The Pain and Policy Studies Group (PPSG) has been involved in evaluating national policies, working collaboratively with colleagues and governments in LMICs from around the world
- PPSG looks at trends, identifies challenges and develops plans to improve the availability of opioids
- PPSG has collaborated with the African Palliative Care Association (APCA), working with stakeholders and governments across the region to improve access to pain management (Namukwaya et al. 2011; Cleary and Maurer 2018)
- PPSG has also worked in India with the central and state governments, to change policy and increase access to essential medicines for pain management (Cleary and Maurer 2018)
- Evaluating policy has been a key aspect of the work of the PPSG International Pain Policy Fellows (Cleary and Maurer 2018)

Regional workshops

- The IAHPC has conducted workshops on the availability and rational use of opioid medications to improve access to pain-relieving medications in LMICs
- Workshops have been undertaken in Latin America with the Latin American Association for Palliative Care (ALCP), the Caribbean and India (International Association for Hospice and Palliative Care 2011)
- These workshops included representatives from El Salvador, Guatemala, Honduras, Panama, Bolivia, Colombia, Ecuador and Peru, as well as the Southern Cone countries

Reviewing the cost of opioids

- The IAHPC also runs the Opioid Price Watch project which aims to present information and generate awareness about availability and access to opioids for legitimate medical use (De Lima et al. 2014, 2018; Pastrana et al 2017)
- Information can be found on the IAHPC website (https://hospicecare.com/what-we-do/projects/opioid-price-watch/)

Increasing access to prescribers

- In Uganda, the narcotics legislation was amended to allow specialist palliative care nurses and clinical officers to prescribe morphine (Fraser et al. 2017)
- Such practitioners undertake either a clinical palliative care course or the Diploma/Degree in Palliative Care, which includes theoretical learning, practical skills and the public health approach
- The programmes are run by Hospice Africa Uganda, with the degree being run in conjunction with Makerere University. More recently, the Mulago School of Nursing and Midwifery (Nampiima Kakonge 2019) has also started running the diploma in clinical palliative care
- An evaluation of nurse prescribing demonstrated that nurses are able to manage pain, and assess and prescribe appropriately, knowing when to ask for help when situations become complex (Downing et al. 2017)

The WHA resolution (WHO 2014), along with the European Association of Palliative Care (EAPC) core competencies for paediatric palliative care (PPC) (Downing et al. 2013, 2014), recognise the need for education in PPC, including pain treatment and prevention, at three levels: (i) the palliative care approach, (ii) general PPC education, and (iii) specialist

PPC education. This education should consider the following.

- The importance of focusing on the resources available within LMICs and how pain in CYP can be successfully managed in these countries.
- Various educational resources and materials have been developed for managing pain in LMICs by regional organisations, e.g. the African Palliative Care Association (APCA), EAPC and the Latin American Association for Palliative Care (ALCP).
- While all three levels of PPC training may not be available in many LMICs, there is a range of programmes that have been developed for managing pain in CYP in different LMICs, e.g. SSA, Latin America, India and Eastern Europe, along with programmes run in HICs that build capacity for LMICs, e.g. the Pain Master Classes and Education in Palliative and End-of-life Care (EPEC) training (Friedrichsdorf et al. 2019).
- The International Children's Palliative Care Network (ICPCN) has developed training on pain assessment and management in CYP across all settings, for use together with the ICPCN Pain App (ICPCN 2019); there are also free e-learning programmes (www.elearnicpcn.org) including one on managing pain (Daniels and Downing 2018), which provide important and accessible basic level training in LMICs.
- The International Association for the Study of Pain (IASP) also has a Pain Education Resource Centre providing on-demand continuing education for pain professionals (IASP 2020).

Specific Issues in LMICs for the Treatment and Prevention of Pain in CYP

While the philosophy and principles of the treatment and prevention of pain in CYP are globally relevant, resources and personnel available vary between settings. The concept of 'total pain' and the principles of treating and preventing pain have been discussed elsewhere in this book, but it is important to identify issues specific to some LMICs.

Assessing Pain in LMICs

- Assessing pain in CYP can be challenging, but in LMICs this process is likely to be more complex.
- Patient, family and health professionals' beliefs and attitudes to pain will impact the assessment and whether a pain assessment is conducted at all, such as the availability of analgesics and cultural and religious beliefs (Box 15.2) (Goucke and Chaudakshetrin 2018), as can be seen in Case Study Part 2.

BOX 15.2   EXAMPLES OF BELIEFS AND ATTITUDES IMPACTING ON PAIN ASSESSMENT

- A nurse working in an LMIC in southern Africa was asked why she did not assess a child's pain. She responded that as she has no access to medications to manage their pain, she could not cope with assessing their pain, identifying they were in pain but helpless to do anything about it.
- Pain may be seen as something that must be endured stoically, or as penance.
- A child may learn that if they say they are in pain they may not be allowed to go home, or they may be given an injection or other unwelcome treatment, leading to further under-reporting of pain.

CASE STUDY: PART 2

Doudi is complaining of pain throughout his leg and is reluctant to move. The first step in managing his pain is to carry out an assessment. Having reviewed the evidence-based approaches to pain assessment discussed in Chapter 6, along with the fact that Doudi lives in an LMIC:

1. What might prevent Doudi from talking about his pain and letting you undertake a full assessment?
2. What additional questions might you want to ask to enable you to get a fuller understanding of Doudi's pain?

Psychological Interventions and Spiritual Considerations for Treating and Preventing Pain in LMICs

The provision of psychological support and interventions for treating and preventing pain in CYP should be standard practice.

- It is essential in helping to reduce depression, anxiety and a sense of helplessness in CYP receiving a plethora of tests and treatments, and may have a role in improving the recovery trajectory (Coakley and Wihak 2017). Without the maturity of speech of adults, these emotions may be expressed as distress, aggression, withdrawal or non-compliance. Withdrawal from school and friends often leads to low self-esteem and decreased social confidence (Boucher et al. 2014).
- For psychological treatment and prevention of pain, child-friendly counselling skills are necessary alongside other therapeutic approaches to communication,

e.g. the use of play with appropriate equipment, drawings and story-telling.

- Young people who are seriously unwell require specific psychological interventions that accommodate the challenges of normative adolescent development. These strategies are vital when a CYP is likely to experience pain.
- The environment must enable honest communication and expression of emotions, while respecting boundaries and age-appropriate expectations. CYP should receive reassurance that they are loved as an integral member of the family and everything possible will be done to keep them comfortable.
- There may be inadequate access to pain medications and limited technological and material resources in LMICs; therefore, psychological interventions that rely on relationships, human contact and innovative techniques become invaluable for promoting resilience, improving functioning on all levels and minimising the risk of psychological comorbidities (Coakley 2016).
- While cognitive behavioural therapy is the psychotherapeutic technique of choice for pain relief for CYP in HICs, a more realistic option in LMICs is to equip parents, caregivers and CYP with coping strategies to manage pain, including play (Box 15.3). Parental/carer involvement and a calm approach are key to the success of informal pain-relieving interventions.
- Simple skills can be taught to enhance relaxation (e.g. correct breathing techniques, mindfulness and guided imagery) and these can reduce the experience of pain (Coakley 2016). Implementing clear sleep hygiene routines and comfortable sleeping equipment as far as possible will help to ensure restful sleep.
- Non-pharmacological distracting techniques show promising results in reducing

BOX 15.3   THE IMPORTANCE OF PLAY

- Play is an integral component in improving a child's psychological well-being, in part due to the sense of normality it can bring and the shift in focus away from their illness and pain (Boucher et al. 2014).
- In LMIC settings where CYP often rely on simple items such as sand, seed pods and discarded cans for toys and creating games, it is possible for CYP to participate in activities that provide fantasy, identify goals or demonstrate aspects of their lives that represent their emotions and perceived losses.
- In this way, play can be helpful in providing an 'emotional holiday' from pain, as well as a useful tool for release of fears (Hunt et al. 2020).
- In settings where poverty determines the quantity and quality of parental time spent with a sick child, it is worth noting that the time for a parent/carer to facilitate play to prevent or treat pain may be limited. Extended family members or community caregivers can be supported to fill this role.

disease may also have an impact – a traditional African perception is that external forces (e.g. witchcraft or revenge) are responsible for disease (Nchako et al. 2018), impacting on both psychological and spiritual considerations for treating and managing pain.

Spiritual considerations, defined as 'that which gives meaning, purpose and connectedness for each unique individual at any age' (Marston et al. 2020, p, 159), are key in LMICs.

- CYP are often influenced in their spirituality and beliefs by their families' beliefs.
- Many families in LMICs will combine traditional religious beliefs and indigenous spirituality and values, such as the concept of Ubuntu in SSA, or the creeds and rituals of the American Indians in Latin America.
- Traditional healers may also play an important part in the care of the CYP and their family, with many individuals seeking the help of a traditional healer before attending a hospital or clinic, therefore connecting the child to the spirits of the ancestors; and utilising traditional healing and cleansing rituals may help in the treatment and prevention of pain.

the experience of pain for CYP exposed to painful procedures. A range of techniques can be used, e.g. singing, massage, use of the magic glove, mobile phone apps, and distraction cards, many of which are available in LMICs.

Cultural issues may also have an impact on the management of pain; e.g., expressing pain may be considered a sign of weakness, and CYP may learn from their parents not to express their pain as they are expected to bear some amount of pain (see Chapter 4 for more information). Likewise, traditional perceptions of health and

CASE STUDY: PART 3

Doudi is in a great deal of pain and does not want to move. On further discussion with Doudi and his family you find the only pain medication they have had access to is paracetamol. This eases the pain for a short period of time. However, his mother says his pain seems to get better when he is sitting outside their hut, on her lap, and watching the birds flying in and out of the tress. When looking at the holistic nature of pain, and using a multimodal approach to treating pain, it is important to consider if there are any psychological or spiritual interventions that could be used to help in the management of Doudi's pain.

1. How might sitting outside watching the birds be helping manage Doudi's pain?
2. In light of this, what other suggestions might you have to help manage his pain from a psychological or spiritual perspective?

Physical Interventions for Treating and Preventing Pain in LMICs

In LMICs where pharmacological options are not always routinely available, non-pharmacological pain-relieving methods (e.g. physical and psychological interventions) are extremely important. Physical interventions are often led by allied health professionals such as physiotherapists, occupational therapists and speech therapists. Although many LMICs will have limited access to allied health professionals, nurses and other health professionals may have basic information on positioning, preventing and managing spasticity, etc. Strategies for implementation include, where possible, supporting families to learn basic movements and massage to help manage their CYP's pain, and ensuring that non-pharmacological interventions are provided alongside pharmacological where possible.

Pharmacological Interventions for Treating Pain in LMICs

Very often health professionals from LMICs will complain that drug availability is the cause of poor pain management as discussed above. However, while this may be a problem, lateral thinking and creativity can help find a solution. By using the WHO principles of pain management (the route, the child, the clock, the ladder), solutions can be found to treat and prevent pain in CYP of all ages. Ascertaining the route for medication to be given is essential, with preference being for the oral route where possible (Box 15.4).

BOX 15.4 ROUTES FOR THE ADMINISTRATION OF MEDICINE TO CYP

Oral

- The simplest and least distressing route in CYP and is used where possible.
- It can be given easily at home, regardless of the situation in which the child and their family are living.
- One of the challenges in LMICs is that often paediatric formulations are not available, and so this may involve dividing and crushing tablets and opening capsules.
- If options are limited, a higher concentration of oral liquid morphine (20 mg/mL) can also be dripped sublingually. Special care must be given to dosing as medication may be swallowed, either increasing or decreasing the potency (Hospice Palliative Care Association of South Africa 2012).

Buccal or intranasal

Very often, if the intravenous preparation of a drug is available, this can be given buccally (dripped between the cheek and gum) or intranasally.

Rectal

- If the oral route is not possible, even via a nasogastric tube, then rectal administration can be considered.

- Some medications have specific rectal formulations (e.g. paracetamol) but there are other medications that can be given rectally.
- If only the intravenous preparation of a drug is available, this can be given using a feeding tube inserted into the rectum.

Subcutaneous

- Many medications can be given subcutaneously using the intravenous preparation.
- This could be by continuous infusion using a syringe driver, but in the absence of this equipment, subcutaneous bolus doses of medication can be given via an indwelling butterfly/cannula. It will need to be flushed with 0.9% sodium chloride after each use.
- Paracetamol cannot be used subcutaneously.
- Syringe drivers are not available in many LMICs, and even where they are, they are not always culturally accepted, hence the need to be creative; e.g., in India they have 'human syringe drivers' where family members are taught to give the subcutaneous medication every four hours.

Ensuring medication is given appropriately for each CYP and regularly by the clock are principles that need to be applied in a similar manner in LMICs. However, challenges may exist when it comes to providing medication via the analgesic ladder, including the following:

- Originally, there was a three-step analgesic ladder. However, the 2012 WHO guideline on persisting pain in children (WHO 2012) removed step 2 (weak opioids) from the ladder, creating a two-step ladder. (Note that the 2012 guidelines have subsequently been withdrawn.)
- Some LMICs do not have access to strong opioids, so step 2 forms an important component of pain treatment, while other LMICs do not have access to weak opioids and so will, by necessity, exclude the second step and progress straight to step 3; therefore, the use of a two-step or three-step ladder often depends on availability of medicines.
- While advocating for access to both weak and strong opioids, clinicians should use whatever medications they have available to manage pain; these may include weak opioids such as tilidine, codeine and tramadol. Response to these drugs should be carefully monitored and co-analgesics used as available.
- In many LMICs the full range of adjuvant (co)analgesics may not be available. Clinicians must be flexible and innovative. Table 15.3 provides a list of widely available and relatively cheap pharmacological options.

Table 15.3 List of widely available and relatively cheap adjuvant analgesic options.

Neuropathic pain	Amitriptyline is effective in most children
	Carbamazepine may help but is sedating and interferes with liver metabolism
Muscle spasm and hypertonia	Diazepam
Cramping abdominal pain	Hyoscine butylbromide
Inflammation, swelling, space-occupying lesions	Prednisone
Pain and anxiety	Clonidine

Table 15.4 Possible options for preventing procedural pain.

	Procedure associated with mild pain	Procedure associated with moderate pain	Procedure associated with severe pain
Local	Topical lidocaine/prilocaine Lidocaine gel	Topical lidocaine/prilocaine Lidocaine infiltration 1%	Lidocaine infiltration 1% Local block: anaesthetist
Analgesia	<6 months: sucrose 24%, breastfeed >6 months: paracetamol, ibuprofen	Oral: tilidine SL, morphine, ketamine Intravenous: morphine, ketamine Intranasal: fentanyl	Consider general anaesthesia
Sedation	Not generally required	Oral: midazolam, ketamine Intravenous: midazolam, ketamine	General anaesthesia

Key: SL = sublingual. Sources: National Department of Health (2017); Nederveld et al. (2017).

- When managing pain (e.g. as in Case Study Part 4) it is necessary to work with what you have available.

Preventing pain where possible is essential, and possible options for preventing procedural pain in LMICs include those found in Table 15.4. (The prevention and treatment of procedural pain is discussed in more detail in Chapter 12.)

CASE STUDY: PART 4

Doudi has been in the hospital for 36 hours and is still in a lot of pain. You have tried giving him paracetamol regularly, which has helped a bit but does not take the pain away or last for very long. You decide you need to change his medication, but only have limited availability of certain drugs (e.g. paracetamol, tilidine and immediate-release morphine tablets). He has advanced disease, and his cancer has spread. You are therefore not able to give him any curative treatment, and he has said he wants to go home and be with his friends and the rest of his family.

1. Using the evidence provided in preceding chapters, and being aware of the limitations of medicines that you have available, how might you manage Doudi's pain?
2. Once you have got Doudi's pain under control, what might you need to do to enable him to go home to the village and remain pain-free?

Summary

- Pain can be effectively managed in CYP in LMICs.
- Access to adequate pain management is a human right and an extremely important public health issue, particularly in LMICs

that have a high burden of communicable and non-communicable diseases, violence and trauma.
- There are considerable barriers to pain management, including lack of effective

national policies and/or implementation, drug and equipment availability, access to training, and human resources.

■ LMICs frequently use research that has been extrapolated from HICs. However, there is much to be learned from other LMICs in evidence and practice.

■ A great deal has already been achieved through advocacy, networking and the development of resources for LMICs. However, the lack of assessment and undertreatment of pain remains a significant problem for many CYP.

■ Clinicians are encouraged to find innovative solutions to managing pain using available resources and up-skilling themselves.

■ There is a need for sustained international pressure on governments and policymakers within LMICs to recognise pain as a serious problem, to ensure progress is made towards preventing and relieving suffering in CYP.

Key to Case Study

Part 1

1. Some of the barriers that prevent Doudi from getting his pain effectively treated may include the following:
   a. Local beliefs about illness, pain and suffering.
   b. Lack of understanding that pain can be managed.
   c. Lack of availability of medicines, including a lack of paediatric formulations.
   d. Lack of trained health personnel to assess and manage Doudi's pain.
   e. Lack of clinical guidelines and protocols, including from the WHO as well as national and local.
   f. Lack of integration of pain management in the health service, with appropriate policies, etc.
   g. Lack of evidence with regard to how to manage pain in CYP in LMICs.
2. Some of these barriers may be overcome as follows:
   a. By working with Doudi and his mother to look at ways to manage his pain, including pharmacological and non-pharmacological methods.

   b. By education and sensitisation of the local community so that they are empowered and informed, and can advocate for access to essential medicines.
   c. By following the WHO guidelines for healthcare planners, implementers and managers, which recognise the importance of pain management in CYP and give guidance as to how to do this.
   d. By sharing and utilising existing guidelines for managing pain.
   e. By educating health professionals with regard to effective pain assessment and measurement.
   f. By advocating to the governments and health services to ensure availability of medicines, including paediatric formulations.
   g. By working to ensure that pain management is integrated into the healthcare system.

Part 2

1. The following factors might prevent Doudi from talking about his pain and letting you undertake a full assessment:

a. Cultural issues with regard to the meaning of illness and suffering including pain.

b. Cultural issues with regard to children speaking up and therefore his mother may speak for him.

c. Fear and anxiety with regard to health professionals/strangers, what is happening to him, etc.

d. Fear of what may happen to him if he talks about and admits he has pain (e.g. staying in hospital, amputation of his leg).

e. Not knowing how to talk about his pain, how to describe it, etc.

f. Not having age-appropriate assessment tools.

g. The fact that he is in a lot of pain and anxiety may mean he is unable to talk about his pain until he is made more comfortable.

h. Your own lack of skills or confidence in communicating with children such as Doudi.

2. Additional questions you might want to ask include:

a. Bearing in mind the issue of total pain, you would need to ask Doudi questions regarding not only the physical experience of pain, but also about psychological, social and spiritual issues.

b. Exploring the meaning and understanding of pain for him.

c. Exploring some of the cultural issues around the meaning of his pain.

d. Where possible explore his social relations, with his parents, his siblings, his friends, and understand how these may impact his pain.

e. Explore other symptoms and issues that might also impact on his pain (e.g. insomnia).

Part 3

1. Sitting outside watching the birds helps Doudi's manage his pain because:

a. This is a form of distraction as his mind is on something other than his pain.

b. Watching the birds helps him to relax and decreases his anxiety.

2. Psychological or spiritual considerations that might help Doudi manage his pain include:

a. Explore with him other interests that he has, which may also be used as distraction and relaxation.

b. Explore his psychological and spiritual responses to his illness and pain to determine what support/counselling may be appropriate.

c. Provide an environment where he feels safe and secure and is able to be honest with regard to his thoughts and feelings.

d. Work with his mother and other carers to help Doudi find ways of coping and managing his pain.

Part 4

1. The following are ways in which Doudi's pain may be managed:

a. Start him on immediate-release morphine tablets if you have the appropriate dosage. Please note that while splitting tablets is not ideal, under the circumstances and if no paediatric formulations are available, this may be the best option.

b. Prescribe the morphine as per his weight and the guidelines provided in other chapters of this book.

c. Review his other medication and give adjuvant pain medication as appropriate and in accordance with the guidelines outlined in other chapters of this book.

d. Utilise both pharmacological and non-pharmacological methods of pain management.

e. Where possible ensure that he is given his medication as prescribed (e.g. four-hourly) and given breakthrough analgesia as appropriate.

f. Teach his parents and caregivers how to give him his medication, the importance of giving it regularly, and how and when to give breakthrough analgesia. Involve Doudi in this as appropriate.

g. Reassess Doudi's pain on a regular basis, changing the dosage according to need and use of breakthrough analgesia, and encourage Doudi to let you know if he is in pain.

2. The following are factors that will enable Doudi to go home to the village and remain pain-free:

   a. Ensure that if he goes home he will have a regular supply of morphine and other medications so that his pain remains controlled. This may not be available locally, so you will need to look at the practicalities of how his caregivers can access the medication (e.g. visiting the hospital as required to pick up the medication).

   b. Prescribe an appropriate amount of medications for him to take home with him. Please note that each country will have a different policy as to how much morphine and other medications you can prescribe; e.g., in some countries this may only be a couple of days, while in others it may be up to two weeks.

   c. Discuss with the family and caregivers how to give his medication. Provide written information, either in words or pictures depending on literacy of his family members, and ensure that they understand how the medication should be given and stored and are able to do this.

   d. Refer Doudi to a home care team, where available, and provide written information for the home care team or other health workers near to where he lives.

   e. Provide the family with information on who to contact and how in case of problems.

Multiple Choice Questions

1. A five-year-old patient suffering from HIV has decreased appetite and is often crying. Do you:

   a. Physically examine the child?

   b. Use toys and locally available play resources to enquire what is upsetting them?

   c. Have a session together with the parents and child to check what is happening?

   d. All the above?

2. A CYP with intractable pain from a neuroblastoma has been referred to your hospital from a rural clinic. They have been prescribed paracetamol to date and your supervisor suggests increasing the dosage of the same medication. Do you:

   a. Comply with their suggestion?

   b. Assess the CYP with a view to changing to available medications on step 2 or step 3 of the WHO analgesic ladder?

   c. Send the CYP back home?

3. The pharmacist at your hospital informs you there is a large amount of morphine in the dispensary which is close to expiry date. You have noticed that most of your health professional colleagues at the hospital are reluctant to prescribe this for pain, and have expressed concerns at giving CYP morphine. Do you:
   a. Encourage the pharmacist to destroy this dangerous drug?
   b. Increase your prescriptions for morphine for CYP even with mild pain?
   c. Initiate an urgent training session to provide accurate information for all health professionals on morphine as an effective pain reliever for moderate to severe pain in adults and CYP?
4. You have limited access to medications at the rural hospital where you work. You have a one-year-old child who needs to have a moderately painful procedure carried out. Do you:
   a. Give them a low dose of oral morphine before the procedure?
   b. Give them sucrose to suck?
   c. Tell the child's parents just to hold them tight so they do not move when they feel the pain?
5. You have a 12-year-old child with cancer in the terminal stages who is unable to swallow. You do not have access to a syringe driver or similar, so do you:
   a. Leave them in pain?
   b. Consider giving intravenous analgesics via the rectal route?
   c. Consider dripping an appropriate amount of oral morphine sublingually?
   d. (b) and (c)?
   e. All of the above?

Online Resources in English and French

There is a wide range of best-practice guidelines and resources for treating and preventing pain in LMICs. Some examples are listed here.

African Palliative Care Association. *Beating Pain: A Pocket Guide for Pain Management in Africa*: https://pos-pal.org/doc15/s19114en.pdf

Worldwide Hospice Palliative Care Alliance. *Palliative Care Toolkit*: http://www.thewhpca.org/images/resources/toolkits/Palliative_Care_Toolkit_2016.pdf

Cairdeas International Palliative Care Trust. Symptom guidelines: https://cairdeas.org.uk/resources/core-resources/core-textbooks

Association for Paediatric Palliative Medicine. APPM Master Formulary: https://www.appm.org.uk/formulary/

Indian Association of Palliative Care, Children's Palliative Care Project. *Training Manual on Children's Palliative Care*: http://palliativecare.in/wp-content/uploads/2014/09/CPC-Training-Manual.pdf

International Association for the Study of Pain. Guide to pain management in low-resource settings: settings: https://ebooks.iasp-pain.org/guide_to_pain_management_in_low_resource_settings

Paliativos Sin Fronteras. *Medecine Palliative Chez les Enfants et Adolescents*. https://paliativossinfronteras.org/producto/medecine-palliative-chez-les-enfants-el-adolescents/

Paliativos Sin Fronteras. *Medicina Paliativa en Ninos y Adolescentes*. https://paliativossinfronteras.org/producto/medicina-paliativa-ninos-adolescentes/

Paliativos Sin Fronteras. *Medicina Paliativa em Crianças e Adolescentes*. https://paliativossinfronteras.org/producto/medicina-paliativa-em-criancas-e-adolescentes/

International Children's Palliative Care Network. *Children's Palliative Care in Africa*: https://icpcn.org/resources/childrens-palliative-care-resources/

International Children's Palliative Care Network. *A Really Practical Handbook of Children's Palliative Care for Doctors and Nurses*: https://icpcn.org/resources/childrens-palliative-care-resources/

PATCH South Africa. *Palliative Care for Children: A Guide for Improving the Quality of Life of Patients and Their Families*: https://bettercare.co.za/palliative-care-for-children/

International Children's Palliative Care Network. *Children's Palliative Care: An International Case-Based Manual*: https://icpcn.org/resources/publications-resources/

World Health Organization. *Guidelines on the Management of Chronic Pain in Children*: https://www.who.int/publications/i/item/9789240017870

References

African Palliative Care Association (2010) *Beating Pain: A Pocket Guide for Pain Management in Africa*. APCA, Kampala.

Boucher, S., Downing, J. and Shemilt, R. (2014) The role of play in children's palliative care. *Children* 1(3), 302–317.

Cleary, J.F. and Maurer, M.A. (2018) Pain and policy studies group: two decades of working to address regulatory barriers to improve opioid availability and accessibility around the world. *Journal of Pain and Symptom Management* 55(2S), S121–S134.

Coakley, R. and Wihak, T. (2017) Evidence-based psychological interventions for the management of pediatric chronic pain: new directions in research and clinical practice. *Children* 4(2), 9.

Connor, S. and Sisimayi, C. (2013) *Assessment of the Need for Palliative Care for Children. Three Country Report: South Africa, Kenya and Zimbabwe*. ICPCN and UNICEF, London.

Daniels, A. and Downing, J. (2018) Increasing access to children's palliative care education through e-learning: a review of the ICPCN experience. *International Journal of Palliative Nursing* 24(7), 351–358.

De Lima, L., Pastrana, T., Radbruch, L. and Wenk, R. (2014) Cross-sectional pilot study to monitor the availability, dispensed prices, and affordability of opioids around the globe. *Journal of Pain and Symptom Management* 48(4), 649–659.e1.

De Lima, L., Arias Casais, N., Wenk, R., Radbruch, L. and Pastrana, T. (2018) Opioid medications in expensive formulations are sold at a lower price than immediate-release morphine in countries throughout the world: third phase of opioid price

watch cross-sectional study. *Journal of Palliative Medicine* 21(10), 1458–1465.

Downing, J., Ling, J., Benini, F., Payne, S. and Papadatou, D. (2013) *EAPC Core Competencies for Education in Paediatric Palliative Care*. Report of the EAPC Children's Palliative Care Education Task Force. European Association for Palliative Care, Milano, Italy.

Downing, J., Ling, J., Benini, F., Payne, S. and Papadatou, D. (2014) A summary of the EAPC White Paper on core competencies for education in paediatric palliative care. *European Journal of Palliative Care* 21, 245–249.

Downing, J., Jassal, S.S., Matthews, L., Britts, H. and Friedrichsdorf, S.J. (2015a) Pediatric pain management in palliative care. *Pain Management* 5(1), 23–25.

Downing, J., Powell, R.A., Marston, J., et al. (2015b) Children's palliative care in low and middle-income countries. *Archives of Disease in Childhood* 101(1), 85–90.

Downing, J., Acuda, W., Adong, D., et al. (2017) Ensuring access to palliative care medicines in Uganda: results of an evaluation into nurse prescribing. In Abstract Book, UCI-PCAU Joint International Conference on Cancer and Palliative Care, 24–25 August 2017, Kampala, Uganda. Available at https://conference.pcauganda.org/abstract-book/

Downing, J., Boucher, S., Daniels, A. and Nkosi, B. (2018) Paediatric palliative care in resource-poor countries. *Children* 5(2), 27.

Downing, J., Rajagopal, M.R., de Lima, L. and Knaul, F. (2020) Universal health coverage and serious health-related suffering: a case for children and young people. In *Children's Palliative Care: An International Case-Based Manual* (ed. J. Downing), pp. 13–24. Springer, UK.

Fraser, B.A., Powell, R.A., Mwangi-Powell, F.N., Nannon, B., Zimmermann, C. and Rodin, G. (2017) Palliative care development in Africa: lessons from Uganda and Kenya. *Journal of Global Oncology* 4, 1–10.

Friedrichsdorf, S.J. and Gomez Garcia, W.C. (2020) Assessment, prevention and treatment of pain in children with serious illness. In *Children's Palliative Care: An International Case-Based Manual* (ed. J. Downing), pp. 65–94. Springer, UK.

Friedrichsdorf, S.J., Remeke, S., Hauser, J., et al. (2019) Development of a pediatric palliative care curriculum and dissemination model: Education in Palliative and End-of-Life Care (EPEC) Pediatrics. *Journal of Pain and Symptom Management* 58(4), 707–720.e3.

Goucke, C.R. and Chaudakshetrin, P. (2018) Pain: a neglected problem in the low-resource setting. *Anesthesia and Analgesia* 126(4), 1283–1286.

Hain, R.D.W. and Friedrichsdorf, S.J. (2012) Pharmacological approaches to pain. 1: 'By the ladder' – the WHO approach to management of pain in palliative care. In *Oxford Textbook of Palliative Care for Children*, 2nd edn (eds A. Goldman, R. Hain and S. Liben), pp. 218–233. Oxford University Press, Oxford.

Harding, R., Simms, V., Penfold, S., et al. (2014) Availability of essential drugs for managing HIV-related pain and symptoms within 120 PEPFAR funded health facilities in East Africa: a cross-sectional survey with onsite verification. *Palliative Medicine* 28(4), 293–301.

Hospice Palliative Care Association of South Africa (2012) Paediatric palliative care guidelines. https://hpca.co.za/Resources/clinical-guidelines/ (accessed 12 October 2022).

Hunt, J., Talawadekar, P. and Friedel, M. (2020) Anticipatory grief and bereavement support. In *Children's Palliative Care: An International Case-Based Manual* (ed. J. Downing), pp. 201–210. Springer, UK.

International Association for Hospice and Palliative Care (2011) IAHPC news. https://hospicecare. com/news/11/04/chair.html (accessed July 2022).

International Association for Hospice and Palliative Care (2020) Opioid Price Watch Project. https://hospicecare.com/what-we-do/projects/opioid-price-watch/ (accessed September 2023).

International Association for the Study of Pain (2020) Pain Education Resource Center (PERC). https://www.iasp-pain.org/Education/Content.aspx?ItemNumber=8610&navItemNumber=8609 (accessed 12 October 2022).

International Children's Palliative Care Network, Worldwide Hospice Palliative Care Alliance, International Association for Hospice and Palliative Care (2018) Palliative care and universal health coverage fact sheet June 2018. https://thewhpca.org/resources/palliative-care-and-universal-health-coverage-fact-sheet-june-2018/ (accessed 12 October 2022).

International Children's Palliative Care Network (2019) ICPCN Pain assessment app helps Huyaam manage her chronic pain. International Children's Edition of eHospice. https://ehospice.com/sa_posts/icpcn-pain-assessment-app-helps-huyaam-manage-her-chronic-pain/ (accessed 12 October 2022).

Ju, C., Wei, L., Man, K.K.C., et al. (2022) Global, regional and national trends in opioid analgesic consumption from 2015 to 2019: a longitudinal study. *Lancet Public Health* 7, e335–346.

Knaul, F.M., Farmer, P.E., Krakauer, E.L., et al. (2018) Alleviating the access abyss in palliative care and pain relief: an imperative of universal health coverage. The Lancet Commission report. *Lancet* 391(10128), 1391–1454.

Marston, J., Abbiati Fogliati, G. and Bauer, R.W. (2020) Spiritual care: In *Children's Palliative Care: An International Case-Based Manual* (ed. J. Downing), pp. 157–166. Springer, UK.

Milani, B., Magrini, N., Wiffen, P. and Scholten, W. (2011) WHO calls for targeted research on the pharmacological treatment of persisting pain in children with medical illnesses. *Evidence-Based Child Health* 6(3), 1017–1020.

Mwangi-Powell, F.N., Downing, J., Powerll, R.A., Kiyaneg, F. and Ddungu, H. (2015) Palliative care in Africa. In *Oxford Textbook of Palliative Nursing*, 4th edn (eds B.R. Ferrell, N. Coyle and J.A. Paice), pp. 1118–1129. Oxford University Press, Oxford.

Nampiima Kakonge, E. (2019) Establishment of the advanced diploma in palliative care nursing. In *Abstract Book. The 2nd Uganda Conference on Cancer and Palliative Care*. PCAU/UCI, Kampala, Uganda.

Namukwaya, E., Leng, M., Downing, J. and Katabira, E. (2011) Cancer pain management in resource limited settings; a practice review. *Pain Research and Treatment* 2011, 393404.

National Department of Health (2017) Pain control. In *Standard Treatment Guidelines and Essential Medicines List for South Africa, Hospital Level, Paediatrics*, pp. 533–539. Department of Health, Pretoria.

Nchako, E., Bussell, S., Nesbeth, C. and Odoh, C. (2018) Barriers to the availability and accessibility of controlled medicines for chronic pain in Africa. *International Health* 10(2), 71–77.

Nederveld, C., Barron, A., Porter, A. and Recicar, J. (2017) Intranasal fentanyl as a pain management modality during dressing changes in the outpatient setting. *Journal of Pediatric Surgical Nursing* 6(2), 43–47.

Pastrana, T., Wenk, R., Radbruch, L., Ahmend, E. and De Lima, L. (2017) Pain treatment continues to be inaccessible for many patients around the globe: second phase of opioid price watch, a cross-sectional study to monitor the prices of opioids. *Journal of Palliative Medicine* 20(4), 378–387.

Population Reference Bureau (2017) World population. Available at https://assets.prb.org/pdf17/2017_World_Population.pdf

Scholten, W.K., Christensen, A.E., Olsen, A.E. and Drewes, A.M. (2019) Quantifying the adequacy of opioid analgesic consumption globally: an updated method and early findings. *American Journal of Public Health* 109(1), 52–57.

Stjernsward, J., Foley, K.M. and Ferris, F.D. (2007) The public health strategy for palliative care. *Journal of Pain and Symptom Management* 33(5), 486–493.

World Health Organization (2011) *Ensuring Balance in National Policies on controlled substances: Guidance for Availability and Accessibility of Controlled Medicines*. WHO, Geneva

World Health Organization (2012) *WHO Guidelines on the Pharmacological Treatment of Persisting Pain in Children with Medical Illnesses*. WHO, Geneva.

World Health Organization (2013) *WHO Essential Medicines in Palliative Care*. IAHPC Press, Houston, TX.

World Health Organization (2014) Sixty Seventh World Health Assembly 2014: Strengthening palliative care as a care component of comprehensive care throughout the life course. Available at https://apps.who.int/gb/ebwha/pdf_files/WHA67/A67_R19-en.pdf

World Health Organization (2018a) *Astana Declaration. Global Conference on Primary Health Care: From Alma-Ata Towards Universal Health Coverage and the Sustainable Development Goals*. Available at https://www.who.int/docs/default-source/primary-health/declaration/gcphc-declaration.pdf

World Health Organization (2018b) *Integrating Palliative Care and Symptom Relief into Paediatrics: A WHO Guide for Health Care Planners, Implementers and Managers*. WHO, Geneva.

World Health Organization (2018c) *Integrating Palliative Care and Symptom Relief into the Response to Humanitarian Emergencies and Crises*. WHO, Geneva.

World Health Organization (2018d) *Integrating Palliative Care and Symptom Relief into Primary Health Care*. WHO, Geneva.

World Health Organization (2019) Universal health coverage. Available at http://www.who.int/health_financing/universal_coverage_definition/en/ (accessed 28 September 2019).

World Health Organization (2020a) *Clinical Management of COVID-19. Interim Guidance*. WHO, Geneva.

World Health Organization (2020b) *Guidelines on the Management of Chronic Pain in Children*. WHO, Geneva

World Health Organization (2021) *Assessing the Development of Palliative Care Worldwide: A Set of Actionable Indicators*. WHO, Geneva.

Zubizarreta, E.H., Fidarova, E., Healy, B. and Rosenblatt, E. (2015) Need for radiotherapy in low and middle income countries: the silent crisis continues. *Clinical Oncology (Royal College of Radiologists)* 27(2), 107–114.

16 Knowledge Implementation and Dissemination: Effectively Moving Forward

Bonnie Stevens, Amelia Swift, and Denise Harrison

Research determining effective interventions for preventing and treating pain has grown substantially over the past decade. Increased knowledge should result in reduced pain and improved outcomes for infants, children and young people (CYP). However, implementing new knowledge in practice is not a straightforward process. Rather, it involves implementation science (IS) and considering the intervention (innovation), the complexities of the implementation process, barriers and facilitators, and the influence of the setting and wider society in relation to pain and its treatment.

Implementation Science

Implementation research was defined by Eccles and Mittman (2006, p. 1) in the inaugural issue of the journal *Implementation Science* as:

> *the scientific study of methods to promote the systematic uptake of research findings and other evidence based practice into routine practice and, hence, to improve the quality and effectiveness of health services and care.*

More recently, the scope of IS has stressed the processes of dissemination and implementation and the importance of partnerships with healthcare organisations – clinical, administrative and educational leaders and clinicians, and patient partners, to ensure minimal divide between research and practice to increase the public health impact of evidence-based innovations. Dissemination captures the spread of evidence-based interventions to targeted audiences (Landsverk et al. 2017). Passive approaches (e.g. written publications, policies or guidelines) are generally less effective than more active engagement of stakeholders (e.g. engaging the child and family in developing a pain plan for the child). Implementation refers to the process of integrating evidence-based knowledge or interventions within a particular context (National Institutes of Health 2010), e.g. educational strategies such as educational outreach.

Implementation (referred to as knowledge translation or KT hereafter; also known as knowledge exchange, knowledge transfer, knowledge utilisation and knowledge mobilisation):

- research evaluating implementation practices
- the growth of novel frameworks
- training of multiple stakeholders

Managing Pain in Children and Young People: A Clinical Guide, Third Edition. Edited by Alison Twycross, Jennifer Stinson, William T. Zempsky, and Abbie Jordan.

- tailoring of interventions to local contexts
- highlighting sustainability and scale-up across healthcare systems.

Existing Gaps in Pain Practice

Gaps remain regarding how to prevent and treat nociceptive (acute) and chronic pain in CYP. The focus has frequently centred on increasing knowledge at the provider level versus the broader systems or organisational level. Reliance on passive education strategies (e.g. lectures, written materials) has often impeded KT strategies that are interactive and dynamic (e.g. educational outreach). Current pain-relieving strategies need to address CYP and family, health professionals (HPs) and organisational needs within the context of inter-professional pain care. Research that reflects the voice of individuals with lived pain experiences, interactive online educational interventions, exploration of the underlying mechanisms of pain and its treatment, and the role of interactive broad-reaching social media interventions is required in mobilising knowledge acquisition and care across multiple contexts.

In this chapter we focus on how IS guides us in transforming new evidence into pain practice change. We review IS frameworks, and how they provide insight into factors (e.g. organisational context) that influence the implementation of pain interventions and implementation outcomes. We present evidence-based education strategies that are parent/carer CYP focused, HP focused and inter-professional and systems focused. Methods to evaluate these strategies (e.g. scoping, realist and systematic reviews) are discussed. We also determine the potential barriers and facilitators for effectively tailoring, implementing and disseminating knowledge.

How Implementation Science Guides Us: Theories, Models and Frameworks

Several IS theories, models and frameworks are found in the literature (Birken et al. 2017). From a survey of 223 IS scientists, over 100 theories from different disciplines were used, typically to identify barriers and facilitators to implementation (Birken et al. 2017). The most commonly used was the Consolidated Framework for Implementation Research (CFIR; Damschroder et al. 2009, 2022a), followed by the Reach, Effectiveness, Adoption, Implementation, and Maintenance (RE-AIM) framework (Glasgow et al. 1999), Diffusion of Innovations (Rogers 2003), and the Theoretical Domains Frameworks (TDF; Cane et al. 2012).

Nilsen (2015) categorised IS theories into the following five categories.

- Process models: guiding processes of translating research into practice.
- Determinant frameworks: identifying factors that influence implementation.
- Classic theories: originating from fields external to implementation science, which can be applied to understand and/or explain implementation.
- Implementation theories: developed by implementation researchers (from scratch or by adapting existing theories/concepts).
- Evaluation frameworks: used to determine implementation success.

Examples of contemporary IS research focused on childhood pain and the theories used to guide them are outlined in Table 16.1.

Table 16.1 Examples of contemporary IS research on childhood pain.

Framework	Description	Example of use
Consolidated Framework for Implementation Research (CFIR) (Damschroder et al. 2009, 2022a)	■ A determinant framework ■ A compilation and integration of 19 previously published theories into a single consolidated framework ■ Five key factors (innovation, innovator, process, inner and outer settings) likely to influence implementation of interventions ■ The CFIR Outcome Addendum (Damschroder et al. 2022b) was proposed to address recommendations from a recent literature review to include outcomes in the framework	Informed the development of a KT intervention, i.e. Implementation of Infant Pain Practice Change (ImPaC) resource, aimed at improving neonatal pain management practices in organisations (Bueno et al. 2020)
Knowledge to Action (KTA) framework (Graham et al. 2006)	■ A process model ■ A dynamic cycle including knowledge synthesis, dissemination, exchange and application, and strategies to facilitate change ■ A knowledge creation funnel represents knowledge inquiry, synthesis, and KT tools and products ■ A knowledge action cycle illustrates the iterative and multiple processes for putting knowledge into action and includes adapting knowledge, assessing barriers, tailoring interventions, monitoring knowledge and sustaining knowledge use	Guided a pilot randomised controlled trial (RCT) aimed at improving use of evidence for vaccination pain in infants (Modanloo et al. 2021)
RE-AIM framework (Glasgow et al. 1999)	■ An evaluation framework ■ Developed for evaluating public health interventions ■ Assesses five dimensions: reach, efficacy, adoption, implementation and maintenance	Used to evaluate a digital health implementation for a chronic pain intervention for children (de la Vega et al. 2020)
Promoting Action on Research Implementation in Health Services (PARIHS) framework (Kitson et al. 1998)	■ A determinant framework ■ Posits that successful implementation of evidence into practice is dependent on the interface of high levels of evidence, context and facilitation ■ A citation analysis of PARIHS (Bergström et al. 2020) included 367 articles that cited at least one of four core articles describing the development or evaluation of the framework (Kitson et al. 1998, 2008; Rycroft-Malone et al. 2002, 2004) ■ The citation analysis did not include the modified integrated iPARIHS (Harvey and Kitson 2016) ■ The key elements of iPARIHS relate to *facilitation*, which is positioned as a 'core ingredient' (Hunter et al. 2020), and thus essential in relation to evidence and context. Facilitation is specified as the facilitator role as well as the process of facilitation	One of the most commonly used frameworks in children's pain research, with 11 of the included studies focusing on pain management in children (Bergström et al. 2020). Year of publications range from 2007 to 2018 and include neonatal and paediatric pain studies. Stevens contributed to six of the included studies as first or senior author, with the most recent being Stevens et al. (2016)

Knowledge Translation Strategies

Evidence-based Education

Parent-focused Knowledge Translation Strategies

Educational strategies have recently involved patients and families. Strategies co-developed with parents can be considered patient targeted and parent mediated, in this case *parent* targeted and mediated (Stacey and Hill 2013). Parent-*targeted* aims at parents' behaviours directly (patient-directed), and parent-*mediated* mediates HP behaviours through information sharing and advocacy to use the strategies during painful procedures. Examples of KT strategies targeting parents during commonly performed painful procedures are outlined in Table 16.2.

More recently, parent-focused KT strategies have used social media. YouTube analytics including reach, acceptability, previous use of pain management strategies and plans to recommend them for future use have been evaluated (Harrison et al. 2016, 2017; Campbell-Yeo et al. 2017; Chambers et al. 2020; Vieira et al. 2020). However, limitations include very low viewer survey response rates and lack of follow-up to determine use of strategies. Vieira et al. (2020), using the Portuguese Be Sweet to Babies video, showed substantially higher survey response rates from viewers who accessed the video from Facebook. This approach may be more effectively completed, compared to embedding surveys within the YouTube videos.

Individual Health Professional Education Knowledge Translation Strategies

Education influences culture, as well as improving knowledge and skills. Despite an expansive evidence base, education targeting HPs has not resulted in widespread improvements in CYP's pain care (Hurley-Wallace et al. 2019). Individual practitioners, particularly those with low perceived authority, are unlikely to be able to challenge embedded practices effectively, therefore explaining why many education programmes designed to improve children's pain practices have limited effect on patient outcomes (AlReshidi et al. 2018). There is increased attention being paid to pain management as an indicator of quality of care. Feedback provided during the quality improvement cycle can provide a powerful incentive to improve knowledge and skills in the team, while also addressing cultural and environmental barriers (Kaye et al. 2020). The educational approaches we advocate below explore pain management in the real-world context (Table 16.3).

Inter-professional Focused Educational Knowledge Translation Strategies

The importance of inter-professional learning initiatives delivered to pre-registration (pre-licensure) HP trainees at all levels and those early in their practice career is undisputed. Table 16.4 outlines five inter-professional educational curricula focusing on pain in CYP that target these populations.

Evaluating Knowledge Translation Strategies

Large numbers of systematic reviews have focused on evaluating the effectiveness of KT strategies in promoting change. Most have focused on HPs and, in general, effect sizes for implementation strategies have been reported as small to moderate. An overview of systematic reviews focused on KT strategies for consumers included 44 systematic reviews (Chapman et al. 2020). The bottom line was that KT strategies should be used in

Table 16.2 Examples of parent-focused KT tools.

Tool	Focus	Tool (link)	Key reference	Details
Power of a Parent's Touch	Neonatal pain	https://m.youtube.com/watch?v=3nqN9c3FWn8&feature=youtube	Campbell-Yeo et al. (2017)	▪ 2 min 40 s video showing parents holding skin-to-skin care and breastfeeding during heel lance ▪ Parent interviews ▪ 13 languages
Be Sweet to Babies	Neonatal pain	https://youtube/L43y0H6XEH4	Harrison et al. (2017)	▪ 4-min videos showing breastfeeding, skin-to-skin care and sucrose during bloodwork ▪ 11 languages
Be Sweet to Babies	Infant vaccination pain	*2 months*: breastfeeding https://youtu.be/FrKmAth4ZGc *6 months*: breastfeeding https://youtu.be/55tejVjzzwE *Sucrose* https://youtu.be/7NDJ463j2iI	Harrison et al. (2016)	▪ Three brief (90-s long) videos showing: (i) breastfeeding a 2-month-old; (ii) breastfeeding an older infant; (iii) sucrose for a 6-month-old ▪ 10 languages
Franck (2nd edition)	Neonatal pain	https://familynursing.ucsf.edu/sites/familynursing.ucsf.edu/files/wysiwyg/Comfy%20PDF%20ENGLISH%20Dec%2017.pdf	Franck (2013)	▪ Multimedia booklet with embedded video clips
Solutions for Kids in Pain (SKIP)	Vaccination pain	https://m.youtube.com/watch?v=KgBwVSYqfps	Chambers et al. (2020)	▪ 2 min 18 s video showing a child telling how parents and HP can help with pain management during vaccinations ▪ 16 languages
Help Eliminate Pain in Kids & Adults (HELP)	Vaccination pain	http://phm.utoronto.ca/helpinkids/resources1.html	McNair et al. (2019)	▪ Series of videos showing evidence-based pain management during vaccination

Table 16.3 Evidence-based educational strategies.

Educational approach	Description and evidence
Enquiry-based learning (EBL)	▪ EBL supports the development of appropriate skills ▪ Successful implementation requires practitioners to frame a question and use a variety of skills to answer it ▪ Malcolm and McGirr (2020) demonstrated how EBL helps an inter-professional group rehearse decision-making in children's palliative care, which improved their confidence in encountering the situation in the clinical world

Simulation	▪ In simulation the practitioner is free to make mistakes and try a range of approaches
	▪ Simulation can:
	    ▪ be low-tech or high-fidelity
	    ▪ be conducted virtually or in a training environment that represents the clinical world
	    ▪ use patient actors, mannequins or virtual humans
	    ▪ be facilitated by tutors or peers
	▪ Valler-Jones (2014) demonstrates how peer-led simulation in care of the critically ill child enabled nursing students to become more confident and competent in working together to solve complex clinical problems
	▪ These skills are essential in increasing the utility of 'classroom'-developed skills being translatable to the real world

Debriefing	▪ Simulation will not yield maximum gains unless it includes debriefing ▪ Skilful facilitators can support the growth in knowledge and learning from emotional responses and biases ▪ There is limited research using simulation for pain management in children ▪ However, Brock et al. (2019) demonstrated the value of the debriefing component of simulation in paediatric palliative care. A 360-degree approach allowed the students to learn from reflection and from commentary and coaching from the parent-actors, and experts
Virtual humans	▪ Vignettes, or case studies, allow learners to explore patient characteristics that can impact their choices ▪ Good practice involves the use of clinicians and other stakeholders to ensure content validity in the development of case studies or vignettes. LaFond et al. (2015) describe how this can be done ▪ Boyle et al. (2019) demonstrated that use of virtual children revealed nurse bias in decision-making related to weight and ethnicity during pain education ▪ Implicit or unconscious bias negatively impacts pain management for CYP (Raphael and Oyeku 2020). The use of virtual tools allows the educator to present the learner with a patient context that approximates problem areas in practice
Real-world learning	▪ Much practice-based pain education involves removing the HP from the clinical area into a classroom ▪ Very few research studies use patient outcomes as a measure of success of a practice-based education intervention ▪ Classroom-based activities yield moderate improvement in knowledge (AlReshidi et al. 2018), but they do not help HP address barriers to effective pain management ▪ Barriers to effective pain management have been remarkably stable over time and mostly involve teamwork and communication (Czarnecki et al. 2011, 2014) ▪ One of the best ways to effect improvement in teamwork and communication has been demonstrated to be inter-professional education strategies

Table 16.3 (Continued)

Educational approach	Description and evidence
Bedside coaching or mentorship	■ Bedside coaching or mentorship in pain-related decision-making for CYP can bring about long-term improvements in attitude, knowledge and behaviours for nurses at the bedside ■ Johnston et al. (2007) used one-to-one coaching to reverse deficits in nursing pain assessment, knowledge and use of non-pharmacological interventions with children in pain
Partnership, empathy and empowerment	■ Many educational approaches dominating the research literature to date have not capitalised on the power of patient or family stories and have not been co-designed with CYP and parents ■ This situation is changing rapidly, as is the accessibility of quality-assured evidence-based materials ■ Communicating Lily's Pain (French 2020; Carter et al. 2021) (https://www.wellchild.org.uk/get-support/information-hub/communicating-lilys-pain/) gives advice for parents and professionals about what to do for their child in pain and provides insight into pain experience of a CYP with a profound cognitive impairment and complex health needs ■ Online resources, e.g. It Doesn't Have to Hurt (Chambers 2021; https://itdoesnthavetohurt.ca/), mark a new chapter in pain research and education, with a clear intent to support knowledge implementation by interweaving personal stories with quality-appraised evidence to produce resources that can be used by HPs, patients and families to improve pain management ■ Similarly, Partnering for Pain (Birnie 2021 and http://partneringforpain.com) harnesses the power of patients, parents and professionals to direct research and education development to address priority problems for children with chronic pain ■ It Doesn't Have to Hurt and Partnering for Pain have a powerful social media presence and a wide reach

combination and repeated over time. Also, a key conclusion from a systematic review that included 21 studies of KT strategies focused on child health research was that there was a lack of methodologically sound research on KT interventions (Albrecht et al. 2016). Only three randomised controlled trials of single KT interventions (two studies used reminders and one used a multidisciplinary clinical team to influence a single screening practice) showed evidence of consistent effectiveness.

Evaluating Social Media

Scoping and systematic reviews have evaluated clinician and consumer focused YouTube videos on pain management education.

■ Farkas et al. (2015) included 25 publicly available online educational videos, most of which were targeted at parents of children and focused on needle pain.

■ A scoping review focused on parent-targeted education regarding infant pain management delivered during the perinatal period included nine studies: six evaluated multimodal educational strategies, including videos, written information, verbal discussion and pictorial information (Richardson et al. 2020).

■ A systematic review focused on KT research targeting parents (Gagnon et al. 2020) and included 12 studies: eight focused on needle-related procedures in infants and six involved videos.

Table 16.4 Inter-professional children's pain educational training initiatives.

KT educational innovation	Description/aim	Focus of KT strategies	Outcomes
Pain In Child Health (PICH) (SickKids, Toronto, Ontario, Canada) https://paininchildhealth.ca	International interdisciplinary training consortium for developing a community of inter-professional scholars in children's pain	Training and mentorship of research trainees in collaboration with research leaders, patients, clinicians, educators and policy-makers. Educational activities include: ▪ Training institutes ▪ PICH2GO conferences ▪ Research lab visits ▪ Monthly online webinars ▪ Mentoring ▪ Trainee awards	PICH has involved 400 trainees from 17 countries in North and South America, Australia, Europe and Asia from psychology, nursing, medicine and pharmacy. Highly rated educational activity
Online Paediatric Pain Curriculum (SickKids, Toronto, Ontario, Canada) https://www.sickkids.ca/en/care-services/centres/pain-centre/#oppc	The Pain Centre and Learning Institute at SickKids has partnered with national/international funding agencies to develop an Online Pediatric Pain Curriculum (OPPC) for entry-level health professionals	The OPPC includes 12 (and one additional in development) interactive educational modules (based on International Association for the Study of Pain (IASP) curricula) developed by international experts: 1. Neurobiology of pain 2. Pain perceptions 3. Epidemiology and taxonomy of pain 4. Pain assessment and measurement 5. Pharmacological pain therapies 6. Non-pharmacological therapies 7. Acute pain management 8. Chronic pain management 9. Pain in palliative care 10. Ethical considerations 11. Pain in low- and middle-income countries 12. Pain in children with intellectual disabilities (autumn 2022) 13. Acute pain in the emergency department (in development)	Since 2016, over 7000 global learners from 10 different countries have accessed the modules. Most (70% nurses) stated the modules improved their knowledge of children's pain and how they work with other health professionals. Almost all rated the modules as acceptable and appropriate and would recommend them to others

University of Toronto Centre for the Study of Pain Interfaculty Pain Curriculum (UTCSP-IPC) http://sites.utoronto.ca/pain/research/interfaculty-curriculum.html	The UTCSP provides inter-professional education for pre-registration (pre-licensure) trainees from dentistry, medicine (including occupational therapy and physiotherapy), nursing and pharmacy through a 20-hour IPC. The UTCSP-IPC is based on the IASP CORE Curriculum (IASP 2012)	The IPC includes: ■ Large group interactive sessions (e.g. patient panel and inter-professional panel) ■ Six to eight concurrent patient-centred research-based medium group sessions ■ Facilitated small inter-professional groups who use patient-oriented case studies ■ Two self-study modules on 'pain mechanisms and manifestations' and 'opioids as a component of pain management, an interprofessional responsibility' ■ Discipline-specific content that individual institutions (e.g. nursing, medicine) provide to their students during a 3-hour session	From 2002 to 2020, approximately 1000 trainees per year completed the IPC, a total of approximately 16 800 trainees. There is a consistent increase in knowledge and skills, and appreciation for working collaboratively with other health professionals on case studies highlighting acute and chronic pain
Pediatric Pain Master Class (Center for Pediatric Pain, Palliative and Integrative Medicine, University of California at San Francisco, Benioff Children's Hospitals) https://www.ucsfcme.com/2022/MMC22100/info.html	The Annual Pediatric Pain Master Class focuses on the prevention and treatment of acute, chronic, neuropathic, visceral and procedural pain through multimodal analgesia. An in-depth review of pharmacology (opioids, non-opioids, adjuvant analgesia), rehabilitation/physiotherapy, psychotherapy, integrative modalities, and regional/neuraxial anaesthesia is included	Faculty (i.e. those teaching the course) includes leading clinicians and researchers in pain medicine and integrative (non-pharmacological) pain care of children. Class is focused on changing practice and developing programmes at participants' home institutions	A total of 651 medics, nurse practitioners and other clinicians from 40 different countries have attended this course, taught by over 30 different members of Faculty

(Continued)

Table 16.4 (Continued)

KT educational innovation	Description/aim	Focus of KT strategies	Outcomes
Pediatric Palliative Care Curriculum and Dissemination Module: Education in Palliative and End-of-life Care (EPEC) (Friedrichsdorf et al. 2019) (Center for Pediatric Pain, Palliative and Integrative Medicine, University of California San Francisco, Benioff Children's Hospitals)	The EPEC-Pediatrics curriculum features training in the skills required to address key domains of children's pain and palliative care. The programme is designed to give children's health professionals the knowledge and skills needed to provide excellent palliative care to their patients and their families. A Spanish version (EPEC) Pediátrico Latino-América is available	Curriculum comprises 22 core palliative care modules, 12 on treatment of pain and distressing symptoms, delivered in a combination of distance online learning and in-person conference sessions. These 'Train-the-trainer' modules provide the 'trainers' (clinicians) with PowerPoint presentations, trigger-tape videos, and a teaching handbook for each module to teach interdisciplinary teams	1356 clinicians from 95 countries were trained by EPEC-Pediatrics Master Facilitators from 2012 to 2021

The findings of these three reviews consistently highlighted that these online resources are perceived as acceptable and feasible. However, there is little evidence relating to whether they are implemented in clinical practice and, importantly, whether the use of such resources leads to short- and long-term improvements in pain management practices.

Organising Knowledge Translation Strategies

Many KT strategies have been explored. The Cochrane Effective Practice and Organisation of Care group organises strategies by target audience (e.g. professional, organisational, regulatory and financial) (Cochrane Collaboration 2018). The Expert Recommendations for Implementing Change (ERIC) project utilised 71 expert stakeholders to organise strategies under nine groups that were individually, group and organisational focused (Powell et al. 2015; Waltz et al. 2015). Examples of strategies within each group and their potential application to CYP's pain are highlighted in Table 16.5.

Evaluating Knowledge Translation Strategies: What Needs Considering?

Implementation scientists have developed a comprehensive list of outcomes for determining

Table 16.5 Implementation strategies from ERIC.

Grouping of strategies	Examples of implementation strategies	Examples of implementation strategies in children's pain
Use evaluative and interactive strategies	■ Audit and feedback ■ Conduct local needs assessment	Conduct an audit to determine frequency of pain assessment and documentation
Provide interactive assistance	■ Facilitation-interactive problem-solving and support	Work with a group of HPs who are having problems changing pain practices
Adapt and tailor to context	■ Tailor strategies	Tailor the pain interventions to address barriers and facilitators (e.g. furniture for skin-to-skin care)
Develop stakeholder interrelationships	■ Identify and prepare champions ■ Visit other sites	Have champions visit a site that has successfully implemented a hospital-wide practice change
Train and educate stakeholders	■ Conduct educational meetings and outreach ■ Develop educational materials ■ Make training dynamic ■ Provide ongoing consultation	Use multiple implementation strategies to address varying learner perspectives and styles, delivered by various HP and patients for young people with chronic pain
Engage consumers	■ Involve patients/consumers as participants ■ Use social media	Include patients and families when implementing pain protocols and procedures. Use social media to communicate new knowledge on pain in children (e.g. SKIP)
Use financial strategies	■ Access funding to facilitate the intervention	Seek funding from foundations and government agencies to support pain education efforts

Source: Powell et al. (2015).

the effectiveness of strategies for implementing new knowledge (Proctor et al. 2009, 2013; Lewis et al. 2015). Some of the most used include the following:

- Acceptability: the KT strategy is acceptable, agreeable, or satisfactory.
- Feasibility: the KT strategy can be successfully implemented.
- Fidelity: the KT strategy is used as prescribed or intended.
- Cost: the impact of an implementation effort on cost.
- Reach: the spread of an implementation initiative.
- Sustainability: the extent to which an intervention is maintained within a setting.

A recent review by Klaic et al. (2022) indicates that the implementability of healthcare interventions is most influenced by acceptability, feasibility and fidelity, especially with regard to sustainability and spreadability. KT outcomes may be valued differently by different stakeholders; clinicians may value acceptability and feasibility, researchers may value fidelity and ease of use, while decision-makers may value implementation costs, sustainability and effective dissemination. Nonetheless, it is important to determine if the KT interventions were successfully implemented and disseminated in the desired context. A new scoping review by Proctor et al. (2023) indicates that acceptability was assessed in more than half of manuscripts and that fidelity, feasibility, adoption and appropriateness were also commonly examined.

The Way Forward

Changing the Statistics

One of the most quoted statistics in IS is 'It takes 17 years to turn 14% of original research to the benefit of patient care' (Balas and Boren 2000).

This is a metric that must change! This gap between research and practice needs to become narrower, and the answer lies within the realm of IS. To date, we have learned from IS that to make successful practice changes, we must consider not only the evidence but the process we use to implement it, the implementer, and the qualities of the context in which it is implemented.

Considering Organisational Context

Organisational context is repeatedly cited by researchers to influence the implementation of evidence-based practices (Li et al. 2018; Nilsen and Bernhardsson 2019). Yet the way to use what we know about organisational context to change knowledge or practice has received little consideration. We know context is important when tailoring KT interventions to organisational needs or implementing KT strategies in healthcare. In an integrative review by Li et al. (2018), organisational culture, leadership, resources, networks and communication, evaluation and feedback and champions were the factors most frequently reported to be associated with implementation success. Just as there is a gap between implementing new knowledge into practice using implementation strategies, there is also a gap between implementation strategies and their use (dissemination) in clinical or other organisational change processes. Unravelling how these factors facilitate or act as barriers in achieving KT outcomes, practice change and child health outcomes is paramount.

Valuing Implementation

Current times reflect a paradigm shift in terms of valuing the implementation of new knowledge as well as its discovery. This shift essentially means we need to carefully evaluate the implementation success of KT interventions using criteria such as acceptability, fidelity, feasibility, cost and sustainability, as well as the intervention effectiveness of the innovation itself. All too often there is little evidence on whether innovations are implemented and disseminated in practice and, more importantly, whether the use of these interventions results in sustained clinical change or, in this case, better pain practices clinically and improved child health outcomes. Ideally, implementation needs to be viewed as an essential component of the research process to ensure effective, affordable and sustainable healthcare practices.

Summary

- The evidence to support effective prevention and treatment of pain in CYP is growing exponentially.
- Reports indicate an ongoing lag in changing HP pain practices at the individual and institutional level, as well as HP facilitation of parental involvement in pain management.
- Failure to effectively implement and disseminate new knowledge on effective pain-relieving strategies results in the continued pain and suffering of CYP.
- We are beginning to better understand the importance of IS in guiding effective practice change within a variety of contexts.
- To optimise knowledge, we need to consider not only effectiveness of the pain-relieving intervention, but the effectiveness of the implementation of the intervention within multiple contexts.
- Context is complex and challenging, and mandates keeping facilitators and barriers at front of mind. We have evidence-based KT strategies at our fingertips, including those that are directed broadly to parent and child partners to make significant change in pain outcomes.
- We need to focus on more effective ways of implementing and disseminating this knowledge to learners, parents and practitioners.

Multiple Choice Questions

1. Which of the following are similar terms for knowledge implementation?
   a. Knowledge translation
   b. Knowledge mobilisation
   c. Knowledge generation
   d. Knowledge utilisation
   e. (a), (b) and (d)
   f. (a), (b) and (c)
2. Which of the following are implementation outcomes?
   a. Acceptability
   b. Feasibility
   c. Cost
   d. Increase in knowledge
   e. (a), (b) and (c)
   f. (a), (b) and (d)
3. What is the aim of patient (parent)-mediated strategies?
   a. Changing parents' behaviours directly
   b. Changing healthcare professionals' behaviours through parents' information sharing and advocacy
   c. Changing healthcare professionals' behaviours directly
   d. Changing parents' behaviours through healthcare professionals' information sharing and advocacy

4. Knowledge dissemination strategies shared via social media avenues have resulted in reported:
   a. Improvements in pain management
   b. Large reach and dissemination
   c. Increased use of effective pain management strategies
   d. Acceptability and feasibility of the knowledge translation tools
   e. (a) and (c)
   f. (b) and (d)
5. The most effective simulation:
   a. Uses a high-fidelity approach
   b. Includes debriefing
   c. Uses patient-actors
   d. Addresses complex issues
6. Pain education should:
   a. Focus on increasing knowledge for the individual practitioner
   b. Take place in a classroom away from the clinical area
   c. Address real-world challenges to effective care
   d. Expose each practitioner's implicit/unconscious bias

ADDITIONAL RESOURCES

- It doesn't have to hurt, http://itdoesnthavetohurt.ca
- Partnering for Pain, http://ww.partneringforpain.com
- SickKids Pain Centre, Online Pediatric Pain Curriculum, https://www.sickkids.ca/en/care-services/centres/pain-centre/#oppc

References

Albrecht, L., Archibald, M., Snelgrove-Clarke, E. and Scott, S.D. (2016) Systematic review of knowledge translation strategies to promote research uptake in child health settings. *Journal of Pediatric Nursing* 31, 235–254.

AlReshidi, N., Long, T. and Darvill, A. (2018) A systematic review of the impact of educational orograms on factors that affect nurses' post-operative pain management for children. *Comprehensive Child and Adolescent Nursing* 41, 9–24.

Balas, E.A., and Boren, S.A. (2000) Managing clinical knowledge for health care improvement. *Yearbook of Medical Informatics* (1), 65–70.

Bergström, A., Ehrenberg, A., Eldh, A.C., et al. (2020) The use of the PARIHS framework in implementation research and practice: a citation analysis of the literature. *Implementation Science* 15, 1–68.

Birken, S.A., Powell, B.J., Shea, C.M., et al. (2017) Criteria for selecting implementation science theories and frameworks: results from an international survey. *Implementation Science* 12, 124.

Birnie, K. (2021) Partnering for Pain. https://partneringforpain.com/ (accessed 22 May 2021).

Boyle, S.L., Janicke, D.M., Robinson, M.E. and Wandner, L.D. (2019) Using virtual human technology to examine weight bias and the role of patient weight on student assessment of pediatric pain. *Journal of Clinical Psychology in Medical Settings* 26, 106–115.

Brock, K.E., Tracewski, M., Allen, K.E., Klick, J., Petrillo, T. and Hebbar, K.B. (2019) Simulation-based palliative care communication for pediatric critical care fellows. *American Journal of Hospice and Palliative Medicine* 36, 820–830.

Bueno, M., Stevens, B., Rao, M., Riahi, S., Lanese, A. and Li, S.-A. (2020) Usability, acceptability, and feasibility of the Implementation of Infant Pain Practice Change (ImPaC) Resource. *Paediatric and Neonatal Pain* 2, 82–92.

Campbell-Yeo, M., Dol, J., Disher, T., et al. (2017) The power of a parent's touch: evaluation of reach and impact of a targeted evidence-based YouTube video. *Journal of Perinatal and Neonatal Nursing* 31, 341–349.

Cane, J., O'Connor, D. and Michie, S. (2012) Validation of the theoretical domains framework for use in behaviour change and implementation research. *Implementation Science* 7, 37.

Carter, B., Young, R. and Munro, J. (2021) Communicating Lily's pain: parents and professionals working together. Available at https://figshare.edgehill.ac.uk/articles/report/Summary_Report_2019-2020_-_Communicating_Lily_s_Pain/13554632

Chambers, C. (2021) It doesn't have to hurt. https://itdoesnthavetohurt.ca (accessed 6 July 2022).

Chambers, C.T., Dol, J., Parker, J.A., et al. (2020) Implementation effectiveness of a parent-directed YouTube video ('It doesn't have to hurt') on evidence-based strategies to manage needle pain: descriptive survey study. *JMIR Pediatrics and Parenting* 3, e13552.

Chapman, E., Haby, M.M., Setsuko Toma, T., et al. (2020) Knowledge translation strategies for dissemination with a focus on healthcare recipients: an overview of systematic reviews. *Implementation Science* 15, 14.

Cochrane Collaboration (2018) EPOC resources for review authors. https://epoc.cochrane.org/resources/epoc-resources-review-authors.

Czarnecki, M.L., Simon, K., Thompson, J.J., et al. (2011) Barriers to pediatric pain management: a nursing perspective. *Pain Management Nursing* 12, 154–162.

Czarnecki, M.L., Salamon, K.S., Thompson, J.J. and Hainsworth, K.R. (2014) Do barriers to pediatric pain management as perceived by nurses change over time? *Pain Management Nursing* 15, 292–305.

Damschroder, L.J., Aron, D.C., Keith, R.E., Kirsh, S.R., Alexander, J.A. and Lowery, J.C. (2009) Fostering implementation of health services research findings into practice: a consolidated framework for advancing implementation science. *Implementation Science* 4, 50.

Damschroder, L.J., Reardon, C.M., Widerquist, M.A.O. and Lowery, J. (2022a) The updated Consolidated Framework for Implementation Research based on user feedback. *Implementation Science* 17(1), 75.

Damschroder, L.J., Reardon, C.M., Wilderquist, M.A.O. and Lowery, J. (2022b) Conceptualizing outcomes for use with the Consolidated Framework for Implementation Research (CFIR): the CFIR outcomes addemdum. *Implementation Science* 17(1), 7.

de la Vega, R., Ritterband, L. and Palermo, T.M. (2020) Assessing digital health implementation for a pediatric chronic pain intervention: comparing the RE-AIM and BIT frameworks against real-world trial data and recommendations for future studies. *Journal of Medical Internet Research* 22, e19898.

Eccles, M.P. and Mittman, B.S. (2006) Welcome to implementation science. *Implementation Science* 1, 1.

Farkas, C., Solodiuk, L., Taddio, A., et al. (2015) Publicly available online educational videos regarding pediatric needle pain: a scoping review. *Clinical Journal of Pain* 31, 591–598.

Franck, L.S. (2013) *Comforting Your Baby in Intensive Care*. Available at https://familynursing.ucsf.edu/sites/familynursing.ucsf.edu/files/wysiwyg/Comfy%20PDF%20ENGLISH%20Dec%2017.pdf (accessed 6 July 2022).

French, C. (2020) Communicating Lily's pain. https://www.wellchild.org.uk/get-support/information-hub/communicating-lilys-pain/ (accessed 6 July 2022).

Friedrichsdorf, S.J., Remke, S., Hauser, J., et al. (2019) Development of a pediatric palliative care curriculum and dissemination model: Education in Palliative Care and End-of-Life Care (EEC) Pediatrics *Journal of Pain and Symptom Management* 58, 707–720.

Gagnon, M.M., Hadjistavropoulos, T., McAleer, L.M. and Stopyn, R.J.N. (2020) Increasing parental access to pediatric pain-related knowledge: a systematic review of knowledge translation research among parents. *Clinical Journal of Pain* 36, 47–60.

Glasgow, R.E., Vogt, T.M. and Boles, S.M. (1999) Evaluating the public health impact of health promotion interventions: the RE-AIM framework. *American Journal of Public Health* 89, 1322–1327.

Graham, I.D., Logan, J., Harrison, M.B., et al. (2006) Lost in knowledge translation: time for a map?

Journal of Continuing Education in the Health Professions 26, 13–24.

Harrison, D., Wilding, J., Bowman, A., et al. (2016) Using YouTube to disseminate effective vaccination pain treatment for babies. *PLoS One* 11, e0164123.

Harrison, D., Reszel, J., Dagg, B., et al. (2017) Pain management during newborn screening: using YouTube to disseminate effective pain management strategies. *Journal of Perinatal and Neonatal Nursing* 31, 172–177.

Harvey, G. and Kitson, A. (2016) PARIHS revisited: from heuristic to integrated framework for the successful implementation of knowledge into practice. *Implementation Science* 11, 33.

Hunter, S.C., Kim, B., Mudge, A., et al. (2020) Experiences of using the i-PARIHS framework: a co-designed case study of four multi-site implementation projects. *BMC Health Services Research* 20, 573.

Hurley-Wallace, A., Wood, C., Franck, L.S., Howard, R.F. and Liossi, C. (2019) Paediatric pain education for health care professionals. *Pain Reports* 4, e701.

International Association for the Study of Pain (2012) Interprofessional Pain Curriculum. https://www.iasp-pain.org/education/curricula/iasp-interprofessional-pain-curriculum-outline/ (accessed 6 July 2022).

Johnston, C.C., Gagnon, A., Rennick, J., et al. (2007) One-on-one coaching to improve pain assessment and management practices of pediatric nurses. *Journal of Pediatric Nursing* 22, 467–478.

Kaye, E.C., Applegarth, J., Gattas, M., et al. (2020) Hospice nurses request paediatric-specific educational resources and training programs to improve care for children and families in the community: qualitative data analysis from a population-level survey. *Palliative Medicine* 34, 403–412.

Kitson, A., Harvey, G. and McCormack, B. (1998) Enabling the implementation of evidence based practice: a conceptual framework. *Quality in Health Care* 7, 149–158.

Kitson, A.L., Rycroft-Malone, J., Harvey, G., McCormack, B., Seers, K. and Titchen, A. (2008) Evaluating the successful implementation of evidence into practice using the PARiHS framework: theoretical and practical challenges. *Implementation Science* 3, 1.

Klaic, M., Kapp, S., Hudson, P., et al. (2022) Implementability of healthcare interventions: an overview of reviews and development of a conceptual framework. *Implementation Science* 17, 10.

LaFond, C.M., Van Hulle Vincent, C., Lee, S., et al. (2015) Development and validation of a virtual human vignette to compare nurses' assessment and intervention choices for pain in critically ill children. *Simulation in Healthcare* 10, 14–20.

Landsverk, J., Brown, C.H., Smith, J.D., et al. (2017) Design and analysis in dissemination and implementation research. In *Dissemination and Implementation Research in Health: Translating Science to Practice*, 2nd edn (eds R.C. Brownson, G.A. Colditz and E.K. Proctor), pp. 201–228. Oxford University Press, New York.

Lewis, C.C., Fischer, S., Weiner, B.J., Stanick, C., Kim, M. and Martinez, R.G. (2015) Outcomes for implementation science: an enhanced systematic review of instruments using evidence-based rating criteria. *Implementation Science* 10, 155.

Li, S.-A., Jeffs, L., Barwick, M. and Stevens, B. (2018) Organizational contextual features that influence the implementation of evidence-based practices across healthcare settings: a systematic integrative review. *Systematic Reviews* 7, 72.

McNair, C., Campbell-Yeo, M., Johnston, C. and Taddio, A. (2019) Nonpharmacologic management of pain during common needle puncture procedures in infants: current research evidence and practical considerations: An update. *Clinical Perinatology* 46, 709–730.

Malcolm, C. and McGirr, D. (2020) Educational needs and preferred learning approaches of the paediatric palliative care workforce: a qualitative exploratory study. *Nurse Education Today* 89, 104417.

Modanloo, S., Dunn, S., Stacey, D. and Harrison, D. (2021) The feasibility, acceptability and preliminary efficacy of parent-targeted interventions in vaccination pain management of infants: a pilot randomized control trial (RCT). *Pain Management* 11, 287–301.

National Institutes of Health (2010) PA-10-038: Dissemination and Implementation Research in Health (RO1). Available at https://grants.nih.gov/grants/guide/pa-files/PAR-10-038.html

Nilsen, P. (2015) Making sense of implementation theories, models and frameworks. *Implementation Science* 10, 53.

Nilsen, P. and Bernhardsson, S. (2019) Context matters in implementation science: a scoping review of determinant frameworks that describe contextual determinants for implementation outcomes. *BMC Health Services Research* 19, 189.

Pain in Child Health. Hospital for Sick Children, Toronto. `https://paininchildhealth.ca` (accessed 4 July 2022).

Powell, B.J., Waltz, T.J., Chinman, M.J., et al. (2015) A refined compilation of implementation strategies: results from the Expert Recommendations for Implementing Change (ERIC) project. *Implementation Science* 10, 21.

Proctor, E.K., Landsverk, J., Aarons, G., Chambers, D., Glisson, C. and Mittman, B. (2009) Implementation research in mental health services: an emerging science with conceptual, methodological, and training challenges. *Administration and Policy in Mental Health* 36, 24–34.

Proctor, E.K., Powell, B.J. and McMillen, J.C. (2013) Implementation strategies: recommendations for specifying and reporting. *Implementation Science* 8, 139.

Proctor, E.K., Bunger, A.C., Lengnick-Hall, R., et al. (2023) Ten years of implementation outcomes research: a scoping review. *Implementation Science* 18(1), 31.

Raphael, J.L. and Oyeku, S.O. (2020) Implicit bias in pediatrics: an emerging focus in health equity research. *Pediatrics* 145, e20200512.

Richardson, B., Falconer, A., Shrestha, J., Cassidy, C., Campbell-Yeo, M. and Curran, J.A. (2020) Parent-targeted education regarding infant pain management delivered during the perinatal period: a scoping review. *Journal of Perinatal and Neonatal Nursing* 34, 56–65.

Rogers, E.M. (2003) *Diffusion of Innovations*. Free Press, New York.

Rycroft-Malone, J., Kitson, A., Harvey, G., et al. (2002) Ingredients for change: revisiting a conceptual framework. *Quality and Safety in Health Care* 11, 174–180.

Rycroft-Malone, J., Harvey, G., Seers, K., Kitson, A., McCormack, B. and Titchen, A. (2004) An exploration of the factors that influence the implementation of evidence into practice. *Journal of Clinical Nursing* 13, 913–924.

Stacey, D. and Hill, S. (2013) Patient-directed and patient-mediated KT interventions. In *Knowledge Translation in Healthcare* (eds S.E. Strauss, J. Tetroe and I.D. Graham), pp. 197–211. John Wiley & Sons, Oxford.

Stevens, B.J., Yamada, J., Promislow, S., Barwick, M. and Pinard, M. (2016) Pain assessment and management after a knowledge translation booster intervention. *Pediatrics* 138, e20153468.

University of California San Francisco (2022) 12th Pediatric Pain Master Class. `https://www.ucsf-cme.com/2022/MMC22100/info.html` (accessed 6 July 2022).

University of Toronto Centre for the Study of Pain Interfaculty Pain Curriculum (UTCSP-IPC). `http://sites.utoronto.ca/pain/research/interfaculty-curriculum.html` (accessed 4 July 2022).

Valler-Jones, T. (2014) The impact of peer-led simulations on student nurses. *British Journal of Nursing* 23, 321–326.

Vieira, A.C.G., Bueno, M. and Harrison, D. (2020) 'Be sweet to babies': use of Facebook as a method of knowledge dissemination and data collection in the reduction of neonatal pain. *Paediatric and Neonatal Pain* 2, 93–100.

Waltz, T.J., Powell, B.J., Matthieu, M.M., et al. (2015) Use of concept mapping to characterize relationships among implementation strategies and assess their feasibility and importance: results from the Expert Recommendations for Implementing Change (ERIC) study. *Implementation Science* 10, 109.

Appendix 1: Drug Dosing Tables

List of Tables

Table A.1 Non opioid analgesia for neonates & infants 0–6 months of age

Table A.2 Opioid analgesics for neonates & infants (0–6 months)

Table A.3 Non opioid analgesia for children and young people older than 6 months

Table A.4 Opioid starting doses for children with acute pain older than 6 months

Table A.5 Starting Doses for Patient (or Nurse)-Controlled Analgesia (PCA) pumps for children in acute pain older than 6 months

Table A.6 Opioid antagonist doses

Table A.7 Adjuvant analgesia for infants, children and young people

Table A.1 Non opioid analgesia for neonates & infants 0–6 months of age (WHO 2020).

Drug	Route	Paediatric Dose	Maximal Dose	Dosing Interval
Ibuprofen*	PO	Infants 3–6 months = 5–10 mg/kg	40 mg/kg/day	6–8 hrs
Paracetamol (acetaminophen)	PO, PR	Neonates 0–30 days = 5–10 mg/kg	20–40 mg/kg/day	4–6 hrs (maximum 4 doses/day)
		Infants 1–3 months = 10 mg/kg	40 mg/kg/day	
		Infants 3–6 months = 10–15 mg/kg	40–60 mg/kg/day	
Paracetamol**	IV	≤10 kg = 7.5 mg/kg	30 mg/kg/day	6 hrs

* For infants < 3 months consult Pain Service **ONLY if rectal or oral administration contraindicated; re-evaluate daily
Key: mg = milligram; kg = kilogram; hrs = hours
Table adapted and used with permission from Stefan J. Friedrichsdorf, Center of Pediatric Pain Medicine, Palliative Care and Integrative Medicine, University of California at San Francisco (UCSF) Benioff Children's Hospitals

Managing Pain in Children and Young People: A Clinical Guide, Third Edition. Edited by Alison Twycross, Jennifer Stinson, William T. Zempsky, and Abbie Jordan.
© 2024 John Wiley & Sons Ltd. Published 2024 by John Wiley & Sons Ltd.

Table A.2 Opioid analgesics for neonates & infants (0–6 months) (WHO 2020).

Drug	Route	Paediatric Dose	Dosing Interval
Morphine	PO/PR/SL	<u>Neonates 0–30 days</u> = 0.075–0.15 mg/kg	6 hrs
		<u>Infants 1–6 months</u> = 0.08–0.2 mg/kg	4–6 hrs
Morphine***	IV/SC**	<u>Neonates 0–30 days</u> = 0.025–0.05 mg/kg	6 hrs
		<u>Infants 1–6 months</u> = 0.1 mg/kg	6 hrs
		Infusion (with PCA bolus of same dose):	
		<u>Neonates 0–30 days</u> = 0.005–0.01 mg/kg/hr	
		<u>Infants 1–6 months</u> = 0.01–0.03 mg/kg/hr	
Fentanyl***	IV/SC**	<u>Neonates & Infants 0–6 months</u> = 0.5–1 microgram/kg	2–4 hrs
		Infusion (with PCA bolus of same dose):	
		<u>Neonates & Infants 0–6 months</u> = 0.5–1 mcg/kg/hr	
Oxycodone	PO/PR/SL	<u>Infants 1–6 months</u> = 0.05–0.125 mg/kg	4–6 hrs

Key: mg= milligram; kg = kilogram; PO = orally, SL = sublingual; PR = rectally; hrs = hours; IV = intravenous; SC = subcutaneous
Administer IV slowly over at least 5 minutes * The intravenous doses for neonates are based on acute pain management and sedation dosing information. Lower doses are required for non-ventilated neonates.
Table adapted and used with permission from Stefan J. Friedrichsdorf, Center of Pediatric Pain Medicine, Palliative Care and Integrative Medicine, University of California at San Francisco (UCSF) Benioff Children's Hospitals

Table A.3 Non opioid analgesia for children and young people older than 6 months.

Medication (route of administration)	Paediatric Dose	Maximal Dose	Dosing Interval	Comment
Paracetamol (acetaminophen)				
Paracetamol (PO/PR)	10–15 mg/kg	<u>6–24 months</u> = 60 mg/kg/day <u>> 2 years</u>: 75 mg/kg/day [max. 4000mg/day acutely, 3000mg chronic use]	4–6 hrs	
Paracetamol (IV)	<u><10 kg</u> = 7.5 mg/kg	30 mg/kg/day	6 hrs	▪ Due to high price use ONLY if PO or PR contraindicated; re-evaluate daily
	<u>≥10kg</u> = 15 mg/kg	60 mg/kg/day	6 hrs	
	<u><50 kg</u> = 15 mg/kg	75 mg/kg/day	6 hrs	
	<u>≥50 kg</u> = 1000 mg	4000 mg/day	6 hrs	

Key: mg = milligram; kg = kilogram; hrs = hours; PO = oral administration, PR = rectal administration; IV = intravenous

Table A.3 Non opioid analgesia for children and young people older than 6 months (Continued).

Medication (route of administration)	Paediatric Dose	Maximal Dose	Dosing Interval	Comment
Non-Steroidal Anti-Inflammatory Drugs (NSAIDs)				
Ibuprofen (PO)	5–10 mg/kg	400–600 mg/dose (2400 mg/day)	6 hrs	
Ketorolac (IV)	<u>6–24 months</u> = 0.25 mg/kg	30 mg/dose	6 hrs	◾ Recommend dosing no longer than five days
	<u>>2 years</u> = 0.5 mg/kg	30 mg/dose	6 hrs	◾ Recommend dosing no longer than five days
Naproxen (PO)	5–6 mg/kg	250–375 mg/dose	12 hrs	
COX-2 Inhibitor				
Celecoxib (PO)	1–2 mg/kg	100 mg	12–24 hrs	◾ If classic NSAIDs contraindicated; safety and efficacy has been established only in children 2 years of age or older and for a maximum of 6 months of treatment in juvenile rheumatoid arthritis.

Key: mg= milligram; kg = kilogram; hrs = hours
Table adapted and used with permission from Stefan J. Friedrichsdorf, Center of Pediatric Pain Medicine, Palliative Care and Integrative Medicine, University of California at San Francisco (UCSF) Benioff Children's Hospitals

Table A.4 Opioid starting doses for children with acute pain older than 6 months.

- Dosing range: Younger children with less pain <u>start</u> on the lower end of the range, older children with severe pain <u>start</u> on the higher end of the dosing range; doses will then be titrated to effect
- Maximum per kg dose capped at 50 kg body weight
- For strong opioids: Rescue ("breakthrough" or "PRN") dose = 10% of total daily dose

Medication (route of administration)	Paediatric Dose	Maximal Starting Dose	Dosing Interval	Comment
Partial mu-receptor Agonists				
Tramadol (PO,SL,PR)	0.5–2 mg/kg	50–100 mg/dose	4–6 hrs	Analgesic ceiling effect: max. 8 mg/kg/day (≥50kg: max. of 400 mg/day)
				FDA BLACK BOX WARNING (2017): Tramadol is contraindicated in children younger than 12 years of age and in children younger than 18 years of age following tonsillectomy and/or adenoidectomy.
Full mu-receptor Agonists				
Morphine (PO,SL,PR)	0.15–0.3 mg/kg	7.5–15 mg/dose	4 hrs	
Morphine (IV,SC)	0.05–0.1 mg/kg	2.5–5 mg/dose	4 hrs	
Oxycodone (PO,SL,PR)	0.1–0.2 mg/kg	5–10 mg/dose	4–6 hrs	

Key: mg= milligram; kg = kilogram; PO = orally, SL = sublingual; PR = rectally; hrs = hours

Table A.4 Opioid starting doses for children with acute pain older than 6 months (Continued).

Medication (route of administration)	Paediatric Dose	Maximal Starting Dose	Dosing Interval	Comment
Fentanyl (IV,SC,SL)	0.5–1 microgram/kg	25–50 microgram	n/a	▪ Due to short half-life, consider starting continuous infusion 0.5–1 mcg/kg/hr (max. 50 mcg/hr), if scheduled analgesia required
Hydromorphone (PO,SL,PR)	40–60 microgram/kg	2000–3000 microgram (= 2–3 mg)	4 hrs	
Hydromorphone (IV,SC)	10–20 microgram/kg	0.5–1 mg	4 hrs	
Multi-mechanistic full mu-receptor Agonists				
Methadone (PO,PR,SL)	0.05–0.1 mg/kg	2.5–5 mg	8–12 hrs	▪ Methadone should not be prescribed by those unfamiliar with its use! ▪ Its effects should be closely monitored for several days, particularly when it is first started and after any dose changes.
Methadone (IV,SC)	0.04–0.08 mg/kg	2–4 mg	8–12 hrs	▪ In paediatrics due to high bioavailability about 80% of the enteral dose appears to be the equianalgesic IV dose (e.g. 1 mg PO = 0.8 mg IV). ▪ Adult recommendations suggest 50% conversion (e.g. 1 mg PO = 0.5 mg IV).

Key: mg= milligram; kg = kilogram; PO = orally, SL = sublingual; PR = rectally, hrs = hours
Table adapted and used with permission from Stefan J. Friedrichsdorf, Center of Pediatric Pain Medicine, Palliative Care and Integrative Medicine, University of California at San Francisco (UCSF) Benioff Children's Hospitals

Table A.5 Starting Doses for Patient (or Nurse)-Controlled Analgesia (PCA) pumps for children in acute pain older than 6 months.

- Dosing range: Younger children with less pain start on the lower end of the range, older children with severe pain start on the higher end of the dosing range. Doses will then be titrated to effect with escalation usually in 33–50% increments both for continuous and PCA bolus dose
- PCA dose usually = continuous infusion (might differ in individual patients)
- Consider adding low-dose naloxone infusion 0.5–2 mcg/kg/hr (max. 25–100 mcg/hr) to treat potential opioid-induced side effects, such as pruritus, nausea, constipation, urinary retention, hallucinations etc.
- For most acute pain conditions treatment with multimodal analgesia can avoid need for continuous infusion

PCA bolus dose	Maximum bolus dose	Continuous infusion (basal rate)	Maximum continuous infusion	Lock-out time	Number of max. boluses
Morphine					
10–20 microgram/kg	500–1000 microgram (= 0.5–1 mg)	10–20 microgram/ kg/hour	500–1000 micrograms/ hour (= 0.5–1 mg/hour)	5–10 minutes	4–6 boluses/ hour
Fentanyl					
0.5–1 microgram/kg	25–50 microgram	0.5–1 microgram/ kg/hour	25–50 micrograms/hour	5–10 minutes	4–6 boluses/ hour
Hydromorphone					
2–4 microgram/kg	100–200 microgram	2–4 microgram/ kg/hour	100–200 micrograms/hour	5–10 minutes	4–6 boluses/ hour

Key: mg= milligram; kg = kilogram
Table adapted and used with permission from Stefan J. Friedrichsdorf, Center of Pediatric Pain Medicine, Palliative Care and Integrative Medicine, University of California at San Francisco (UCSF) Benioff Children's Hospitals

Table A.6 Opioid antagonist doses (Kraemer 2009; Portenoy 2008; Miller 2011; Monitto 2011).

Medication (route of administration)	Indication	Dose
Naloxone IV	Pruritus/urinary retention	0.25–1 microgram/kg
	Sedation	2–4 microgram/kg
	Respiratory depression	10–15 microgram/kg
	Low-dose infusion for prevention of Opioid-induced ADRs	0.5–2 microgram/kg/hour (max 100 microgram /hr)

Key: kg = kilogram

Table A.7 Adjuvant analgesia for infants, children and young people.

Medication (route of administration)	Paediatric Dose	Max. dose (for patients > 50 kg)	Dosing Interval	Comments/Side Effects
Gabapentinoids				
Gabapentin (PO)	5 mg/kg (titrated up to 20 mg/kg)	300 mg (titrated up to 1200 mg)	8 hrs	▪ In school-age children may start at lower doses to reduce risk of initial sedation ▪ Do NOT give PR (missing active transporter = no absorption) ▪ Infants < 1 year: 4.5 mg/kg/dose Q6h (titrated to effect to max. of 18 mg/kg/dose)
Pregabalin (PO)	1 mg/kg (titrated up to 6 mg/kg)	50 mg (titrated up to 300 mg)	Twice a day	▪ In school children start at lower doses to reduce risk of initial sedation ▪ No data for infants ▪ May be given PR
Alpha-Agonists				
Dexmede-tomidine (IV)	0.2 mcg/kg/hour (titrate to max. 2 microgram/kg/hr)	10 microgram (titrate to max. 100 mcg/hour)	Continuous infusion	
Clonidine (PO, transdermal)	1–6 microgram/kg	50–150 microgram	4–6 hrs	▪ Transdermal application usually 1:1 conversion to total daily enteral dose
NMDA-Channel Blocker				
Low-dose Ketamine (IV)	1 microgram/kg/ minute (titrated to 5 mcg/kg/ minute) [= 60–300 mcg/kg/hour])	3 mg/hour (titrated to 15 mg/hour)	Continuous infusion	▪ Conversion to PO ketamine 1:1 (i.e. divide total daily dose by 6 and administer 4 hourly PRN or scheduled)

(Continued)

Table A.7 (Continued)

Medication (route of administration)	Paediatric Dose	Max. dose (for patients > 50 kg)	Dosing Interval	Comments/Side Effects
Tricyclic Antidepressants (TCA)				
Amitriptyline (PO)	0.1 mg/kg (titrated to max. 0.5 mg/kg)	5 mg (titrated to max. 25 mg)	Once at night	▪ Despite the name, medication NOT potent as an antidepressant ▪ Consider ECG to rule out QTc-prolongation ▪ Stronger anticholinergic side effects (including inducing sleep) than nortriptyline ▪ For infants > 3 months
Nortriptyline (PO)	0.1 mg/kg (titrated to max. 0.5 mg/kg)	5 mg (titrated to max. 25 mg)	Once at night	▪ Despite the name, medication NOT potent as an antidepressant ▪ Consider ECG to rule out QTc-prolongation ▪ For infants > 3 months

Key: mg= milligram; kg = kilogram; PO = orally, IV = intravenous; PR = rectally, hrs = hours

Table adapted and used with permission from Stefan J. Friedrichsdorf, Center of Pediatric Pain Medicine, Palliative Care and Integrative Medicine University of California at San Francisco (UCSF) Benioff Children's Hospitals

References

FDA (2017) Drug Safety Communication: FDA restricts use of prescription codeine pain and cough medicines and tramadol pain medicines in children; recommends against use in breast-feeding women. Available at: https://www.fda.gov/drugs/drug-safety-and-availability/fda-drug-safety-communication-fda-restricts-use-prescription-codeine-pain-and-cough-medicines-and [Accessed 16th May 2023]

Fisher E, Villanueva G, Henschke N, Nevitt SJ, Zempsky W, Probyn K, Buckley B, Cooper TE, Sethna N, Eccleston C. Efficacy and safety of pharmacological, physical, and psychological interventions for the management of chronic pain in children: a WHO systematic review and meta-analysis. Pain. 2022 Jan 1;163(1):e1–e19. doi: 10.1097/j.pain.0000000000002297.

Kraemer, F.W. & Rose J.B. (2009). Pharmacologic management of acute pediatric pain. *Anesthesiology Clinics*, 27(2), 241–268. doi: 10.1016/j.anclin.2009.07.002.

Portenoy, R.K., Thomas, J., Moehl Boatright, M.L., Tran, D., Galasso, F.L, Stambler, N., Von Gunten, C.F. & Israel, R.J. (2008). Subcutaneous methylnaltrexone for the treatment of opioid-induced constipation in patients with advanced illness: a double-blind, randomized, parallel group, dose-ranging study. *Journal of Pain and Symptom Management*, 35(5), 458–468. doi: 10.1016/j.jpainsymman.2007.12.005.

Miller, J.L., & Hagermann, T.M. (2011). Use of pure opioid antagonists for management of opioid-induced pruritus. *American Journal of Health-system Pharmacy*, 68(15), 1419–1425. doi: 10.2146/ajhp100475.

Monitto, C.L., Kost-Byerly, S.K., White, E., Lee, C.K.K., Rudek, M.A., Thompson, C. & Yaster, M. (2011). The optimal dose of prophylactic intravenous naloxone in ameliorating opioid-induced side effects in children receiving intravenous patient-controlled analgesia morphine for moderate to severe pain: a dose finding study. *Anesthesia and Analgesia*, 113(4), 834–842. doi: 10.1213/ANE.0b013e31822c9a44.

World Health Organization (2020). Guidelines on the management of chronic pain in children. World Health Organization, Geneva.

Answers to Multiple Choice Questions

Chapter 2

1c, 2b, 3a, 4c, 5d

Chapter 3

1b, 2c, 3d, 4c, 5b

Chapter 4

1a, 2c, 3d, 4a

Chapter 5

1d, 2c, 3b, 4d, 5d

Chapter 6

1c, 2b, 3d, 4c, 5c

Chapter 7

1d, 2b, 3b, 4c, 5c

Chapter 8

1e, 2a, 3b, 4e, 5c

Chapter 9

1c, 2d, 3a, 4b

Chapter 10

1d, 2d, 3c, 4d, 5b

Chapter 11

1c, 2a&d, 3c, 4b

Chapter 12

1e, 2c, 3c, 4b, 5d

Chapter 13

1a, 2a&c, 3b, 4b&c, 5c

Chapter 14

1b, 2d, 3d, 4b, 5d

Chapter 15

1d, 2b, 3c, 4a, 5d

Chapter 16

1e, 2e, 3b, 4f, 5b, 6c

Index

Notes: Page numbers in italics denote figures and those in bold denote tables; page numbers followed by "*b*" denote boxes.